Health Education in the Elementary School

5th edition

CARL E. WILLGOOSE

Boston University

W. B. SAUNDERS COMPANY   1979
Philadelphia   London   Toronto

W. B. Saunders Company: West Washington Square
Philadelphia, PA   19105

1 St. Anne's Road
Eastbourne, East Sussex BN21 3UN, England

1 Goldthorne Avenue
Toronto, Ontario M8Z 5T9, Canada

Library of Congress Cataloging in Publication Data

Willgoose, Carl E

Health education in the elementary school.

Includes index.

1. Health education (Elementary)   I. Title. [DNLM:
   1. Health education.   2. School health services.
   QT200.3 W714h]

LB1587.A3W49 1979   372.3'7   78–32133

ISBN 0–7216–9368–7

Health Education in the Elementary School   ISBN   0–7216–9368–7

Last digit is the print number: 9   8   7   6   5   4   3   2   1

Preface
to the Fifth Edition

The health status of both the individual and society is made known by a variety of advances in human enlightenment and fulfillment. Accompanying this is a sometimes subtle but nevertheless real rise in the *spirit* of the local community and the nation itself.

Expressing this spirit may represent the ultimate state of wellness. Moreover, there is increasing evidence that Western civilization, contrary to the agonizing writings of Spengler and others, is moving toward a fullness of expression and enrichment. The state of wellness is being advanced because comprehensive school health programs are increasing and community health education efforts are reaching larger audiences. A maturation that is demonstrated in a number of ways is occurring. With the enactment of Public Law 94–317 establishing the Office of Health Information and Health Promotion under the Assistant Secretary of Health in HEW, and the Bureau of Health Education in the U.S. Public Health Service in Atlanta, there emerged a noticeable public and professional commitment to health education. When such major happenings occur, there usually follows new expectations for performance and accountability. This is exactly where elementary classroom teachers enter, with their interest, enthusiasm, and professional understanding.

In the belief that there is no person in the public school system in a better position to make a significant contribution to the health of schoolchildren than the classroom teacher, this edition sets forth several means to an end.

The early chapters are concerned with the general topic of school health and the health status of the child. They stress the detection and referral role of the teacher and the unique opportunity to function efficiently with the school health service personnel and other health-related groups in the community. Then follows a discussion of the school environment and its bearing on general behavior and learning. No attempt has been made in these early chapters to be complete in dealing with school health services and healthful school environment. These are major areas of study in themselves. They are briefly presented here so that the elementary school teacher can see the relationship they have to total school health and their connection with health instruction in and about the classroom.

The major part of the book is specifically concerned with health instruction and the movement away from health teaching as a "do-gooder" activity to a carefully organized and programmed part of the total school curriculum. It is designed to furnish the elementary school teacher with a quantity of orderly and practical information to be of help in planning, carrying out, and evaluating health teaching. The concern is for inner-city children as well as those from rural and suburban areas. The direction throughout the text is toward a broad program of essential health topics, taught in a warm and effective style that will not only transmit ideas but also clarify student values and affect student behavioral patterns.

CARL E. WILLGOOSE

Contents

4 HEALTHFUL AND SAFE SCHOOL ENVIRONMENT, 90

5 NORMAL GROWTH AND DEVIATIONS FROM NORMAL, 106

6 THE HEALTH INSTRUCTION PROGRAM, 124

The Nature and Scope of Health Education

The world is too much with us; late and soon
Getting and spending, we lay waste our powers;
Little we see in nature that is ours;
We have given our hearts away, a sordid boon!

—Wordsworth, 1807

We believe that the conditions of perfect health, either public or personal, are seldom or never attained, though attainable;—that the average length of human life may be very much extended, and its physical power greatly augmented;—that in every year . . . thousands of lives are lost which might have been saved;—that tens of thousands of cases of sickness occur, which might have been prevented . . . that these preventable evils require an enormous expenditure and loss of money, and impose upon the people unnumbered and immeasurable calamities, pecuniary, social, physical, mental, and moral, which might be avoided;—that means exist, within our reach, for their mitigation or removal;—and that measures for prevention will effect infinitely more than remedies for the cure of disease.[1]

—Lemuel Shattuck, 1850

As the Industrial Revolution advanced and vast numbers of people moved from the English countryside into the cities, Wordsworth lamented that man was out of tune with nature. The ugliness of the era caused him to yearn for the past. However, the forces of greed and dehumanization led to the birth of the modern public health movement and the initiative to overcome illness and despair. Interestingly, it was Shattuck's leadership a few decades later that promoted confidence in the concept that the *prevention of illness* could become a reality—a concept that is generally accepted today as valid and of high priority.

---

[1]Shattuck, Lemuel. *Report of the Sanitary Commission of Massachusetts.* Boston: Dutton and Wentworth, State Printers, 1850, p. 10.

ACHIEVING HIGH-LEVEL WELLNESS

By predicting and controlling the total environment, the doubts of individuals like Wordsworth can be resolved. To do this one must set as a personal goal the ultimate expansion of *awareness* of both self and surroundings. The heightened awareness of men and women is advanced when there is a real desire to raise the level of health to a maximum level—a level that will make it possible to struggle through life seeking not only to survive but also to achieve a certain happiness "not by acquiescing with what is but by struggling for something else, not by accepting but by doing, not by receiving but by giving, not by rest but by activity."[2]

When individuals are sensitive to the preciousness of life and the potentialities of a fully awakened human being, they will consider high-level wellness worthy of serious attention. This is not an easy objective to attain. After all, the partly ill body can adjust to almost any kind of abuse and deprivation and still manage to survive at a subclinical level and may even succeed at accomplishing some goals. Even close brushes with death frequently fail to bring about needed changes in lifestyle. For example, the men in one study who survived heart attacks and gave up smoking at the advice of their physicians had wives who showed no change in smoking practices despite the life-threatening attacks their husbands had suffered. Cracking the tough crust of personal behavior and lifestyle is the challenge. Unfortunately, behavior is so rooted in social customs and other variables that altering disease-producing behavior is frequently difficult. In a Maryland study 47 per cent of the people interviewed said that they did not use seat belts in their autos. This behavior was significantly higher among females and among persons with less than a high school education or a low income.[3] The non-use of seat belts was also more common among those who felt powerless to change some aspect of their lives.

Obviously, achieving high-level wellness relates to how much people believe that they can exercise change over their lives. Harvey Cox said as much in his book *On Not Leaving It to the Snake;* people, not circumstances, are responsible for directing their futures, and one should embrace the prophetic view that things can be different.[4]

THE TOTAL VIEW OF HEALTH

It is literally impossible to expect to achieve a state of high-level wellness if children and adults continue to take the narrow view and think of health simply as a condition in which there is no immediate ache, strain, or infection. It is for this very reason that the World

---

[2]Lawton, Shailer U. and Rogers, Frederick Rand. *Educational Paths to Virtue-I.* Newton, Mass.: Pleides Co., 1937, p. 47.

[3]Helsing, Knud J., et al. "What Kinds of People Do Not Use Seat Belts?" *American Journal of Public Health, 67*:1043–1049, November, 1977.

[4]Cox, Harvey G. *On Not Leaving It to the Snake.* New York: Macmillan Publishing Co., 1967.

Health Organization of the United Nations defines health in a comprehensive way as "a state of complete physical, mental and social well-being, and not merely the absence of disease and infirmity."[5]

The real meaning of the WHO definition is to be found in the direction it gives to life and living. Implied is that human health potential is on a continuum, with near death at one end and optimal health at the other. It is frequently a fluctuating state. Hoyman classifies health status into five levels.[6]

Referring to health in terms of high-level wellness, Dunn defines it as "an integrated method of functioning which is oriented toward maximizing the potential of the individual."[7] Burt carries this further by examining the potential in terms of lifestyle conditions and components (see Fig. 1–1). He wants to learn how a person thinks, makes choices, copes with life crises, handles risks, relates to people, and what kind of a consumer he or she really is.

The observation that a state of health has far-reaching consequences was clearly illustrated by Julian Huxley, when he said that ". . . the highest and most sacred duty of man is seen as the proper utilization of the untapped resources of human beings."[8] Involved

---

[5]Constitution of the World Health Organization, *Chronicles of the World Health Organization, 1*:29–43; Geneva: World Health Organization, 1947, p. 3.

[6]Hoyman, Howard S. "Our Modern Concept of Health," *Journal of School Health, 32*:253–264, September 1962.

[7]Dunn, Halbert L. "What High-Level Wellness Means," *Health Values, 1*:9–16, January/February 1977.

[8]Quoted by Theodosius Dobzhansky in *Biological Basis of Human Freedom.* New York: Columbia University Press, 1956.

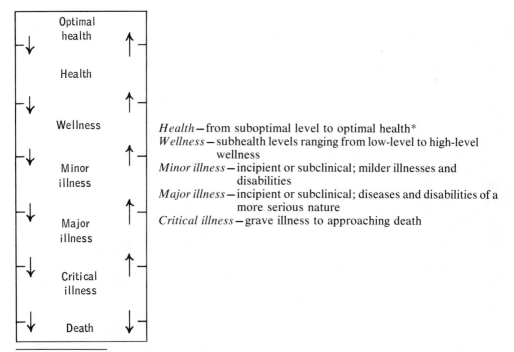

Health —from suboptimal level to optimal health*
Wellness — subhealth levels ranging from low-level to high-level wellness
Minor illness — incipient or subclinical; milder illnesses and disabilities
Major illness — incipient or subclinical; diseases and disabilities of a more serious nature
Critical illness —grave illness to approaching death

---

*The level at which an individual's living approaches his full desirable potentialities (e.g., Dr. Albert Schweitzer, Grandma Moses, Konrad Adenauer).

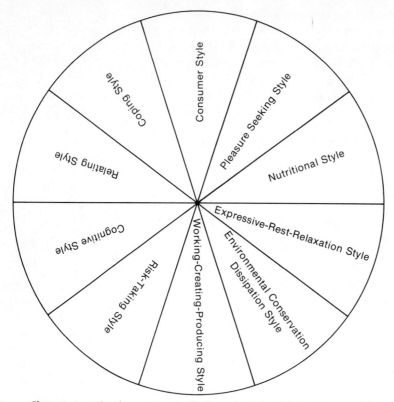

Figure 1-1. Lifestyle components affecting potential well-being. (Courtesy John J. Burt, University of Maryland.)

here is the whole of one's capacity for expression. It is multidimensional—anthropological, biological, psychological, economic, and even political. This gives support to the concept of an "ecology of health" in which all human relationships between a community and its environment are health-related. Moreover, there is a personal responsibility of the individual for his or her own health and the health of the community. As far back as the seventeenth century, John Donne expressed this viewpoint beautifully when he stated: "No man is an Island, entire of itself; every man is a piece of the Continent, a part of the main . . . any man's death diminishes me, because I am involved in mankind."

HEALTH FROM PAST TO PRESENT

Through the years there has been overwhelming support for government and school-community programs designed to raise the health of the citizenry. Strong recommendations have come from groups such as the American Medical Association, the American Pediatric Association, the American Public Health Association, the Educational Policies Commission of the National Education Association, and the White House Conference on Health. It was at this conference that both private and public health physicians reported that "educated patients" are much better patients; they understand something about their own health, follow the recommendations of their physicians, and recover sooner from illness.

The concern for health, welfare, and survival has not always been so noticeable and scientific as it appears to be today.

The gradual decrease over the centuries of magic, guesswork, incantation, and superstition, together with the corresponding rise in applied scientific knowledge, represents a magnificent process of slow evolution. Sound ideas were practiced side by side with unsound treatments and rituals. As in all ages of humanity, only a minority knew the truth, and they had to work uphill in the face of customs, habits, and ignorance. In prehistoric times and even today in some parts of the world, evil spirits were "scared away" because of the general belief that they caused sickness. Yet these same prehistoric people discovered that certain herbs and other plants were quite good for numerous disorders. As far back as 4500 B.C. along the Nile in Egypt, Imhotep was practicing medicine in Luxor and Karnak. By 2500 B.C., surgical operations were being performed with the "help" of Thoth, the god of medicine. Today, thousands of Egyptians in the same region wear the scarab beetle charm about their necks to ward off disease and encourage fertility.

The constant struggle for light over darkness has been, and always will be, a continuing one. This is well demonstrated by early Hebrew law relating to communicable disease, isolation, quarantine, and cleanliness. Two books of the Bible—Leviticus and Deuteronomy—are rich in illustrations of early health recommendations and practices. This is further illustrated by a 500 year period of ancient Greek and Roman history (300 B.C. to A.D. 200). It was Hippocrates who taught that each disease arises from a natural cause. It was the Athenian youth who took good care of their bodies and worshipped the goddess Hygeia under the guidance of priest-physicians. It was Galen, the Greek physician and writer, who experimented widely in physiology but was looked down upon by the Roman citizens of the period. Yet the Romans were really interested in health and developed many practical surgical instruments to be used on wounded gladiators and soldiers. They made more progress in sanitation, plumbing, and sewer construction than almost any other civilization over the years. The Roman aqueduct is still considered a masterpiece of engineering.

During the disease-ridden Middle Ages, advancement in hygiene and medicine was somewhat retarded. Hospitals were organized for the care of the sick, but it was not until the tail end of the fifteenth and the beginning of the sixteenth centuries that scientific advancements began to be noticeable. By the seventeenth century Leeuwenhoek and his microscope opened a previously invisible world to man. Witchcraft reached a new high, but alchemy slowly gave way to chemistry. By the middle 1700's all physical and biological sciences were making great strides. Scientists were no longer hidden for protection but were looked upon with some degree of respect. Uncleanliness was everywhere, in the streets, in the hospitals, and in the homes.

In the nineteenth century a variety of medical discoveries and changes in hygienic practices took place. In the face of high death rates from infectious diseases, a number of significant discoveries occurred. Some of these were the clinical thermometer, the stethoscope, the x-ray, radium, the antiseptic method, and anesthesia. It was proved once and for all that communicable diseases are caused by microorganisms that enter the body from without, that insects carry malaria and yellow fever, and that the universal practice of healthful living not only improves one's resistance to tuberculosis and other diseases but also improves total health.

The twentieth century, building upon the past, has produced much of what is known and practiced today. Health promotion activities may go down in history as the greatest single contribution of the twentieth century. Federal, state, school, and community health programs have flourished. Ordinary men and women have not only felt the impact of this but have also actually taken part in the promotion program. They have had a hand in hospital organization, maternal education, the mental health movements, and school health education. They know something about heart disease, allergies, psychological stress, cancer, brain surgery, obesity, disease-carrying insects, blood transfusions, the science of nutrition, longevity, *Streptococcus* and *Staphylococcus* bacilli, antibiotics, tranquilizers, sodium fluoride and fluoridation, and countless other items related to disease. Their dollars have supported the fight to bring poliomyelitis under control, to pursue the cause of multiple sclerosis, muscular dystrophy, and coronary occlusions. Their personal sacrifices on the local level to raise money for the Community Chest or United Fund or to give blood have given them an insight into and appreciation for the place of health in modern society.

THE NEED FOR EDUCATION FOR HEALTH

The more complex civilization becomes, the less valid instinctive behavior is, and the more one must depend upon the processes of education for guidance.

It is not difficult to make a long list of the reasons *why there is a need for health education.* Some of the more significant reasons are as follows:

The Changing Times

Nothing stands still. Change, like night and day, is an absolute. And Western civilization, in addition to reaping the sweet fruits of progress, is suffering from the spoils. In a society where speed, status, comfort, and economic success are high marks of achievement, it is not uncommon to find men and women who cannot adjust to the increasing pressures. They keep plugging along, lacking an apparent sense of values. Some become overfed and underactive. And, while others become complacent and simply vegetate from year to year with few goals in life to stimulate the best in them, still others literally "burn" themselves out in a life packed with situations generating insecurity, fear, anxiety, worry, jealousy, anger, and hatred. Resulting tensions refuse to stay bottled. They make their presence known in headaches, indigestion, gastrointestinal upsets, restlessness, sleeplessness, irritability, and fatigue.

Society today is anything but peaceful and serene. Even with a careful education for health, it is most difficult to achieve balance in living and to obtain an attitude of mind conducive to total well-being. Western civilization is characterized by the spectacle of people fighting for perfection while knowing little about where they are headed. The effort all too often does not produce the peace of mind they seek. Instead, our way of life results in higher levels of cholesterol causing coronary disease, increased gastric secretions causing ulcers, elevated blood pressure levels causing cerebral hemorrhage, and a high degree of frustration leading to mental breakdown. Reduced to its simplest terms, survival depends on the physical-mental-spiritual balance. Moreover, it depends on how one *travels* toward the goals of life, perhaps more than whether or not one ever arrives.

Value Illness

The concern for health by official bodies and professionals in health-related fields is at an all-time high. This does not mean that the average citizen is well informed or has permitted his value system to be changed to any substantial degree. Although individual health status has improved, there are still thousands of people suffering from what Maslow refers to as "value illness."[9] This is the negative element behind drug addiction, alcoholism, illegitimacy, corruption, graft, and numerous irregularities in all walks of private and public life. The adult citizen *knows* what to do but is not *moved* to the state of doing it. This is illustrated continually in the field of health behavior where knowledgeable individuals are simply indifferent to the consequences of their own acts. Their own moral principles and standards of right and wrong actions somehow do not compel them to act in keeping with what they know is best.

Norman Cousins, editor of the *Saturday Review,* cites an alarming example of this value illness when he discusses a doctor friend who is a heavy smoker.[10] The doctor reports that he did not need all the government publications to convince him that smoking can cause cancer or bronchitis or various forms of heart disease. The evidence was admittedly plain to him in his daily visits to the hospital wards. Moreover, he was able to reinforce his feelings by noting that he had seen enough lung surgery to recognize the difference between the pink healthy tissue of the non-smoker and the discolored tissue of smokers. Yet, he could not give up smoking himself.

Here, says Cousins, is a problem far more serious than the

---

[9]Maslow, Abraham H. *Toward a Psychology of Being.* Princeton, New Jersey: D. Van Nostrand Co., Inc., 1962.

[10]Cousins, Norman, "The Danger Beyond Smoking," *Saturday Review,* January 25, 1964.

problem leading up to it. Involved here are the ultimate questions a society has to ask about itself. Cousins asks: "What are the basic values of its people? How much sensitivity do they have to the fragility and preciousness of life? What connections do they see between a respect for life and health development of the society itself?"

World-Wide Conditions

Ultimately the thoughts of all people must be geared to conditions the world over. More people live in mud huts than in any other type of dwelling; more travel by foot (or by burro) than any other way; most have a life expectancy less than half that of the people in the United States; most mothers see half their children die before reaching maturity; more people get sick who do not have a physician's help available than those who have even rudimentary medical care. In short, most of the world's peoples are in the "have not" stage. It is encouraging, however, to know that evidence is available to indicate that in the long run improved health practices in one area of the globe have a favorable effect on other areas. This is also true in terms of health education ideas, for these ideas spread sometimes as quickly as new vaccines, sanitary practices, and wonder drugs.

The effectiveness of the World Health Organization is demonstrated by the large number of countries embarking upon health protection and education programs. Some of the world goals and accomplishments in a single year's time are impressive.

Improved communication and transportation have brought the people of the world closer together. Consequently, the health and welfare of other people is more the worry of the ordinary citizen than ever before. Although people may value their individuality, they are still not separate from the universal self—the oneness of humanity. In fact the healthiest people alive today owe their enviable status to the practices of friends and neighbors. In a complex society the welfare of the majority is directly affected by the welfare, knowledge, and understanding of the minority. In short, education for health is the concern of the individual on both a local and a world-wide basis.

Contemporary Health Care

The health care system is in trouble because of the soaring costs of medical attention and the increasing health problems in society.[11] The public is acutely aware of the difficulty. A Cadell public opinion poll taken in late 1977 showed that 46 per cent of the public want increased governmental spending for health care. This was followed by slightly lower percentages favoring aid to the elderly and education.

Between 1976 and 1977 health care expenditures in America went up from approximately $140 billion to $160 billion a year, with $10 billion alone going to long-term care for Medicare patients. It

---

[11]Ehrbar, A. J. "A Radical Prescription for Medical Care," *Fortune*, February 1977, p. 165.

is estimated that this steady increase over the decades will reach $200 billion by 1980. These figures exceed the growth in expenditures for other goods and services by a considerable amount. The greatest health care increases since 1970 have occurred in hospital and nursing home care. Although better controls over the health care delivery system and improved insurance coverage are needed, the ultimate remedy is to prevent a large share of human disease and deprivation.

American Health Statistics

The health of the American people is well on the rise and has been for some time. Much of this is due to vast achievements in medical research, spectacular progress in the field of antibiotics, and an increase in health maintenance organizations.

In addition to these medical factors, a large share of credit should be given to public health and school health practices. The reduction in the tuberculosis death rate, for instance, represents one of our finest accomplishments. At the start of the century the annual

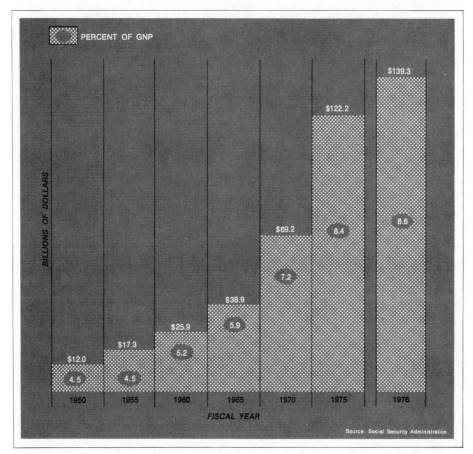

Figure 1-2. National health care expenditures and per cent of gross national product, 1950–1976. (U.S. Department of Health, Education, and Welfare, 1977.)

death rate in the United States from tuberculosis was 194 out of 100,000 persons. Today it is less than four. Such a favorable picture has been brought about by a number of factors and not solely by medical care and research. It is related to items such as better housing, improvement in nutrition, public health education, and a generally higher standard of living. The significance of education is further illustrated by the death rate from appendicitis; it has been reduced approximately 60 per cent over a 20 year period, due primarily to an enlightened public—a public that does not run for a cathartic every time there is a stomach or abdominal pain.

It is true that health in America is becoming a "social accomplishment." The death and sickness rates for practically all infectious diseases are down. A decline of 80 per cent in maternal death rates was recorded over the last two decades. Life expectancy is the highest ever. Moreover, it is positively correlated with level of education. Under the mortality rate prevailing around the year 1900, the expectation of life at birth for the total population was not quite 50 years. By 1930 the figure had risen to 60 years; in 1955 it was 69.5 years. According to the National Center for Health Statistics it rose to about 72 years by 1977. The lowest life expectancy rates are in the South where there are more poverty and minority populations. The highest for both sexes are in Hawaii. As in earlier years, white females have the best record of longevity. In 1955 it was 73.6 years, while in 1977 it was 76 years. Thus, since the turn of the century almost 25 years have been added to the expected lifetime.

Recently the California Department of Health demonstrated a positive relationship between engaging in health practices and longevity. The seven practices studied involved getting seven to eight hours of sleep a night, eating breakfast, rarely eating between meals, maintaining desirable weight, engaging in physical exercise, drinking moderately or not at all, and not smoking. Life expectancy increased consistently for men and women at three different ages with the number of health practices observed (see Figure 1–3). The

AVERAGE REMAINING LIFE EXPECTANCY FOR HEALTH PRACTICE GROUPS: CALIFORNIA HUMAN POPULATION STUDIES			
	Number of Health Practices		
Ages	*0–3*	*4–5*	*5–6*
Men			
45	21.6	28.2	33.1
55	13.8	20.2	25.0
65	10.6	13.7	17.4
Women			
45	28.6	34.1	35.8
55	20.0	25.1	27.8
65	12.4	17.3	19.8

Figure 1–3. Life expectancy increases in keeping with personal health practices. (Courtesy Research Digest of President's Council on Physical Fitness and Sports, Washington, D.C.)

Figure 1–4. Infant mortality rates continue to decline in U.S. (National Center for Health Statistics.)

reduction in over-all mortality during the present century is concurrent with the rapid reduction in newborn deaths. However, there is room for improvement in the survival chances of the newborn. Although the United States has the lowest infant mortality rate it has ever experienced—less than 15 deaths per 1000 live births (Figure 1–4)—it still ranks behind several countries of the world. The Scandinavian countries rank at the top.

Medical science has made spectacular progress in the last 20 years. The danger of infection through surgery has been greatly reduced. Low cost vaccines are very effective against serious illness. Regular medical examinations and early treatment prevent disease and disability in thousands of individuals. Vast numbers of people who would have died of these same diseases two decades ago today leave hospitals well. The average stay in the hospital for an appendectomy is five and a half days; it was 14 days 20 years ago.

Significant Health Problems

The degenerative diseases of the adult population frequently have their roots in the day-to-day health practices of children and youth. Proper practices, established early in life, tend to reduce mortality and morbidity rates at all age levels. Childhood deaths, however, represent a significant statistic, particularly in the five to fourteen year age period (see Fig. 1–5).

Some of the more prominent health problems are as follows:

Cardiovascular diseases rank first among the leading causes of death in the United States, Canada, and Western Europe. More than half of all deaths each year are attributed to these diseases. The male statistic is higher than that for the female prior to age sixty (see Fig. 1–6). Coronary arterial disease has become less prevalent because people are beginning to know enough to watch their weight and limit their consumption of fats, to seek diversion and tension-free recreation to attain a sound attitude of mind, and to engage in a moderate amount of physical activity. Mortality and morbidity from heart disease are two to three times as high among people who do not

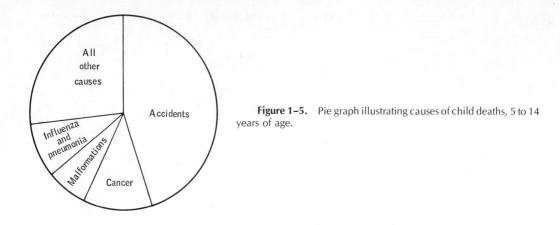

Figure 1–5. Pie graph illustrating causes of child deaths, 5 to 14 years of age.

realize the importance of physical activity and fail to get regular exercise. From the Framingham Heart Study, where there has been continuous evaluation of 5127 adults in one community since 1949, it has been shown that there is a clear association of coronary heart disease with age, elevated blood pressure, serum cholesterol, overweight, cigarette smoking, and lack of physical exercise. This is confirmed by the results of a study of 88 per cent of the entire community of Tecumseh, Michigan, where it was discovered that the maintenance of desirable body weight is an effective method of controlling blood cholesterol levels. Of major importance is the increased attention being given to hypertension by numerous groups, many of which are related to the National High Blood Pressure Education Program. There are a million deaths a year involving hypertension in 26 million Americans. Another 235 million are

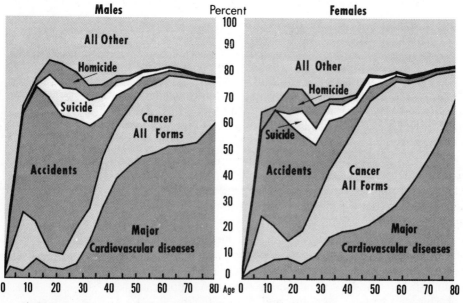

Figure 1–6. Per cent of deaths from selected causes, 1977. (Metropolitan Life Insurance Company, *Statistical Bulletin,* April 1977.)

borderline cases. The program is succeeding in bringing about public awareness of the problem (see Figure 1–7). While 50 per cent of hypertensives were undiagnosed in 1971, over 70 per cent are currently aware of their problem. Especially helpful have been the workplace on-the-job programs that detect and sometimes treat this usually symptomless disease.

Mental illness is a multidimensional problem that affects people in all walks of life. Approximately 20 million people are affected. As a disease entity it ranges from those who are simply unhappy, hard to live with, and poorly adjusted to their world. Mental patients occupy 50 per cent of all the hospital beds in the United States. According to a Harris poll of some 500 physicians, about 90 per cent of their patients suffer from hypochondria and psychosomatic ailments—derived chiefly from problems such as loneliness, insecurity, family conflicts, the pressure of raising children, the stress of overwork, burning the

Figure 1–7.   High blood pressure poster for school and industry. (U.S. Department of Labor, Washington, D.C.)

candle at both ends, and fear of failure. Boredom and monotony rank high as underlying factors contributing to poor mental health.

Another serious outcome of inadequate mental health relates to the all-time high national divorce-marriage ratio—the number of divorces granted per 1000 new marriages. The average figure is now 500; in some states it is well over 500. This rise in broken marriages to over 1 out of every 2 is considered alarming by many, but is dismissed by others as just a trend toward easier divorce due in part to "no fault" laws that recognize "irreconcilable differences" as the only grounds needed.

Children are especially involved. About 400 out of 100,000 children under age 18 require psychiatric care as out-patients each year. Moreover, mental disorders are considered a significant factor in numerous physical illnesses, are strongly associated with suicide, and are often found to be implicated in accidents. In addition to causing considerable suffering and family disruption, mental illness exacts a financial toll of several billion dollars a year for health care and several billions of dollars more in annual loss to industry.

Because of better treatment and rehabilitation, there has been some decline in the number of patients. This advance has been offset by the number of people seeking treatment sooner. Also, the alcoholic, the retarded, and the brain damaged are being served.

Poor health in a society has many manifestations. Suicide, for example, was the cause of over 25,000 deaths in the United States in a recent year. This fact in itself should prompt more attention to the type of behavior that leads to an individual's self-destruction. But the suicide figure does not tell the whole story of suicide. For every successful suicide there are ten unsuccessful attempts for various reasons. Because of the moral and religious stigma attached to suicide, many such cases are undoubtedly not recorded. Also, it is difficult to determine what percentage of other violent deaths, including the thousands of automobile deaths, is caused by a conscious or subconscious desire to end life. Medical and safety authorities are almost unanimous in the belief that some percentage of all categories of violent death are in reality suicides. Moreover, almost half the suicides occur within three months of an emotional crisis, and about 40 per cent of the men and 20 per cent of the women kill themselves because of ill health. The rising rate has led to the recognition of a major medical and public health problem. Existing suicide prevention centers have been effective in saving lives each year and have demonstrated the importance of public education in detecting the potential suicide. Many suicides can be averted if unusual depression or signs of mental illness are recognized and properly treated.

The suicide rate for younger people in the age groups from 10 to 19 has been rising steadily, but the number of persons involved is relatively low. Among males and minority groups the incidence is higher. Divorcees in the general population are three times as suicide-prone as married men. With young people, part of the problem stems from poor communication, especially with parents.[12]

---

[12]Frederick, Calvin J. "Suicide in the United States," *Health Education,* 8:17–22, November/December 1977.

The need for a formal educational approach to prevent and reduce poor mental health is evident. Experience has taught that preventive mental health services can reduce mental illness, alcoholism, divorce, suicide, emotional disturbances, juvenile crime, and employment problems.

The real solution is to *prevent* the disorders through the combined efforts of lay and professional people. This is not easy, for our way of life with its emphasis on personal status, speed, and materialism tends to produce individuals with a disturbed sense of values. Balance in living is frequently difficult to attain. Large numbers of people are basically unhappy. They are looking for relief—"a way out." Only a few years ago the pharmaceutical industry spent more money on developing new tranquilizers, stimulants, sedatives, and analgesics than on any other kind of drug. Even earning a living fails to satisfy large segments of the population, as thousands of production time workers make good wages but suffer from the "worker blues" and the "blahs." The frustrations and resentments that pile up at the workbench move along into the family circle, the neighborhood council, the polling place, and the social gathering. The worker cannot change the personality, the lack of self-esteem, the sense of impotence, and the boredom—in short the patterns imprinted by the job—as easily as a pair of overalls are shed.

Alcoholism and drug addiction are primarily symptoms of poor mental health. The nation's No. 1 "drug problem" is alcohol. It is estimated that there are 10 million alcoholics in the United States out of the 95 million who drink. One in every 18 beginning drinkers will become an alcoholic. Untreated alcoholism shortens life 12 years and contributes to many types of fatalities—with at least half of the nation's traffic deaths involving drunken drivers. In combination with tobacco smoking, alcohol contributes to cancer of the mouth and tongue. Heavy drinkers cost the nation many dollars a year in lost work time, property damage, health and welfare costs, and do incalculable damage to personal and family life (a leading cause of separation, divorce, desertion and emotional problems).

The heavy use of alcohol by women during pregnancy may result in a pattern of abnormalities in the offspring, termed the fetal alcohol syndrome, which consists of specific congenital and behavioral abnormalities. In a Boston study of 600 pregnant women who were heavy drinkers (two to three drinks a day) the risk associated with birth was double. Moreover, it was made clear that abnormalities and defects were associated with the alcohol itself and not factors such as poor nutrition.[13]

The alcoholism problem will be helped when there is wide discussion of drinking patterns and the responsibilities of those who drink. Cultural attitudes have much to do with practices. Evidence suggests that the behavior which accompanies drinking under abstinence and permissive conditions differs significantly.

A Department of Health, Education, and Welfare study of fourth, fifth, and sixth grade children indicated that 45 per cent considered

---

[13]U.S. Department HEW, Public Health Service, Alcohol, Drug Abuse, and Mental Health Administration, IFS No. 39, September 8, 1977.

themselves users of alcohol. By the fourth grade the majority of students already had had at least one experience with alcohol.

Many young drug addicts start with alcohol and graduate to opiates by age 18. Also, it is felt that the management of heroin addiction may be influenced by alcohol use. Faced with the staggering number of 700,000 heroin addicts, many private and public associations are seeking preventive measures as well as controls. The highest per capita use in late 1977 was in San Francisco, followed by Los Angeles, Phoenix, Detroit, San Diego, and Chicago.

According to the National Institute of Mental Health, marihuana use has increased and may well prove to be an enduring cultural pattern. Actually, some 36 million people have tried the weed, and more than half have quit using it—which may reflect increasing age and acceptance of adult responsibilities. Although the safety margin appears high and the drug seems to be more socially acceptable than other more potent narcotics, research findings show evidence of a number of negative side effects to the individual user. An achieved "high" on marihuana tends to impair responses ranging from driving to intellectual and interpersonal functioning. Unfortunately, users ignore side effects for major effects.

Cancer, a malignant neoplasm, is killing about 500,000 Americans a year. It is the second most frequent cause of death in the United States, Canada, and virtually all the countries of Western Europe. It is calculated that about six out of every 24 persons will develop cancer; of this number two will be saved, one will die who could have been saved, and three will die who cannot presently be saved. Significantly, the high death rate could be reduced by 33 per cent if proper treatment were started in time. Recent studies show that a high percentage of people treated early for cancer live for many years. Although there are 33,000 deaths a year from breast cancer alone, the survival rate has been improving. Among women of all ages combined and all stages of the disease, 62 per cent survive for five years, 49 per cent survive for 10 years, and 44 per cent survive for 15 years. Increased emphasis on breast self-examination has been a major factor in discovering 90,000 cases a year. In 1977, 94 per cent of breast cancers were discovered by women themselves. Incidentally, only two out of ten breast lumps are malignant or cancerous, with the potential of spreading. There has been a long-term decline in cancer of the uterus attributed to educational programs for women and widespread use of the Pap test.[14]

Getting the public to accept the fact of cancer openly and getting them to do something about it in time are primarily health education jobs. Today, pregnant women discuss it in mothers' classes, and children discuss it in the schoolroom. Posters like the one in Figure 1–8 help to get the message across. In lung cancer, the single biggest problem is a lack of knowledge of how to motivate smokers to stop smoking and to forestall young people from acquiring the smoking habit. Simply telling them that 12 times as many smokers as nonsmokers die of emphysema is not the answer. Educational programs

---

[14]Metropolitan Life Insurance Company, "Cancer Survival Among Women," *Statistical Bulletin, 58*:7–9, October 1977.

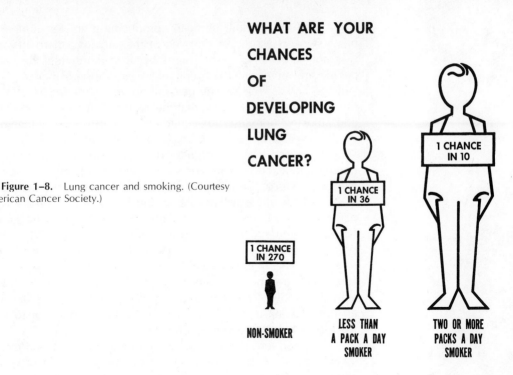

WHAT ARE YOUR CHANCES OF DEVELOPING LUNG CANCER?

1 CHANCE IN 270

NON-SMOKER

1 CHANCE IN 36

LESS THAN A PACK A DAY SMOKER

1 CHANCE IN 10

TWO OR MORE PACKS A DAY SMOKER

Figure 1–8. Lung cancer and smoking. (Courtesy American Cancer Society.)

in the schools, coupled with the efforts of the U.S. Public Health Service and the National Clearinghouse for Smoking and Health, may prove helpful during the next several years.

In addition to causing cancer, coronary heart disease, chronic bronchitis, and emphysema, cigarette smoking cuts several years off the life expectancy of millions of Americans. Smokers at every age pay a high risk price—22 per cent of heavy smokers can expect to be hospitalized during any given 24-month period as compared with only 14 per cent of non-smokers.

Fatalities from ulcers, particularly gastric ulcers, are three times as high among smokers as among non-smokers. A less well-known statistic is that mothers who smoke tend to have more premature babies. In one study of 2000 pregnancies, fetal mortality of babies born of mothers who smoked was 79 per 1000 as against 41 per 1000 for non-smoking mothers.[15]

Although 30 million Americans and Canadians have quit smoking for a very good reason, smoking among young people continues to increase, most dramatically among young girls. For example, the percentage of regular smokers for boys aged 12 to 14 has increased about 40 per cent since 1968. During the same period it has increased seven times for girls of the same age group.

It was hoped that with the discontinuance of cigarette advertising on television the practice of smoking would drop off. It did for a

---

[15]Oschsner, Alton. "The Health Menace of Tobacco," *American Scientist*, 59:246–252, March/April 1971. Further confirmed by American Cancer Society Statistics in 1977.

while, and then it built up again, producing a greater number of heavy smokers. Moreover, the effect on the smoking patterns of youth was not particularly great. This is because the actions of young people are more affected by people around them—their parents, siblings, and especially their peers. If no one in the family smokes, there is a very good chance that the student will not smoke. In the end, smoking for many young children is a positive choice that must be discussed in terms of self-image and social identification.[16]

The over-all *physical fitness* of youth is another concern of parents and teachers. Youngsters frequently lead a rather sedentary existence. Research indicates that civilization plays strange tricks. Many of the youth of the land are lacking the physical wherewithal to participate in vigorous, growth-stimulating activities. They simply have not been exposed to first rate health and physical education programs. Muscular weakness and lack of physical fitness are linked to a life lacking in muscle-building chores, with rich foods, bus and automobile transportation, more spectator rather than participation activities, more TV viewing, less walking, labor-saving devices, apartment living, and lack of adequate play space. Education to meet the loss of fitness is a constant need.

The need for proper programs of physical activity and movement exploration is of paramount concern to teachers of young children. Adults can hardly be expected to change their sedentary ways of living if in their early years of formal education they did not acquire an appreciation for physical skills and the need for regular exercise throughout a lifetime. Walking and bicycling, according to the late heart specialist, Dr. Paul Dudley White, are simple and practical exercises that should be a part of one's plan of normal living.

It has been demonstrated by the President's Council on Physical Fitness and Sports that physically underdeveloped children can be readily identified and given vigorous developmental activity to increase their level of physical fitness. A project involving over 200,000 schoolchildren in five states revealed that where a school had a physical education program prior to its selection in the project, the average physical fitness test failure was 25 per cent. In schools that had no program, however, the average rate of failure was 46 per cent. In all schools, swift improvement was achieved when below-average students were given individual attention.

Further related to the capacity for physical activity are *overweight* and *obesity,* both of which can be controlled to some extent in spite of any genetic predisposition toward being heavy. Coupling sound nutrition practices with pleasant physical activity is most effective in modifying overweight conditions when it is started in the pre-teen years. Moreover, the frequently severe discrimination against obese youngsters and adults can be reduced, and the ugly mental picture that young obese people have of themselves at the very time their own self-image is forming can be improved. Too many obese children are passive and altogether too dependent on their

---

[16]See especially the clear discussion presented by Bernard Mausner and Ellen S. Pratt, *Smoking: A Behavioral Analysis.* Elmsford, N.Y.: Pergamon Press, 1971.

parents. Both young people and adults need to know that it is to their advantage to reach a desirable or "ideal" weight and stay there the rest of their lives. However, about three out of five men in their fifties are overweight; half of the women beyond the age of 40 are more than 10 per cent above their desirable weight.

Millions of people have *poor teeth.* In fact, about 95 per cent of the population suffers from this condition. The average number of unfilled cavities is five per head. Also, 26 million people have lost all of their teeth. Obviously, the American mouth is a disaster area that could be improved if gum stimulators and toothbrushes were properly used. The high rate of periodontal disease, caused by an accumulation of tartar which results in swelling and inflammation (68 million adult Americans have this disorder), is largely due to the fact that early symptoms are ignored and neglected.

Tens of thousands of children have serious difficulties with their teeth. The National Health Survey has indicated that half the children in the country under 15 have never been to a dentist. It is true that poverty, ignorance, and indifference have something to do with dental decay statistics, but there are numerous examples of well-educated parents with moderate to high incomes whose children's teeth are no better than the average.

By the time the average child reaches school, he or she has three carious teeth. At age 12 or 13 it rises to five permanent teeth attacked by caries. The decay rate rises sharply in the intermediate grades and is associated with poor academic achievement and high absence frequency. By the age of 16 years the average youth has seven decayed, missing, or filled teeth involving 14 tooth surfaces. It is evident, too, that fluoridation of the water supply is highly significant. Yet, large numbers of people continue to resist a move in this direction because of entrenched beliefs and general misinformation. Although the effectiveness of water fluoridation has been amply demonstrated, this procedure is only now beginning to have the impact that might be expected. When large cities such as New York, Chicago, Philadelphia, Baltimore, Cleveland, Washington, St. Louis, and Detroit fluoridated their water, the results in terms of healthier teeth were significant.

Fluoridation of the drinking water not only reduces tooth decay up to 70 per cent but it also is a tremendous money saver. This financial saving is dramatically illustrated by the findings of a two-city study in New York State, where the mean cost for dental care per child in Kingston (non-fluoridated water) was more than double that in Newburgh (fluoridated water).

The benefits from public water fluoridation programs greatly reduce the hazard of malocclusion, especially of severe malocclusion, which may be regarded as physically handicapping. Also, research is beginning to indicate that fluorides slow the course of periodontal disease by retarding bone destruction. Rheumatoid arthritis and osteoporosis—abnormal porousness of bone—are lower in areas where there is a high fluoride content in the water.

It has been conservatively estimated that if all the dentists devoted their time exclusively to filling teeth, five years would be required to take care of the backlog alone. Education aimed at getting more people to see their dentists regularly must involve both the general public and the school personnel. Only a cooperative effort in the years ahead will improve the situation to any degree.

Accident statistics overwhelm the average reader. *Accidents* are the greatest threat to life and limb in childhood and call for education of the public through school and community health agencies. This is recognized today as a necessity if one is to survive in a society demanding ever-increasing human adaptability.

Fifty-two million people a year are injured in some kind of an accident, and another 105,000 are killed.

Accidents are the chief cause of death in children ages five to 14 years.

Over four million non-fatal injuries occur annually in and about the home.

Sports and recreation account for approximately 5200 fatalities and a great many more serious injuries annually.

More than 8000 people die by drowning each year. Over half the people in the U.S. cannot swim well enough to save themselves in an emergency (National Safety Council).

Motor vehicle accidents take over 50,000 lives a year and inflict disabling injuries on an additional 1,800,000 persons in the United States. Another 1,500,000 are injured but not disabled. The use of seat belts and shoulder straps and the reduction in the mandatory speed limit to 55 miles per hour has brought about a decline in automobile accident statistics.

Socially maladjusted individuals are more likely to be involved in accidents than are those without such difficulties.

The National Safety Council estimates that if seat belts were used consistently by all drivers and passengers, the incidence of serious injury could be reduced by one third and between 8000 and 10,000 lives could be saved annually. However, few parents when driving regularly lock car doors and secure children in seat belts.

Seventy-five million bicycles ridden in the United States today are connected with an annual loss of 800 lives. Four out of five such fatalities are believed to be associated with the disregard of safe practices. Safety authorities estimate that between 120,000 and 150,000 persons sustain disabling injuries in such mishaps in a single year.

Firearm accidents claim a toll of about 2400 lives a year. Snowmobile injuries have increased spectacularly, chiefly because of poor judgment by the operators.

Annually some 1500 pedestrians, five to 14 years of age, are killed in traffic. Injuries, which are a better indicator of the seriousness of the problem, show that 50,000 schoolchildren are injured in pedestrian accidents every year.

Burns kill more children than do all forms of cancer and infectious diseases. In addition to fatalities, severe human suffering can occur from a burn injury. Through a combination of factors— environmental hazards, deficiencies in knowledge, and movements of personal stress or distraction—a healthy person can be permanently disfigured and physically impaired.

A great number of accidents still occur in the workplace, caused chiefly by unsafe conditions and unsafe acts.[17] The current approach to accident causation is through safety research that analyzes job tasks, workplace surroundings, and human behavior (see Figure 1–9).

Accidental ingestion of medicines causes most accidental poisonings in children, and aspirin heads the list. Children under five who swallowed aspirin were the victims in one fourth of all cases of accidental poisoning reported in a recent year to the National Clearinghouse for Poison Control Centers.

Animal bites, a significant urban public health problem, represent about half of the total of other reportable accidents and diseases in some large cities—with children under 15 years of age being the major victims.

The need for education for safe living is great indeed. It must begin early with children. While adults have a high incidence of motor vehicle and firearms accidents and often discuss ways of reducing them, it becomes most difficult to talk to the excitement-loving, venturesome youngsters who are repelled by the idea that being safe means avoiding unnecessary risks. So they have needless accidents while pursuing their day-to-day activities.

---

[17]Stilkind, Jerry. "Why Do Accidents Happen?" *Job Safety and Health,* 5:4–9, April 1977.

Figure 1–9.   Safety inspections at the workplace. (U.S. Department of Labor, Occupational Safety and Health Administration.)

Childhood curiosity, like childhood enthusiasm, needs guiding. For example, every 24 hour period more than 800 children in the United States are poisoned by their own curiosity, which impels them to gulp aspirin and sleeping pills, sip floor polish and kerosene, and swallow kitchen detergents, rubber cement, and cosmetics. Children consume pesticides too. Out of 111 deaths reported in one study 51 per cent occurred in children under 10 years of age. Children, it has been said, will eat just about anything—and there are some 15,000 substances which are, to some extent, poisonous.

The *problems of aging* are many. People are living longer; the population is growing older. It is not at all unrealistic to base training of children now in school on the probability that a high percentage will live past 90 and many beyond 100 years. This will place increased value on the continuous application of proper health knowledge all through the years. Interestingly, people who live to a ripe old age have some practices in common. Charlie Smith, a bona fide 130 year old Southerner, uses his body and mind as much as possible and stays clear of stressful situations. Shirali Mislinov of Azerbaidzhan (Republic of USSR) at 167 years of age has never been obese, competitive, over-ambitious, or gluttonous for the delights of food and has always practiced a certain self-control. In America more than two fifths of all persons 65 years of age and over are limited in activity by chronic conditions, primarily heart disease, arthritis, and rheumatism. Some 26 per cent are undernourished and 25 per cent are anemic. Interlocking services are needed to respond to the complications of aging, but preventive medicine and health education during the active years need more attention.

The effects of *environmental pollution* are shocking. As the ecological balance is slighted and technological progress is championed by the many, the pollutants tend to increase, causing huge economic losses and lowered health for mankind. Fortunately, the environmental movement has come of age. The industrialists are beginning to stop further damage to the living space. Large numbers of people are rallying behind the Commoner "laws" of ecology. (1. Everything is connected to everything else, and 2. Everything must go somewhere.)[18] And as difficult as it is to comprehend, the human mind is attempting to understand the complexity of ecological processes.

Partially related to the pollution problems are sheer numbers of people taking up space, having certain needs, and creating a number of dysfunctions—a number of which lead to overcrowding, dehumanization, tension, and violence and severely challenge the earth's carrying capacity. Some of this is not new. Over a century ago the educator-poet Edwin Markham wrote, "Why build the city glorious if man unbuilded goes . . ." He was purposely directing his words to the core of societal issues now accepted as part of environmental health. In his widely known poem, "The Man with the Hoe," he made the individual person the symbol of the exploited classes throughout the world, and focused on the social and economic abuses of the day. He didn't bring about much change. The abuses to

---

[18]Commoner, Barry. *The Closing Circle.* New York: Alfred A. Knopf, 1971.

life, limb, and spirit are still part of the scene, as too many people remain unaware of the powerful relationship between their environment and well-being.

Although the air is getting cleaner, dozens of large cities suffer from radiation, smoke, smog, fumes, and chemicals. Research findings of the U.S. Environmental Protection Agency indicate that 200 million tons of air pollutants enter the atmosphere every year in the form of carbon monoxide, sulfur oxides, nitrogen oxides, hydrocarbons (unburned chemicals), particulates (smoke, fly ash, dust, and so on), and photochemical smog. Generally, the greater the air pollution the greater the number of deaths. Air sampling stations show that the automobile is still a top-ranking culprit which produces one half of the contaminants found in the air. Other methods of transportation rank second, followed by the petroleum industry, combustion of fuels, use of organic solvents, metals, chemicals, incineration of refuse, and minerals.

Severe air pollution triggers illness and may bring about premature death to thousands of people. Even "ordinary" levels of air pollution can cause coughing, sneezing, wheezing, and suffering.

Figure 1–10. Winter smog in Phoenix, Arizona. Note diminishing visibility in background.

Short-range discomfort may be followed by long-range disease. Bronchitis, emphysema (a deteriorating lung condition sometimes marked by heart enlargement and impairment of heart action), and lung cancer are more prevalent in areas of high air contamination. Studies carried out in four distinct geographical areas of the United States, involving 20,472 children and adults, clearly linked excessive, acute respiratory disease with communities heavily polluted with sulfur dioxide and suspended sulfates. Pollution exposure of three years or longer was an important component in increased risk for acute respiratory disease.[19] A careful check of total deaths in New York City by day of occurrence indicates periodic peaks in mortality which are associated with periods of high air pollution. Temperature inversion conditions and low wind speed permit air pollution to build up to high levels.

Although it is known that cigarette smoking and air pollution are separate causes of emphysema, it has now been shown that the combined effect is even more deadly. Smoking, however, has a greater chance of influencing emphysema than air pollution, for it has been found that the percentage of emphysema is higher among moderate smokers not exposed to pollution than non-smokers exposed to pollution.

Cleaning up America's polluted waters is a task for government at all levels and for industry in every community. The Council on Environmental Quality reports that rivers and waterways are gradu-

---

[19]French, Jean G., et al. "The Effect of Sulfur Dioxide and Suspended Sulfates on Acute Respiratory Disease," *Archives of Environmental Health, 27*:129–134, September 1973.

Figure 1–11. Breakup of the Tanker *Argo Merchant* off Nantucket, spilling 7.3 million gallons of heavy fuel oil. (U.S. Coast Guard.)

ally becoming cleaner. Lake Erie is again producing many tons of fish. Education of the citizen is required if water pollution control programs are to continue to be implemented. Man has made numerous bodies of water so bacteria-ridden that he cannot drink it, so oily and irritant that he cannot swim in it, so unsupportive of life that he cannot fish in it, and so malodorous and filled with refuse and old junk that he cannot contemplate its once natural beauty. Even the oceans are threatened by indiscriminate dumping practices and accidental oil spills (see Figure 1–11).

Today, even noise pollution is a health hazard in industry and in the community. Exposure to severe noise causes hearing loss, changes in cardiovascular blood pressure, pulse rate, and breathing, gastrointestinal motility, and endocrine gland excretions and interferes with the process of thinking and learning. Noise does not need to be deafening to be dangerous; exposure to noise levels of 85 decibels for more than five hours a day may lead to a gradual loss of hearing. A noise of 160 decibels, however, can rupture the eardrum. Only an educated consumer will demand a reduction in noise levels in the home or on the street. Slowly the public is beginning to regard a good environment as a *natural right*—as are civil rights and the right to education. René Dubos is fully supportive of this view when he says that the environmental movement cannot be merely a fad, ". . . because history shows that there has never been a lasting retreat from the recognition of a natural right of man."[20]

Absenteeism everywhere has been slowly climbing. The annual rate for industrial absenteeism is approximately 7 per cent, an all-time high. The acute diseases such as colds and upper respiratory illnesses account for half of the current absenteeism; chronic debilitating disease accounts for the other half. Because of this, more than ten billion dollars a year is drained from the economy. Studies among high absentees show that they tend to be unhappy, discontented, egocentric, and generally unhealthy. Thousands of workers suffer from the "blues" and "blahs" associated with unrewarding, routine production line work that frequently pays well but leaves the worker in a state of chronic fatigue and stress at the week's end. Conversely, the worker with few absences tends to be happy and contented, outgoing, and reasonably well.

In New York City 65 per cent of school absences are caused by health problems. Preventable school absences in this one city cost several million dollars annually in state aid.

Sex-Related Problems

There is a massive accumulation of evidence to indicate that one of the foremost health-related problems of the century is the widespread lack of knowledge and understanding of human sex and sexuality.

Since 1958 the venereal disease rate has increased 500 per cent to become pandemic, despite the fact that it should be common

---

[20]Dubos, René. "Progressive Degradation," *World Health,* July 1975, p. 15.

knowledge that syphilis and gonorrhea can be cured with penicillin. Reported cases of gonorrhea have more than doubled in the past several years. (Note distribution in Figure 1–12.) Much of the increase has been among children between the ages of 12 and 19 years. Moreover, in the past decade the incidence of congenital syphilis in children under 10 years of age rose by 168 per cent. Society has been slow to act. In 1940 the U.S. Surgeon General could not even use the word syphilis in a radio broadcast. Almost 35 years later the word still causes adults to blush and sixth graders to ask what it is. In New York City, where syphilis doubled among teenage boys in an eight-year period, a study showed that 32 per cent did not know that it could be cured, and 60 per cent did not know that venereal disease is transmitted through sexual intercourse. Keeping sex information "under wraps" has been exactly the wrong thing to do.

Since 1940 teenage marriages have risen 500 per cent, and studies indicate that 50 to 80 per cent of teenage wives are pregnant at the time of marriage. The divorce rate in such marriages is three times as high as that for individuals married after 21. Interestingly, the proportion of brides who are pregnant at marriage decreases as the level of education increases.[21]

Births to the nation's mothers aged 15 and younger climbed by 75

[21]Tillack, Warner S., et al. "A Study of Premarital Pregnancy," *American Journal of Public Health, 62*:676–679, May 1972.

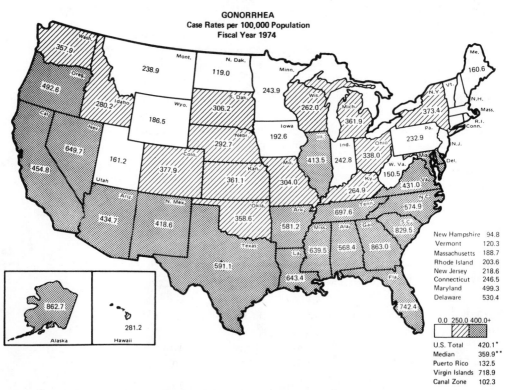

Figure 1–12. U.S. distribution of gonorrhea by states. (U.S. Public Health Service.)

per cent between 1960 and 1977. More than 50 per cent of the 21 million people between the ages of 15 and 19 years have had sexual intercourse. So have about one fifth of the 13 and 14 year old boys and girls. Of the one million teenage pregnancies about 325,000 were terminated by a legal abortion. Most are out-of-wedlock pregnancies, which are still on the increase. Moreover, they are the most common cause of school dropouts. Studies show that very few of these girls understand conception and the sex function. Unfortunately, upper elementary youngsters learn history from Miss Jones, mathematics from Mr. Smith, and sex education from the gang at the corner of Main and State Streets.

In view of the large number of unwanted teenage pregnancies and the increasing desire to amend the situation through abortion, one is compelled to support the view of Goldstein from the University of California Medical Center:

> The greater good is to be gained in viewing abortion for what it is—a poor, very poor method of remedying a failure of contraception. And generally, failure of contraception is a failure of education, just as surely as delay in seeking advice and help to obtain an abortion is a failure of education.[22]

Although unwed mothers and pregnant girls are being helped and children with venereal disease are being treated, very few school systems are providing a comprehensive sex education curriculum for students of both sexes in grades one to 12. Only one fifth of states requiring health education mandate sex education in the schools and only three in ten teach about contraception and boy-girl relationships. This is most unfortunate, for this is a society in which chaperones and supervision of youth are unfashionable, the young people are left on their own with easy access to privacy, children of all ages are totally vulnerable to the onslaughts of commercial exploitation of sex, news media report all kinds of sordid sexual occurrences, and sex misinformation comes from many questionable sources. Until this void is filled with a quantity and quality of factual knowledge, the young person will continue to remain very defenseless about sex. Studies show that boys and girls do not want sexual license; they crave information and explanations. They seek standards which will help them understand the role of sex as a part of their total personality. And they want to talk about it—in the way that they talk about any other topic in the school curriculum. Kirkendall, in calling for sex education, makes this need quite clear when he says:

> The chief determinant of sexual conduct is not factual information but the general feeling of satisfaction and worth which the individual has been able to develop about himself as a person. One's pattern of sexual behavior is a reflection of one's total life pattern. An individual who feels he is accomplishing something with his life . . . will not be driven by guilt, anxiety or compulsion to engage in sex with little regard for what it means to other persons or to his total situation. In other words, he is in a position to direct and manage his sexuality.[23]

---

[22]Goldstein, Phillip and Stewart, Gary. "Trends in Therapeutic Abortion in San Francisco," *American Journal of Public Health,* 62:695–699, May 1972.

[23]Kirkendall, Lester A. "Sex Education," *Discussion Guide No. 1,* published by Sex Information and Education Council of the U.S., October 1965, p. 9.

Considerably more attention will be given to program planning in the area of sex and family living education in Chapter 8.

Superstitions

There is a wide variety of superstitions in existence throughout the world. They are based in some cases on old wives' tales and in other cases on pure magic. Rich and poor alike believe them, and contrary to what might be expected they are a part of the daily existence of the bright scholar as well as of the dull and ignorant. Superstitions are difficult to combat because they are concealed beneath the veneer of education. It has been succinctly stated that man surveys the world about him, clutching science with one hand, hoping for its benefits, yet holding firmly with the other hand to the superstitions of the ages. One sees the figure of Samuel Pepys, famous diarist of the 1600's, headed for home with a rabbit's foot in one pocket and a copy of Hooke's "Book of Microscopy" in the other.

Gullibility

This is a nation of healthy people. It is also a nation of tub thumpers, pill takers, television addicts, neurotics, and helpless individuals. Probably more people are "lost" in terms of what to do for themselves along health lines than most people realize. Newspaper advertising on the one hand and television ads on the other keep heads turning from this product to that product like a mass of humanity watching a tennis match. Americans have been accused of buying everything and anything if it is supposed to be "good for you." Nearly 20 billion pills are consumed each year. This averages out to about one hundred pills annually for every man, woman, and child in the country. Most pills, of course, are taken out of necessity and render an important service in conquering or checking disease and improving personal efficiency. Millions of pills and gallons of patent medicines are devoured for imaginary illnesses brought on by gullibility. Parents are gullible and so are their children; they require a better understanding of health.

Fads, Diets, and Quackery

Mature people are sometimes like the classmates of the little girl in the fourth grade who comes to school with a pretty red ribbon in her hair. Before the week is out, half of her girl friends in the class will be seen sporting attractive ribbons in their hair.

On almost any street in the community, friendly neighbors spread the word that something helped them with their aches and pains. Some people subject themselves to such things as vitamin pills, steam baths, spinal manipulations, or blackstrap molasses and yogurt simply because their friends think it good for them. No thought of securing qualified medical attention has entered their minds. Reducing fads cost the public 100 million dollars a year. Too often overweight folks seek only an easy way to lose weight. Instead of exercising they would rather deaden the appetite with an amphetamine pill (which is not an effective treatment for obesity). People want to swallow a pill, suck a skim milk or lemon juice wafer or chew mint-flavored gum, eat what they please, and still lose weight. They do not know that it may even be harmful. For example, diabetics and individuals with high blood pressure or heart disease should take tablets only upon the advice of a physician. People are always waiting for the "miracle drug," and if tranquilizing drugs work for one person's illness, the attitude of the person on the street is often: "Why won't it work for my troubles, too?"

Combine ignorance with a frantic desire to overcome pain and illness and the stage is set for the development of unproven and usually bizarre nostrums. In this respect cancer, arthritis, and other baffling diseases for which there is no sure cure have always been a fertile ground for the quack and charlatan. The Hoxsey treatment in the 1940's, the Krebiozen "cancer serum" of the 1950's, and the more recent Laetrile claims for curing cancer are examples. Unfortunately, what actually cures illness and what doesn't is frequently difficult to ascertain. A placebo will relieve pain if the patient really believes in it. And in a debilitated patient, a little rest and tender loving care can be a more effective cure than almost anything else. Providing proof of quackery, therefore, is complicated.

Cults and quackeries may be more serious than fads, for they tend to confuse the public as to their relationship with science. People practicing certain cults and quackery often believe they have a "cure," and they make what they have to offer sound powerfully scientific, especially to the person who is in need of help. Quacks are hard to place behind bars because they often claim that they are not dispensing medicines. As long as they do not prescribe drugs or practice surgery, they seem to be safe in many states today. But their influence in spreading health misinformation is great indeed. Public and school health education can do much to curtail fads, cults, and quackeries.

Misconceptions

"The trouble with people is not that they don't know . . . but that they know so much that ain't so."

—Josh Billings, 1818–1885

People are under all kinds of common misconceptions. Some border on superstitions; others are more acceptable and easy to believe, such as "it is impossible to cure any cancer." One of the biggest misconceptions in our society today relates to the topic of who is qualified to practice medicine. Thousands of unsuspecting people have little idea of the meaning of "Dr." or "M.D." They assume that these letters refer to specialists of comparable ability. Yet, in some places, almost anyone can hang up a sign in the front yard with "Dr." written on it.

A rather extensive list of harmful misconceptions about health and safety was compiled by Dzenowagis from information given by sixth grade schoolchildren.[24] As in his later studies, he points to the needs for health education in a convincing manner. Children in this grade had erroneous beliefs, and they had trouble discriminating among truths, half-truths, and falsehoods. In studying family health practices in Kentucky, an urgent need to integrate health education into the health care delivery system was found. Far too many people accepted sickness and disability as part of their lives. They were unhappy and pessimistic about the state of their health but didn't know how to improve it.[25]

The Extremes—Indifference Versus Neurotic Behavior

People seem to vary in their attitude toward health on a scale all the way from a state of indifference with too little concern for health to a state of over-concern to the point of neurotic behavior. Somewhere between the two lies the area of the moderate attitude.

Indifference is closely allied to gullibility and ignorance. It is a negative factor that has always retarded the wheels of progress. It is more common in adults, whose minds are less flexible, than it is in children, who tend to be openminded. It evaporates slowly when human enlightenment takes hold. Indifference to common health practices is illustrated rather well by the story of the nurse-teacher who called on Mary's mother to tell her about the little girl's long standing case of head lice. After the nurse had spoken to her for several minutes, the mother simply gazed out across the fields, shrugged her shoulders as if to dismiss the whole business and said, "Well, everybody has a few."

The other extreme is neurotic behavior. A growing number of adults are becoming almost neurotic about their health. They sometimes join cults, become food faddists, and practice any health fancies which suit them at the moment. These people thrive on all the loose bits of information on psychosomatic illnesses that float about in their community. Moreover, their imaginary difficulties sometimes become real, and then their neurotic behavior relates to something more serious.

HEALTH ACTIVATION AND SELF-CARE

In late 1976 Congress enacted Public Law 94–317, an Act which gave the Department of Health, Education, and Welfare considerable freedom to provide health education and disease prevention activities. It is aimed directly at consumers and what they can do for themselves, together with governmental support mandating certain promotional practices.

---

[24]Dzenowagis, Joseph G. "Prevalence of Certain Dangerous Safety Misconceptions Among a Group of Sixth-Grade Children," *Journal of School Health,* 33:26–32, January 1963.

[25]Carlton, Bill. "Is Community Research Effective in Establishing Health Education Programs?" *Health Education,* 8:10–12, March/April 1977.

Currently there is a strong effort to activate an educational approach to health care that emphasizes self-care and self-help. The focus is on what individuals can do personally and how they can establish a "health partnership" with professionals. For too long the consumer has leaned almost entirely on the "providers" of cure and care. Such a mental set is quite incongruous with the concept of responsibility for self-care. Dubos was aware of this when he said that ". . . to ward off disease or recover health, men as a rule find it easier to depend on healers than attempt the more difficult task of living wisely."

The concept of caring for one's own health and making decisions about health matters is contributing to the emerging ethic regarding the legitimacy of lay initiatives in health matters, both official and non-official, at local, state, and national levels. There are more lay people today attending open forums and hearings having to do with health than ever before. The growing concern with medical self-help, information on nutrition and the environment, coping with life situations, and prevention of common illnesses and emergencies is being demonstrated from Canada to Texas.

Closely related to the self-care program is *patient education—* "a process by which patients and/or those responsible for their care (1) are taught their roles in the maintenance of health and the treatment of disease, and (2) are motivated to carry out their identified responsibilities."[26] Involving the patient in his or her health care away from a setting of acute illness is becoming an acceptable practice—one that depends heavily upon an informed patient. Quality patient education not only improves health care and fosters a better use of physicians' consultation time but also elevates the spirit of the recuperating individual and advances the healing process.

EDUCATION DEFINED

A proper definition of education includes some reference to aims, purposes, or goals. The word "education" comes from the Latin word *educere,* meaning "to lead forth" or "to lead out." It refers to the drawing out of a person something latent or potential. It suggests a change in some particular direction. Education, therefore, may be defined toward certain preconceived goals. Thus, education is anything but haphazard. There is a well-defined purpose expressed through clearly stated aims and objectives.

EDUCATIONAL AIMS AND OBJECTIVES

Principles, not men—when men desert principle, may they be deserted by the people.

—Courier of New Hampshire, 1802

---

[26]Definition as set forth by the American Group Practice Association, Alexandria, Virginia 22314.

There has always been a high degree of respect in this country for the person with an avowed purpose.[27] One of the most famous remarks used year after year at commencement exercises was made by Leland Stanford who said, "the world stands aside for the man who knows where he is going."

In education, as in other fields of endeavor, one needs to know where he or she is going. Direction is always important. One must possess a personal philosophy of life that is fundamentally sound. Like Maxwell Garnett, most people believe that human societies should aim toward the fulfillment of some far-reaching purpose.[28] Such a point of view, coupled with an interest in education, equips the individual with the basic ideas to formulate the aims and objectives of education.

Most purposes of education make a definite reference to healthful living. In 70 B.C., Cicero proclaimed to his subjects in Rome, "In nothing do men more nearly approach the gods than in giving health to men." Centuries later, in 1550, Rabelais said, "The aim of education is not so much to fill thee with learning as to train both thy mind and thy body. . . . Without health, life is no life." In 1690, John Locke made his much quoted statement: "A sound mind in a sound body is a short but full description of a happy state in this world; he that has these two has little more to wish for; and he that wants either of them, will be but little the better for anything else."

The essential purposes of education have not varied to any great degree in a century of time. What Herbert Spencer wrote in 1860 on the question, "What knowledge is of most worth?" does not depart significantly from modern goals. His ends of education were concerned with life and health, earning a living, family rearing, citizenship, and leisure.

In 1898 Nicholas Murray Butler, president of Columbia University for 43 years, again asked the old Spencerian question. He acknowledged Spencer's science in education approach and went on to point out that the most enduring knowledge must ultimately relate to things of the spirit.[29] A major contribution of Butler's was that he viewed a proper education as one in which the practical aspects could be linked to the things of the spirit. This means that health education must be both reasonable and emotional if it is to penetrate the mind of the student and be significant in the spiritual life that constitutes humanity's full stature.

As far as health education is concerned, most sets of purposes stress health as the primary aim. Recently the National Education Association once again reemphasized health as a cardinal principle of education.[30] They also point to the need for education for leisure,

---

[27]For a clear-cut illustration of singleness of purpose, see Abraham Lincoln's straightforward letter to Horace Greeley on the Saving of the Nation. (Willgoose, Carl E. "Health: The Fundamental Objective," *Education,* 68(8):451, April 1948.)

[28]Garnett, J. C. Maxwell. *Education and World Citizenship.* Cambridge, England: The University Press, 1921. p. 315.

[29]Butler, Nicholas Murray, *The Meaning of Education, and Other Essays and Addresses.* New York: The Macmillan Co., 1898.

[30]National Education Association Bicentennial Committee. "The Seven Cardinal Principles Revisited," *Today's Education,* 65:57–72, March 1976.

an item that concerns physical and mental health to a great degree and probably has as much to do with the survival of humanity as any other aim.

THE ULTIMATE SCOPE OF HEALTH EDUCATION

It may be seen in the preceding objectives of education that agreement has been reached by educational philosophers stressing the need for health education in the schools. The ultimate scope of health education is a broad one. Thus, each person, in order to satisfy his or her own needs and, at the same time, contribute his or her share to the welfare of society must possess:

1. Optimum organic health consistent with heredity and the application of present health knowledge.
2. Sufficient coordination, strength, and vitality to meet emergencies as well as the requirements of daily living.
3. Emotional stability to meet the stresses and strains of modern life.
4. Social consciousness and adaptability with respect to the requirements of group living.
5. Sufficient knowledge and insight to make suitable decisions and arrive at feasible solutions to problems.
6. Attitudes, values, and skills that stimulate satisfactory participation in a full range of daily activities.
7. Spiritual and moral qualities that contribute the fullest measure of living in a democratic society.

If we learn anything at all from the present condition of adult mankind, it should be that the problems, diseases, and inadequacies of the moment did not suddenly appear; rather, they emerged gradually, having had their roots established during the early elementary school years. This is to say that the backaches, ulcers, gastrointestinal pains, hypertension, obesity, chronic fatigue, coronary thrombosis, and the neurotic and psychotic behavior related to anxiety, apprehension, worry, fear, hatred, and jealousy are all tied directly to a *pattern of living* and level of understanding obtained during the formative years. A sense of values early in life, coupled with the proper skills and knowledge, sets the stage in more ways than one. The part played by health education in this period can be most productive.

QUESTIONS FOR DISCUSSION

1. Comment on the view that the government works against itself when it supports tobacco farmers on the one hand and wages a continuing battle against tobacco smoking on the other. What are the facts and implications?

2. What is the relationship of physical efficiency to total health?

3. How can we get citizens in the community interested in, concerned with, and involved in school health programs?

4. What is happening in your community relative to the control of air pollutants? Water pollutants? The control of traffic accidents?

5. Are there ways in which health professionals in the community can influence health instruction practices in an elementary school?

6. How has the World Health Organization contributed to child health on an international level?

SUGGESTED ACTIVITIES

1. Dobzhansky, writing in *Mankind Evolving: The Evolution of the Human Species* (Yale University Press, 1962, pp. 346–347), points out that "nature and nurture" work together. Hoyman writes about the same thing. So does Dubos. (See references listed at end of the chapter.) Look over an article or two which pertains to human ecology and health. Prepare a written paragraph on what you have read and another one setting forth your comments.

2. Survey a number of persons in health-related professions (public or private) and find out how they feel about education as a means of preventing poor health. Are they concerned about venereal disease or cardiac statistics, or something called "value illness"? Compare your findings with those of several of your classmates.

3. Compare the several positions with regard to population growth and its bearing on human health and welfare. Do official governmental figures substantiate the views of demographers and ecologists? What is the view of the conservationist?

4. Investigate current health care practices in a community of your choice. Where are the opportunities for self-help? How much patient education is being done? What is the general attitude toward preventive medicine and health promotion through community health education?

5. Among others, William Curran is a spokesman for the rights of individuals for a healthful environment. He regards the role of public health law as an important tool in bringing about these rights (see Selected References). However, he feels uncomfortable about mandating health practices and would prefer that citizens accept personal responsibility for their actions. What are your comments relative to the *balance* between (1) legislation to improve health and (2) voluntary actions on the part of the citizenry?

6. In his utopian book, *The Shape of Things To Come*, H. G. Wells assumed that scientific thinking, modern-day engineering, and public education, by their intrinsic worth, would prepare a kind of future that would be approved of by the educated middle-class citizen. Later, when he wrote *Mind at the End of Its Tether*, Wells became disillusioned as he noted that Nazi Germany scored higher on scientific rationalism, engineering, and public education than did any other European nation. Take a moment to examine this observation. Do educational goals and programs need very careful definition as they relate to a civilization? Write out some specific implications for educators and others who build a society "close to the heart's desire."

SELECTED REFERENCES

Boyd, Velena. "The High-Level Wellness Approach to Health." *Health Values,* *1*:63–65, March/April 1977.

Bucher, Charles A., Olsen, Einar A., and Willgoose, Carl E. *The Foundations of Health.* 2nd ed., Englewood Cliffs, N.J.: Prentice-Hall, Inc., 1976.

Buonomano, Louise and Buonomano, Vito D. "Contemporary Health Care: Problems and Projections." *Dental Survey, 53*:9–14, September 1977.

Callahan, Joseph F., and Clark, Leonard H. *Foundations of Education: Planning for Competence.* New York: Macmillan Publishing Co., 1977, Chapter 3.

Carrell, Alexis. *Man the Unknown.* New York: Harper and Brothers, 1936.

Commoner, Barry. *The Closing Circle.* New York: Alfred A. Knopf, 1971.

Curran, William J. "Direct Advertising to the Public: Free Speech, Risks and Benefits," *American Journal of Public Health, 67*:56–57, January 1977.

———————. "A Constitutional Right To A Healthy Environment," *American Journal of Public Health, 67*:262, March 1977.

Dubos, René. *Man Adapting.* New Haven: Yale University Press, 1965.

Frederick, Calvin J. "Suicide In The United States," *Health Education, 8*:17–21, November/December 1977.

Galli, Nicholas. *Foundations and Principles of Health Education.* New York: John Wiley & Sons, Inc., 1978.

Gershenson, Charles P. "Child Maltreatment, Family Stress, and Ecological Insult," *American Journal of Public Health, 67*:602–603, July 1977.

Haven, Brent Q. *Self-Destructive Behavior: A National Crisis.* Minneapolis: Burgess Publishing Company, 1972.

Higginson, John. "A Hazardous Society," *American Journal of Public Health, 66*:359–364, April 1976.

Hoyman, Howard S. "An Ecological View of Health and Health Education," *Journal of School Health, 35*:110–123, March 1965.

Kegley, Charles F., et al. "Cocaine: Old Drug, New Problems," *Journal of School Health, 47*:600–602, December 1977.

Leff, S. V. *From Witchcraft To World Health.* New York: The Macmillan Company, 1957.

Levi, Lennart. *Society, Stress and Disease.* New York: Oxford University Press, 1976.

May, Rollo. *Man's Search For Himself.* New York: Dell Publishing Company, 1953.

McIntire, Matilda A., et al. "Safety Packaging—What Does the Public Think? *American Journal of Public Health, 67*:169–172, February 1977.

McKenna, Ken. "If Creeping Boredom Is Your Work Problem," *Today's Health, 50*:43–46, August 1972.

Milio, Nancy. *The Care of Health In Communities.* New York: Macmillan Publishing Co., 1975.

Rosen, George. "History and Health Care," *American Journal of Public Health, 67*:326–327, April 1977.

Ross, Helen S. "Redefining The Future of Health Education," *Health Education, 7*:5–6, July/August 1976.

Salk, Jonas. "What Do We Mean By Health?" *Health Education, 9*:14–16, January/February 1978.

Simonds, Scott K. "Health Education Today: Issues and Challenges," *Journal of School Health, 47*:584–593, December 1977.

Stone, Stephen E. "The Meaning of Health," *Health Education, 8*:2–4, May/June 1977.

Vincent, Roland G. "A Fence or an Ambulance," *Journal of School Health, 37*:369–373 October 1967.

Willgoose, Carl E. "Providing for Change: New Directions," in Read, Donald E. (ed.) *New Directions In Health Education.* New York: Macmillan Publishing Co., 1971, pp. 1–17.

——————— "Health, Welfare, and Religious Freedom," *School and Society,* *73*:198, March 31, 1951.

———————*Health Teaching in Secondary Schools,* 2nd ed., Philadelphia: W. B. Saunders Company, 1977, Chapter 1.

The Elementary
School Health
Program

2 _____

> Look to this day!
>   for it is life,
> the very life of life.
>   In its brief course
> lie all the verities and
>   realities of your existence.
> The bliss of growth
>   The glory of action
> The splendor of achievement
>   For yesterday is but a dream,
> and tomorrow is only a vision;
>   But today, well lived,
> makes every yesterday
>   a dream of happiness,
> And every tomorrow a vision of hope,
>   Look well, therefore, to this day.
>
> *—Salutation to the Dawn*
> Translated from the Sanskrit

From the early era of the soothsayer to the psychiatrist's couch of the present, optimum health has depended upon the intricacies of one's way of life—the predominant lifestyle. Thus, the enlightening expression from Sanskrit calling attention to "...today, well lived" is the very essence of wisdom. For indeed, the way one lives at the moment determines all tomorrows. Getting this message across at an early age is an educational challenge.

JUSTIFICATION FOR SCHOOL HEALTH PROGRAM

As a society comes of age it strives for excellence instead of quantitative growth. Dubos says as much when he speaks of the "mature society" as one that is not only stable in numbers and in material production but also in "ecological equilibrium with the resources of the Earth."[1] Along with this comes the development of a far greater sense of personal and collective responsibility, which tends to ensure a proper *quality of life*. As a sensitive historian, Dubos

[1]Dubos, René. *A God Within.* New York: Charles Scribner's Sons, 1972.

wants humanity to be aware of the past and to consider human welfare in the future in a more humane way. What better justification could there be for improving the health of the citizenry through the creation of well-planned programs of health education in the schools?

There are numerous justifications for a total health maintenance and education effort in the schools. For one thing there is a considerable body of evidence available to support the premise that failure to develop optimum health puts a limit on genius. *Mens sana in corpore sano* is not a new expression. The quality of the mind is made known through the competent actions of the body. A lowered health status reduces one's ability to perform—as a genius or as a moron. People approach their potential mental capacity only when they are capable of transforming their thoughts into actions. The same is true of learning. Thorndike's law of readiness simply means that the individual pupil must be ready to learn. He or she must be organically sound, mentally alert, and emotionally able to receive the most from the total school curriculum. A pain in the stomach, an earache, or some other bothersome factor is a distracting stimulus. Whereas an adult can say to a stomach ache, pain, or emotional problem, "Get thee behind me," the primary grade pupil simply cannot ignore it. The ability to learn is directly impaired, and the student will not respond as well as his or her contemporaries, either in the classroom or anywhere else.

The Educational Policies Commission of the National Education Association has stated repeatedly that an educated person understands the basic facts concerning health and disease; the educated person protects his own health and that of his dependents; and an educated person works to improve the health of his community. Social accomplishments and well-being are closely related in any community because charity consists of being able to give of oneself without thought of return. And in the school, social accomplishment as well as academic accomplishment is ever-dependent on good eyesight and hearing, freedom from disease and handicapping defects, emotional stability, and a satisfactory rate of growth. The broadly conceived school health program is as concerned with these things as it is with classroom instruction. The focus today is on disease prevention. There is wide acceptance of the concept that the cancers and afflictions of humankind represent educational rather than medical failures. Thus, preventive medicine and education have much in common. This idea is expressed in the following verse:

" 'Twas a dangerous cliff, as they freely confessed,
    Though to walk near its crest was so pleasant;
But over its terrible edge there had slipped
    A duke, and full many a peasant.
The people said something would have to be done,
    But their projects did not at all tally.
Some said, "Put a fence 'round the edge of the cliff";
    Some, "An ambulance down in the valley."
The lament of the crowd was profound and was loud,
    As their hearts overflowed with their pity;

But the cry for the ambulance carried the day
    As it spread through the neighboring city.
A collection was made, to accumulate aid,
    And the dwellers in highway and alley
Gave dollars or cents—not to furnish a fence—
    But an ambulance down in the valley.
The story looks queer as we've written it here,
    But things oft occur that are stranger.
More humane, we assert, than to succor the hurt,
    Is the plan of removing the danger.
The best possible course is to safeguard the source;
    Attend to things rationally.
Yes, build up the fence and let us dispense
    With the ambulance down in the valley.[2]

In the School Health Study it was verified that school children display much ignorance about general health and well-being. This "major weakness in the educational system," as it was called by the writers of the study, prompted them to say that the best place for health instruction is in the school—chiefly because the school is the only agency that can keep pace with the rapid advance of medical science and that can teach the child the causes of health problems so that he or she can engage in intelligent health practices.[3]

HISTORY OF SCHOOL HEALTH MOVEMENT

The history of public health programs is as old as the Egyptian and Hebrew civilizations. But the history of the school health movement is much more recent. Certainly, one of the reasons for this is that, in the centuries gone by, humanity had only a slight regard for the growth and development of youth. It was a man's world; women and children were strictly secondary. Although formal education was fostered in many places, health maintenance and promotion were not the concern of the school.

The school health movement has a European heritage. In 1790 Benjamin Thompson, known as Count Rumford, started a school lunch program for underprivileged children in Bavaria. About this time Johann Peter Frank wrote scientific articles on the topic of school hygiene. Other eminent scientists of the day such as Rudolph Virchow (1821–1902) and Henry P. Bowditch (1840–1911) advocated medical examinations of schoolchildren and studies on their growth and development. In England, in 1832, Edwin Chadwick studied child employment conditions and became interested in the schools. Theophile Roussel followed somewhat the same pattern in France. Great writers such as Victor Hugo, Charles Reade, and Charles Dickens were influential in starting a school health move-

[2]Tussing, Lyle. *Psychology for Better Living.* New York: John Wiley & Sons, Inc., 1959, pp. 18–19.

[3]School Health Education Study. *School Health Education: A Call for Action.* Washington, D.C., 1965.

ment. It was Hugo, in 1865, who established a school lunch program for poor children on the Isle of Guernsey. It became so popular that by the early 1900's half the cities in Germany had lunch programs for schoolchildren.

In the United States interest was growing in the areas of school health. In 1842, Horace Mann, Secretary of the Massachusetts Board of Education, wrote in the *Common School Journal,* "So intimately are all parts of the human constitution connected and so vitally do the mental and moral depend upon the physical power, that we can understand either only by studying them in connection with others. For this reason, the knowledge of laws of structure, growth, development, and health of the body is essential to a comprehension of the corresponding particular in the phenomena of the mind." These words carried a great amount of weight. It is not strange, therefore, that by 1885 the American Association for Physical Education was formed. Prominent medical doctors from this group advocated scientific programs of physical activity and hygiene in the schools. By 1894 the Boston schools were ready to begin the first regular medical inspection program in America. Chicago, New York, Philadelphia, and others followed. Interest grew and numerous health agencies were born that had a potent effect on school health efforts. Notable among these was the formation in 1912 of the Children's Bureau of the Federal Security Agency, an organization set up to investigate subjects relating to child life and welfare. Shortly thereafter in 1918 the American Child Hygiene Association was formed.

From about 1900 to 1915 a continued effort was made in the schools to give medical examinations and control communicable diseases. Public health practices improved in many communities and influenced the promotion of child health. Some schools taught hygiene courses consisting chiefly of anatomy and physiology. At first the teaching emphasis was on health knowledge as pure subject matter. It became apparent after a while, however, that the educator must appraise the quantity and quality of the health information in terms of its effect on attitudes and practices of students. As far back as 1910 men like Luther H. Gulick and R. Tait McKenzie stressed the need for appraisal in school health.

Following World War I, school health programs accomplished a great deal. Research was done illustrating the benefits of properly constituted programs. In 1922, Claire E. Turner, working with Mary Spencer, carried out his now famous Malden, Massachusetts, school health demonstration project. Over a two year period they compared the children of three fourth grades, three fifth grades, and three sixth grades in two school buildings with a control group of similar grade school children in two other schools.[4] A health education program was developed with the experimental group and data were collected concerning growth, health status, and health habits. The demonstration not only was successful, but also because it was widely publicized it caused other promoters of school health to "take heart" and begin health instruction in the grades.

---

[4]Turner, Claire E. "Malden Studies in Health Education and Growth," *American Journal of Public Health, 18*:1217–1230, 1928.

The most thorough research into the status of health education and the needs of youth was started in 1961 and completed in 1965 by the School Health Education Study.[5] The findings indicated that health content is repetitious throughout the grades and without consideration for the problems of youth. Numerous weaknesses in health knowledge were also reported. Similar studies in Georgia and Kansas done ten years later reemphasized the existing shortcomings.

The School Health Curriculum Project (Berkeley Project), supported by the Bureau of Health Education, the American Cancer Society, the American Heart Association, the American Lung Association, and others, focused on the elementary and junior high schools. It included intensive teacher preparation and extensive classroom teaching resources. Since its inception over ten years ago, it has been adopted by more than 300 school districts in 30 states.

Today, school health is an integrated phase of the total school program. This has come about chiefly from a rising interest in the welfare of children, an increase in associations dedicated to improving the nation's health, White House Conferences, and the funds of philanthropic organizations. In addition, considerable credit should go to organizations such as the American School Health Association, American Public Health Association, American Alliance for Health, Physical Education, and Recreation, and the Joint Committee on Health Problems in Education of the National Education Association and the American Medical Association.

LEGAL FOUNDATIONS FOR SCHOOL HEALTH PROGRAMS

One of the first laws created for the protection of schoolchildren was passed in 1833 in France. It made public school authorities responsible for the health of schoolchildren. Other European laws followed in Austria, Sweden, Germany, and Russia.

Horace Mann's agitation for the study of health science, then termed "physiology and hygiene," resulted in Massachusetts, in 1850, becoming the first state to require hygiene by law as a compulsory subject in all the public schools. A number of other legal enactments occurred at about the turn of the century. Instruction about alcohol and narcotics was required by 1890 in all states. Many states required physical education before 1900. In 1899 teachers in Connecticut were required to test the vision of their pupils. A school dentist was hired in Reading, Pennsylvania, in 1903. By 1933 the Nebraska State Supreme Court had decreed that the control of the pupil's health during school hours was the responsibility of the school personnel. This is indeed a big responsibility, and the schools have accepted it in the spirit of service.

Today most states have legal foundations for their school health programs. Many of these are in the form of rules and regulations of

---

[5]Sliepcevich, Elena M. "Health Education: a Conceptual Approach." *School Health Education Study,* Washington, D.C., 1965.

state education commissions. The laws in states such as Minnesota, Pennsylvania, Ohio, and New York are particularly clear in setting forth the need for proper attention to health. In fact, it was New York legislation in 1967 (Critical Health Problems Act) mandating the teaching of health education in all schools that set in motion what Bedworth describes as ". . . a wave of public awareness stretching across the country resulting in many more states enacting similar legislation."[6]

PUBLIC AND PRIVATE AFFIRMATIONS

In 1975 Congress enacted Public Law 93–641, the Health Planning and Resources Development Act, which restructured and reconstituted the federal health planning system and, significantly, specifically included disease prevention and health education among the responsibilities of the new Health Systems Agencies.

Then in 1976, Congress enacted Public Law 94–317, the Consumer Health Information and Health Promotion Act, which integrated the services of a broad range of educational and promotive health authorities. Much of the activity and control was assigned to the Bureau of Health Education at the Center for Disease Control in Atlanta.

Also in 1976 a private sector-based National Center for Health Education was established with the goal of avoiding duplication of the health promotional work of existing public and private agencies. Much of this organization's work has dealt with self-help and self-care programs, over-the-counter medications, and helping to reduce malpractice claims by educating people about the limitations of medicine, health research, and the evaluation of current health education activities.

Both the American Academy of Pediatrics and the American Public Health Association have publicized the concept of health education as a continuing process, from conception to death, and have emphasized that such education must be comprehensive and integrated in all community planning for health. Their concern is for sequential programs, kindergarten through grade 12, that should result in a "health-educated consumer citizen who adopts a health-promoting lifestyle . . . and influences public policy and planning on health care issues."[7]

SCHOOL HEALTH ORGANIZATION

Paramount to the success of a health program in any school system is the organization of health activities, personnel, facilities, and time. With a school population exposed to many subject matter

---

[6]Bedworth, David A. "State Health Education Program Revisited," *Health Education, 8*:29–30, January/February 1977.

[7]APHA Policy Statement. "Health Education and Public Health," *The Nation's Health,* September 1977, p. 12.

areas, it becomes increasingly difficult to meet all the health objectives with ease. Yet, efforts in most places are regularly intensified to improve health through preventive and remedial measures.

Health education is an applied science concerned with relating research findings in health to the lives of people. It narrows the gap between what is known and what is practiced. It is what Will Durant calls "preventive medicine in the classroom." If we say that *health education is the sum of experiences that favorably influence practices, attitudes, and knowledge relating to health,* it is readily seen that we are dealing with something that occurs at all times and in all places in the school.[8] Hence, all school personnel and every area of the curriculum have a part in health education to some degree. The organization of these varied efforts into a sound working program is the job of the school administrator.

School health education is essentially a three-pronged process. It consists of health services, a healthful school environment, and health instruction. Definitions of these terms have existed for decades.[9]

Health services "comprises all those procedures designated to determine the health status of the child, to enlist his cooperation in health protection and maintenance, to inform parents of the defects that may be present, to prevent disease, and to correct remediable defects."

Healthful school living "is a term that designates the provision of a wholesome environment, the organization of a healthful school day, and the establishment of such teacher-pupil relationships as make a safe and sanitary school, favorable to the best development of living of pupils and teachers."

Health instruction "is that organization of learning experiences directed toward the development of favorable health knowledges, attitudes, and practices."

The prevalent point of view is that the term "health education" should be reserved for the teaching or instructional part of the school health program. In this manner the pupil has no difficulty attaching a suitable name to the course; it can be called health education.

RESPONSIBILITY OF THE CLASSROOM TEACHER

There is no person in the school system better suited to make a significant contribution to the health of schoolchildren than the classroom teacher in the elementary school. He or she alone occupies the key position for improving child health. With the teacher's interest, enthusiasm, and understanding, the school health program moves ahead. Without his or her support, however, the program is limited.

---

[8]This definition of health education is the one agreed upon by the Joint Committee on Health Problems in Education of the National Education Association and the American Medical Association. The report, *Health Education,* 6th ed., may be obtained from the National Education Association, Washington, D.C.

[9]Health Education Section, Committee Report, American Physical Education Association. *Journal of Health and Physical Education,* December 1934.

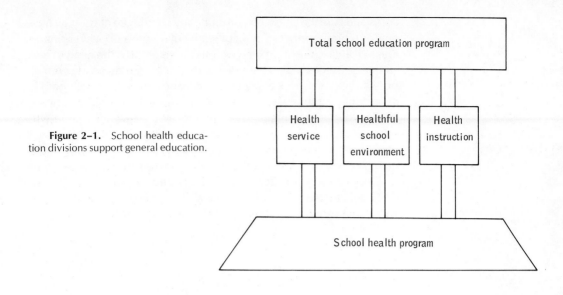

Figure 2–1. School health education divisions support general education.

The role of the classroom teacher is unique; no other person sees the child as the teacher does. He or she can readily compare the student's appearance and actions today with what they were yesterday or a month ago. Or the child can be compared with the other 25 children in the classroom who are about the same age. This provides the alert teacher with a vantage point that neither the parent nor family physician can match. Thus, every classroom teacher has a potentially powerful capacity for building sound health (Figure 2–1). The extent to which this is accomplished will depend upon many things—administrative support, a warm personality and feeling for children, and the power of careful observation.

HOW THE CLASSROOM TEACHER PROMOTES HEALTH

The classroom teacher promotes health in a number of ways:

By Cooperating with the School Health Services Personnel

Children should be properly prepared by the teacher for a visit to the school physician or nurse for periodic physical examinations. Teachers must take a positive approach to the examinations by saying to their pupils, "The doctor is coming to see how many healthy boys and girls we have." Learning to visit medical personnel and come away happy is an education in itself. Any experience that is satisfying or "feels good" to children is effective in terms of their future behavior. The nurse, the physician, and the dental hygienist should be their friends.

By Detecting Abnormalities and Referring Them to Proper Authorities for Appropriate Follow-Up and Correction

The teacher who uses the "eyes to see" can observe a variety of items related to the onset of poor health. The child with frequent colds and sore throats, who is continually sniffling in class, may have any one of a number of difficulties involving the upper respiratory area. Likewise, the child who squints to see or turns the head to hear simple questions may be in need of medical aid right away. Numerous children who appear to be well often need medical attention. The child who exhibits signs of emotional upset that may be missed entirely by the parents may be spotted by the teacher as one who behaves differently from the group and needs individual attention. It should be remembered that the younger the person, the more readily he or she responds to pain or other distracting stimuli. The response may be in the form of a series of incidents leading to poor scholarship. The pupil, for example, who scores well on a test of learning aptitude yet produces work in class that is hardly better than average is the kind of pupil who bears watching.

By Making the School Environment Pleasant and Desirable for the Pupils

The school, to be at all effective, must be the kind of place a child wants to go to. The classroom is made more inviting by the teacher, who regulates physical items such as temperature, ventilation, lighting, and seating. His or her own attitude toward the students has much to do with the health and happiness of the class. There are numerous children who dislike school and show this by coming down with "morning sickness," a psychosomatic disease that mysteriously disappears on Saturdays, Sundays, and holidays.

By Providing Health Instruction in the Classroom

Teaching is done both formally and informally. In this respect, the teacher seldom misses an opportunity to refer to the child's health and welfare. Health as a topic is also correlated with other materials. The teacher's task is to teach it with the aim of changing practices and attitudes.

THE TEACHER'S HEALTH

Teaching can be an exhausting activity. Many grade-school teachers complain of getting too little exercise and sleep and cite stress as their biggest health problem. The effective teacher is one who possesses the vitality to do the job expected and has a little reserve left at the close of the day for personal enrichment activities. According to reports and opinions, personality maladjustments are responsible for failure in teaching more often than physical disorders. Even the admirable teacher who loves children, is intellectually alert, and gets along well with others will be limited in expression and enthusiasm proportionate to the degree of physical and mental health.

The health status of the teacher has another significant bearing on education. This relates to the image the teacher presents to the pupils. The sick teacher with a sour disposition can hardly practice what he or she preaches. Whether we care to admit it or not, teaching is a process of making little images of the teacher in the minds of the pupils. Very little effective health education can be expected from the image of a teacher suffering from complaints such as chronic fatigue, gross overweight, nagging headache, low back pain, irregular teeth, and a negative, complaining attitude toward life. Thus, in teaching young people, the importance of the example of personal health and well-being cannot be underestimated.

RESPONSIBILITY OF THE ELEMENTARY SCHOOL ADMINISTRATOR

The practice of accepting primary responsibility for school health is not the same in each community. Essentially it boils down to the question of whether the school controls all the health education or whether it is the responsibility of the local or county health department. In a number of places the city or county health depart-

Figure 2–2. Academic performance and health status can be detected by the classroom teacher. (Courtesy Joe Di Dio, National Education Association.)

ment is responsible for school health services. In fact, county school health planning committees are formed and composed of school and county health personnel and interested citizens. These committees, meeting with county school superintendents and county health officers, initiate desirable health programs in the schools. By and large, however, the trend throughout the country is to place full responsibility for school health and health education with the school administrator and board of education. In the larger cities the administrator may appoint a school health director.

The classroom teacher will find the elementary school principal most helpful, especially if he or she engages in many of the following activities:

1. Provides for health services and "sets the stage" for the work of physicians, dentists, nurses, psychologists, dental hygienists, and teachers of the handicapped.
2. Is concerned with safe and sanitary building construction and the activities of the school custodial staff.
3. Is interested in the preparation and personal health of teaching personnel.
4. Promotes in-service education for medical personnel and classroom teachers.
5. Obtains adequate funds for the program.
6. Maintains lines of communication between school and community agencies.
7. Arranges for periodic nurse-teacher conferences and meetings of health councils.
8. Meets with parents to secure adequate treatment for all children.
9. Initiates a total school safety program.
10. Assists classroom teachers in securing necessary facilities, materials, and time for health instruction.
11. Provides leadership to school feeding programs.
12. Conducts studies relative to school absences and health problems.

It is interesting to note that in one large city school system, the Los Angeles City Schools, the results of a thorough survey indicated several ways in which school administrators could help improve the existing health education effort. In planning and coordinating the health program of the individual school, it was suggested that greater use be made of health councils. It was also felt that more use should be made of the school environment in health teaching experiences. Moreover, administrators were urged to develop teacher guides in health education at each grade level, offer more in-service health education, and do a more thorough job of planning the health instruction program.

In many school systems today there is a health education coordinator who helps health teachers set goals and competencies for students to achieve, develops elementary activities and teaching aids, and evaluates programs. Frequently this person organizes in-service health-related courses to meet local needs.

INNER CITY HEALTH PROBLEMS

Urban problems can best be understood by understanding the nature of urban communities, for solutions to urban problems tend to be only as good as the problem-solver's grasp of the nature of urban communities.[10]

In recent years the wide variety of conflicts, frustrations, and unhappiness in the urban areas has been uppermost in the thoughts of leaders of government, medicine, social welfare, and education. Hardly an issue or problem is not in some way a health concern.

One thing is for certain: the lowered health status of inner city children, together with other negative variables such as low income and less than adequate family care, frequently results in increased absences and poor school performance. The background for much of this may be blamed on the early years. When there is inadequate nutrition at the infant stage, growth is compromised. The brain fails to synthesize protein, and consequently suffers a decrease as great as 20 per cent in the number of cells. Thus, severe malnutrition, which is found frequently in the depths of the inner city as well as in isolated rural areas, results in decreased learning ability and retarded growth, maturation, and personal productivity. Moreover, poor child-rearing practices contribute a negative psychological dimension that hinders effective learning. It has also been demonstrated that inner city families change their place of residence a great deal; this in itself creates numerous non-utilizers of health care.

Low income persons spend more days in bed as a result of illness or injury than do high income persons. Young children in low income families spend twice as many days in bed because of illness and injury than do young children from high income families.

Ethnic groups have particular problems. The ills of the Spanish-speaking population are often unreported. Illness and premature death are generally more common for blacks than they are for whites. Among the Chinese in San Francisco the incidence of children with vision problems, dental caries, and immunization deficiencies is especially high. Reaching these needy people is difficult to do, for they "hole up" in their crowded, noisy, polluted, insensitive, incomprehensible, push-button world. To reach these groups with the health and education message is, at times, all but impossible because of the breakdown of the neighborhood concept. A return to definable neighborhoods is needed. There is great merit in preserving an Italian North End, an Irish-Polish South Boston, a Chinatown, a black Roxbury, or any enclave that "feels" comfortable to its residents and has some compatible common denominator, not necessarily ethnic or religious.

One reason that low socioeconomic status and poor health go together is that there is a lack of concrete information among the disadvantaged about the causes and treatment of diseases and the availability of health services. When medical advice is wanted it is generally sought from friends and neighbors rather than from a

---

[10]Dentler, Robert A. *Urban Problems: Perspectives and Solutions,* Chicago: Rand McNally, 1977, p. 1.

physician or health center personnel. The result is that children are denied medical treatment until a relatively late stage of illness. Many black people know nothing about sickle cell anemia, a genetic disease affecting the red blood cells—for which a medical checkup is a must. Large numbers of families of all races and persuasions will listen to some extent to what the schools have to say. Unfortunately, urban bureaucracies are to blame for much of the deterioration of city schools, but the potential for change is ever-present.[11] If some 150-odd compensatory education schemes have been tried and have been either totally or partially unsuccessful, it is probably because the disadvantaged children continue to be *locked into total environments* which are inhibiting models of behavior. It is today obvious that health status and health practices will change very little through the usual hit-or-miss school health efforts. Only a calculated attempt by school personnel to move outside the school and penetrate the community with innovative health education programs will meet with any measurable degree of success.

THE NEEDS OF CHILDREN: POLITICAL, ECONOMIC, AND FAMILY OVERTONES

The Carnegie Council on Children, after a five year study, concluded that what is needed to improve the welfare of children is a national family policy based on the premise that supporting child health means supporting the parents. Economics, politics, and the sociology of the family play a major part in child welfare. Also involved are emotions, attitudes, and the meaning of life and community.

Child health cannot be promoted solely by school teachers and families. Other issues, particularly politics and the government's concern for family economics, are intimately related to the health of children. Fully one quarter to one third of all American children are born into families with financial strains so great that the children will suffer fundamental deprivations. Ultimate health decisions are largely outside most parents' ability to affect because of the profound influence of the economic system on the family. Despite several decades of helping families through innovative school programs, expanded medical services, Head Start programs, and family counseling centers, the effect has been fragmented and family problems still exist.

Since unhealed social and economic ills degrade family life, the welfare of children becomes a political matter. In short, family and child health probably are affected more by the labor market and social justice in the nation than they are by a particular health lesson in the classroom or the routine pediatric examination. No wonder the question is frequently raised as to whether prevention of illness for certain people is a myth. There are, after all, numerous preventive

---

[11]For suggestions for change see Atron Gentry, et al. *Urban Education: The Hope Factor*. Philadelphia: W. B. Saunders Co., 1972.

measures that are alien to the cultural frame of reference that plays such an important role in daily living patterns.[12]

CONTRIBUTIONS OF PHYSICAL EDUCATION TO THE SCHOOL HEALTH PROGRAM

Physical education may be defined as a process of changing behavior toward certain preconceived educational goals, primarily through large muscle activity. Health is advanced by increasing the child's vigor, strength, and endurance. Through a broad and varied program of physical activities in the elementary grades, organic growth is stimulated, fundamental physical skills are developed, social efficiency is promoted, and attitudes toward recreation and leisure time are planted like seedlings in the slowly maturing bodies of young people.

Elementary physical education activities such as simple games, movement exploration, sport skills, mimetic activities and story plays, rhythms and dances, and self-testing stunts are full of meaning to the growing child. When properly taught, their contribution to total health, through the avenue of improved physical efficiency and social emotional behavior, is not insignificant.

In recent years each president from Eisenhower to Carter has made a personal effort to promote a national awareness of the need for physical fitness. The President's Council on Physical Fitness and Sports has done much to improve existing programs of physical education. Significantly, where programs have been initiated or improved, levels of individual pupil fitness have risen, resulting in an increase in personal vigor and stamina for the many activities of the

---

[12]Spector, Manuel. "Is Prevention Myth or Reality," *Health Education,* 8:23–26, July/August 1977.

Figure 2–3. Vigorous activity in the elementary school.

school day. Moreover, it is not uncommon to find a corresponding rise in levels of achievement and social accomplishment (Figure 2–3).

Physical activities, by their very nature, are health teaching activities. They are as much a part of the school health program as are food tasting parties or health services. They need to be taught with purpose and understanding. Merely turning children loose on a playground twice a day, day after day, to "blow off steam" is not physical education. In fact, it represents an example of a situation where a unique opportunity is being missed. True, the children will find some relief from the academic activities of the classroom, but they will be denied the chance to learn the skills and develop the attitudes that are so much a part of a good physical education program. This is not to be treated as a haphazard activity, for physical education is not just aimless movement; it is part of the educational process. Moreover, physical condition is being increasingly equated with mental efficiency and intellectual productivity rather than with games and sports alone. Unfortunately, not everyone realizes this. In a recent study carried out by the Bureau of Health Education in Atlanta, it was found that among the essential health topics and practices poorly understood by both children and adults was the relationship of physical exercise to the optimum maintenance of health and well-being.

Elementary teachers who feel somewhat unprepared in the physical education area or who lack the skill and knowledge to carry on even a partial program of purposeful activity, should do one or two of the following things:

1. Visit a class where a good program of suitable activities is being taught and observe how it is done. In most communities there are at least one or two especially successful teachers in this area.
2. Visit the school or community library and search the existing books for appropriate games, dances, and self-testing stunts.
3. Write the nearest elementary teacher preparation institution for program help.
4. Contact the state educational department's supervisor of elementary physical education. He or she either will pay a visit, arrange for the teacher to visit a school, or will send written suggestions.

In many schools classroom teachers work closely with physical educators not only in the improvement of motor skills but also on individual pupil posture, muscular strength, and remedial exercises.

PRESENT AND FUTURE TRENDS VERSUS PAST PRACTICES IN SCHOOL HEALTH

As education has grown more scientific over the decades, medical and educational workers associated with school health have concerned themselves with the scientific aspects of health status, health knowledge, and health behavior. This is reflected in current trends and practices, especially when compared with the practices of several decades ago. Some noteworthy examples follow.

Present Trends

1. Physical examinations of schoolchildren are given in less haste and are more thorough. Better use is made of the physician's time. No longer are 60 to 80 children examined an hour.
2. Screening examinations for hearing and vision losses, together with weighing and measuring of pupils, are popular appraisal activities carried on with objective measures.
3. Classroom teachers cooperate with school nurses, dental hygienists, and other medical personnel in an effort to determine the health status of the child. Many teachers have special training to improve their observation of health abnormalities.
4. Schools have effective health service departments designed to evaluate the *total* school health effort.
5. Health councils operate in a democratic way to determine health status and analyze health behavior. Case studies are frequently run on individual children.
6. The objective is to evaluate the child as accurately as possible and then see that something is done about his or her needs. Family accountability has been reemphasized.
7. Health teaching is done from the viewpoint of a child's needs and interests, and factual information is used to bring about maximum understanding. Individual differences and lifestyles are recognized in the discussion of the total life cycle from conception to death.
8. There is increased use of evaluation techniques designed to measure health attitudes and health practices.
9. Health concepts are being directed toward the acquisition of skills for individual responsibility for health, with a high priority on self-development and self-care.
10. Health education is concerned with community resources and is carried on by concerted action of home, school, and public and private agencies.
11. There is increasing recognition that the emotional health of the teacher influences the emotional tone of the classroom.

As one looks to the future, it becomes quite clear that the impact of professional, public, and voluntary health organizations is such that it will only be a few years before all states implement legislation requiring direct health instruction for all children. There will be a properly *balanced* curriculum with adequate scope and sequence which does justice to all major health problems rather than singling out any one popular problem for overemphasis. The need will be met for greater numbers of school health coordinators or curriculum specialists to work with classroom teachers and for a continuing in-service program to keep teachers up-to-date with rapidly changing health concepts and to encourage creative teaching. Already, health teaching is moving at an accelerated speed from a "do-gooder" activity to a carefully organized and programmed part of the total school curriculum.

QUESTIONS FOR DISCUSSION

1. How likely is the elementary classroom teacher to put across the general concept that wellness is a life-long personal investment?

2. What is the relationship between physical activity and health instruction in the promotion of health?

3. Observe an elementary school and its health education program. After comparing your findings with others, what are common observations?

4. If health observation of school children is an art, do you think it possible to train the elementary teacher so that a high level of proficiency may be obtained?

5. Discuss the role of the teacher's health in relation to teacher employment and retention practices. Should a teacher object to a physical or mental examination? To what extent is a physical handicap a negative attribute when it comes to teaching efficiency?

SUGGESTED ACTIVITIES

1. In Robert Dentler's book on urban problems he raises several issues relative to teaching success in depressed areas where social, economic, and political considerations are paramount (see Selected References). After reading his comments, do you think that teaching with any degree of success is possible in an urban area?

2. Alfred North Whitehead wrote that ". . . you may not separate the seamless coat of learning." In short, every classroom teacher as well as health professional is a health teacher to some extent. What are the implications here for school-community cooperation? Look into this relationship in a specific locality.

3. Find out the health education requirements for your state. Is health instruction required in the elementary or middle schools? If so, how much time has been legislated? If not, is any move being made to bring about a change in state requirements?

4. In the short book by Irene Schram, *Ashes, Ashes, We All Fall Down*, the story is told of some fifth grade children being exposed to terrifying situations (see Selected References). Read the book and compare the story to real-life situations where one must survive under similar or worse threats. Are there health implications here?

SELECTED REFERENCES

Anderson, C. L. *School Health Practice.* 6th ed., St. Louis: C. V. Mosby Co., 1977.

Aubrey, Roger F. "Health Education: Neglected Child of the Schools," *Journal of School Health,* 42:285–289, May 1972.

Dentler, Robert A. *Urban Problems: Perspectives and Solutions.* Chicago: Rand McNally College Publishing Co., 1977.

Dropkin, Stan, and Schwarcz, Ernest. *Contemporary American Education.* New York: Macmillan Publishing Co., 1977.

Dubos, René. *Man, Medicine and Environment.* New York: Praeger Publishing Co., 1968.

Etzioni, Amitai. "Human Beings Are Not Very Easy to Change," *Saturday Review,* June 3, 1972.

Galli, Nicholas. "Foundations of Health Education," *Journal of School Health, 46*:158–165, March 1976.

Gay, John, et al. *Current Health Problems,* Philadelphia: W. B. Saunders Co., 1978.

Hilton, Ernest. "Early Childhood Education: A Sense of Urgency," *Instructor, 62*:15, September 1972.

Logston, Bette J., et al. *Physical Education for Children: A Focus on the Teaching Process.* Philadelphia: Lea & Febiger, 1977.

McClendon, E. J. "America's Health in Two Centuries," *Journal of School Health, 47*:271–274, May 1977.

Oberteuffer, Delbert, Halverson, Orvis A., and Pollock, Marion B. *School Health Education.* 5th ed., New York: Harper & Row, 1972, Chapter 2.

Price, James H. "The Health Education Coordinator," *Health Education, 8*:40, January/February 1977.

Schaller, Warren, and Nemir, Alma. *The School Health Program.* 4th ed., Philadelphia: W. B. Saunders Co., 1976.

Schram, Irene. *Ashes, Ashes, We All Fall Down.* New York: Simon & Schuster, 1972.

Taub, Alyson, and Clarke, Vivian P. J. "Training Elementary School Leadership Teams for Health Education," *Journal of School Health, 47*:615–618, December 1977.

Vannier, Maryhelen. *Teaching Health in Elementary Schools,* 2nd ed., Philadelphia: Lea and Febiger, 1976, Chapter 2.

Willgoose, Carl E. *Health Teaching in Secondary Schools,* 2nd ed., Philadelphia: W. B. Saunders Co., 1977, Chapter 2.

—————, "Saving the Curriculum in Health Education," *Journal of School Health, 43*:19–23, March 1973.

The Scope of School Health Services

3

_____

What we need to do is define all measures taken . . . as transitional to a saner, fairer, more human lifestyle.

—Margaret Mead[1]

How do the schools help children achieve a more human and healthful lifestyle? How are health problems and school performance associated with learning and academic success? To a great extent the over-all task of school health services is to answer these questions successfully so that the student will realize his or her full potential in school.

There is a complex relationship between pupil performance and health status. For example, in Gary, Indiana, where there are 35,000 schoolchildren, a recent profile of high school students revealed that a staggering 46 per cent had not attained sixth grade level proficiency in writing, reading, and mathematics. A thorough examination of these students indicated that they had a greater than normal number of visual and hearing defects and other health abnormalities that could interfere with learning. To prevent a repetition of such occurrences, school nurse practitioners were employed to work with social workers to carefully examine children early in the elementary school years and to single out those with health problems.

No attempt will be made in this chapter to go into all the details of school health services. But it would be remiss of the author if he failed to give the elementary school teacher an opportunity to understand the function and some of the activities of this operation.

School health services are well defined procedures that are established:

1. To appraise the health status of pupils and school personnel.
2. To counsel pupils, parents, and others concerning appraisal findings.
3. To encourage the correction of remediable defects.
4. To assist in the identification and education of handicapped children.
5. To help prevent and control disease.
6. To provide emergency service for injury or sudden sickness.

It may be seen from these precise definitions that school health

_____

[1]Mead, Margaret. "This Time There Is No Enemy," _AAAUW Journal,_ 67:6, April 1974.

services embrace a considerable amount of school activity. This is to be expected, for the services are educationally sound and defensible. Not only do they contribute to the realization of educational aims, but they help minimize the hazards of attending school and make it possible to adapt school programs to individual capacities and needs. Also—and this is sometimes not recognized by many teachers and parents—there are potential educational values inherent in health service activities. Through these activities children become informed of their health assets and liabilities and develop lasting attitudes toward physicians, dentists, nurses, and other health personnel. They also stand to gain two especially important understandings that may affect future behavior:

1. The need to establish a lifelong practice of having one's health status evaluated at regular intervals.
2. An appreciation of the value of professional services, methods, and techniques.

A COMPREHENSIVE FUNCTION

The most recent White House Conference on Children placed a high priority on the development of a nationwide network of comprehensive health services for children. Health care delivery systems were to be improved, with an emphasis on the development of preventive and curative health services. Schools and other community agencies were to strive together to improve deficiencies that would otherwise impede scholastic performance.

What is practiced today varies considerably. Big cities with greater resources do more. Even in small school systems much goes on under the leadership of school health services personnel. A good part of this cuts across other school lines and involves considerable cooperative effort between school and community. The kinds of services performed can be extensive. In a statewide public school study in California, for example, the percentage of time given to a wide variety of school health services activities is shown in the table on the following page.

The degree to which a particular health services organization becomes involved in many of these kinds of activities depends upon local understandings and leadership. It requires much cooperative effort in and out of the school. It also depends on the background of the families of the schoolchildren. In one elementary school study of visits to the health office it was discovered that there were significantly greater numbers of visits among older children, black students, children from families in which the mothers had been hospitalized for illness during a previous year, and among those with lowest academic achievement.[3] Also, those elementary grade pupils

---

[2]Hazell, Joseph W. et al. "Intermediate Benefit Analysis—Spencer's Dilemma and School Health Services," *American Journal of Public Health,* 62:500–565, April 1972.

[3]Van Arsdell, William et al. "Visits To An Elementary School Nurse," *Journal of School Health,* 42:142–146, March 1972.

Direct Health Service Programs	Per cent
Minor first aid	7.6
Vision screening	6.5
Hearing screening	4.7
Major emergency care	3.7
Health communication (information exchange with health professionals, pupils, parents, teachers, and community)	3.7
Emotional development (developmental diagnosis, behavioral problems, and mental health)	3.7
Absence due to illness (investigation of absence by health-service personnel)	3.4
Dental (screening and care)	2.3
Health services planning and evaluation	2.3
Drug Abuse (resource support of education and management of drug reactions)	2.3
Communicable disease (exclusions, readmissions, and immunizations)	2.1
Referral physical examination (as needed rather than as scheduled or required)	1.8
Chronic disease (allergies, diabetes, etc.)	1.5
Periodic physical examination (scheduled or required)	1.0
Immunization identification (determination of pupil status regarding required immunizations)	1.0
TB screening	0.8
Other health service programs	1.8
Health service components of other programs for:	
Nutrition (food or food service)	17.7
Educationally handicapped and mentally exceptional (contributions to programs)	11.2
Physically exceptional (components of programs for pupils with hearing, speech, vision, or orthopedic problems as well as for home and hospital instruction)	6.3
Physical education (services for other than athletics, sports, or physically handicapped)	3.4
Health education (personnel as resources)	3.1
Athletics and sports	2.6
Environment (safety and sanitation)	1.8
Remedial physical education (health service components of programs for the physically handicapped)	0.8
Pregnancy (health service components only)	0.3
Other purposes	2.6
Grand Total	100.0

who are less well-accepted by their peers tended to make more visits to the school nurse.

The so-called "watchdog function" of the school health services crew is helped measurably by cooperative teachers who enthusiastically report what they are able to observe in the classroom and about the school. However, this function is made more difficult by examples of ignorance and indifference found in the homes. For instance, in her study of school nursing procedures, Dorothy Basco found that there is considerable need for parent education—particularly relative to childhood diseases and important symptoms of illness.[4] Par-

---

[4]Basco, Dorothy. "Epidemiologic Analysis in School Populations as a Basis for Change in School Nursing Practice," *American Journal of Public Health*, 62:491–497, April 1972.

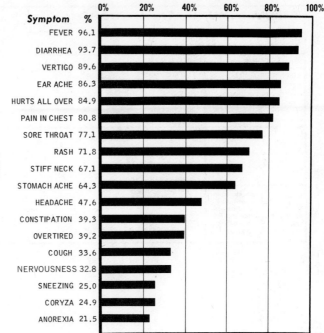

Symptom	%					
		0%	20%	40%	60%	80%	100%
FEVER	96.1					
DIARRHEA	93.7					
VERTIGO	89.6					
EAR ACHE	86.3					
HURTS ALL OVER	84.9					
PAIN IN CHEST	80.8					
SORE THROAT	77.1					
RASH	71.8					
STIFF NECK	67.1					
STOMACH ACHE	64.3					
HEADACHE	47.6					
CONSTIPATION	39.3					
OVERTIRED	39.2					
COUGH	33.6					
NERVOUSNESS	32.8					
SNEEZING	25.0					
CORYZA	24.9					
ANOREXIA	21.5					

Figure 3–1. Per cent of parents who would keep child home for selected symptoms. (Courtesy Dorothy Basco and *American Journal of Public Health.*)

ents will send children to school when they are really ill enough to stay home. In the Basco study it was shown that almost all parents would keep their child at home if he or she had a fever or diarrhea, but less than one third would do so in cases of respiratory infections causing coughing and sneezing (see Figure 3–1). Similar findings were reported in a North Carolina study of mothers' perceptions of mild illness in children and their perception of the worth of school health services activities.[5]

IMMUNIZATION PROBLEMS

Another example of the need for a vigilant health services operation is the immunization program, which requires both careful monitoring and greater publicity. Currently about 20 million children under the age of 15 lack adequate immunization against one or more of the communicable childhood diseases. In 1963, not long after the polio epidemic of the fifties, 80 per cent of the younger children in the U.S. had received vaccinations. Just ten years later this figure had dropped to 60 per cent, reflecting a growing lack of concern. By 1977 the National Immunization Commission was calling for a major effort to immunize 90 per cent of all children against polio. Forty-six states have laws requiring specific immunizations before school entry is permitted, but in Ohio, one of the states having such laws, 60 per cent of the primary grade children were inadequately immunized.[6]

---

[5]Slome, Cecil, et al. "Should James Go to School? Mothers' Responses to Symptoms," *Journal of School Health, 47*:106–110, February 1977.

[6]Anthony, Nicholas et al. "Immunization: Public Health Programming Through Law Enforcement," *American Journal of Public Health, 67*:763–764, August 1977.

FAMILY IMMUNIZATION RECORD ❀ Metropolitan

■ Ask your doctor when shots are due.
■ When shots are given, have your doctor enter dates under child's name.

SHOTS FOR ▼	CHILD'S NAME ▶				
• DIPHTHERIA • TETANUS • WHOOPING COUGH One immunization (one shot each date) can immunize for all three if doctor recommends.	AT AGE 2 MOS.*				
	2 MOS. LATER				
	2 MOS. LATER				
	12 MOS. LATER				
	BOOSTER 4-6 YRS. OLD				
• POLIO One oral immunization each date.	AT AGE 2 MOS.*				
	2 MOS. LATER				
	2 MOS. LATER				
	12 MOS. LATER				
	BOOSTER 4-6 YRS. OLD				
•MEASLES •MUMPS •RUBELLA (German measles) { Triple immunization (one shot for all three). Measles booster at 15 mos. if first immunized before 1 year.	AFTER 1 YEAR OLD				
	AFTER 1 YEAR OLD				
	AFTER 1 YEAR OLD				
	*For children already beyond infancy, don't delay. See your physician and start series now.				

DETACH AND SAVE CARD FOR REFERENCE.

Figure 3–2. Immunization record card for school-home use. (Courtesy Metropolitan Life Insurance Company.)

A similar enforcement problem concerns measles, a disease that dropped from 400,000 cases a year before 1968 to a low of 22,000 in 1974.[7] Then because of indifference there was a 62 per cent increase by early 1978. Although measles in most children is not dangerous, its complications can be severe. Most serious is inflammation of the brain (encephalitis), which develops in one of every 1000 measles cases. Approximately one fourth of all measles encephalitis patients die, another one fourth develop mental retardation, another one fourth suffer later convulsive disorders, and the remainder recover without adverse effects. Schools and cooperating insurance organizations have helped to stress the need for family immunizations (see Figure 3–2).

HEALTH APPRAISAL

As in all evaluation processes, the more scientific the appraisal, the sooner the purposes of the program may be reached. The total health status of a child may be appraised in a number of ways. Health histories, teacher and nurse observations, screening tests, medical and dental examinations, and psychological examinations represent the more common appraisal activities. These appraisals serve the medical personnel, the classroom teachers, and the pupils. They help the teachers understand their pupils, and they help the pupils appreciate the findings in relation to themselves. The results of appraisals are also valuable to groups and individuals concerned with health counseling.

Some of the more important appraisal activities will be reviewed:

---

[7]Metropolitan Life Insurance Co., "Measles, Mumps, and Rubella," *Statistical Bulletin,* 58:3–4, November 1977.

Health Histories

These are of particular concern to both medical personnel and classroom teachers. Just as history usually helps one to understand the present better, so the past diseases and defects of a pupil help everyone to understand his or her present status. Good teachers generally ask, "What makes Johnny tick?" It helps to know, therefore, what communicable diseases, immunizations, major operations, or injuries Johnny has had. In some schools today, classroom teachers help maintain health history records by noting pupil health behavior items.

This kind of record is especially valuable when kept up-to-date and referred to when children behave strangely or appear to be in need of special counseling. It is a functional instrument for the exchange of information between the classroom teacher, the school nurse, and the school physician concerning the pupil's health. In California, for example, a particularly useful Health Insert is used with the California Cumulative Record system. It is an integral part of the individual's cumulative record and provides specific information concerning needed adjustments in the school program. It is transferred from school to school and was designed so that a minimum amount of time need be spent in keeping it up-to-date.

Routine Medical Examinations

The chief purposes of these examinations are to determine health status and to solve any problems that arise. Their value is recognized in most states by a law requiring periodic examinations of every child in school. When the examination is not conducted by the family physician, it must be done by the school physician. The compulsory medical examination of all school children, however, has not always been effective. For one thing, the schools have ended up performing the "lion's share" of the examinations, thus missing the obvious advantage of having the family physician examine the child.

The routine medical examination should be a thorough one. To be worth the energy put forth, it must allow the physician time enough to observe the whole child: the behavior characteristics, nervous reflexes, speech characteristics, nutritional status, and temperament, as well as the more typical items having to do with blood pressure, heart rate, respiratory function, and assessment of sensory abilities. For almost two decades the American Public Health Association has had standards calling for a maximum of 12 examinations per hour—at least five minutes per child. This rule was brought about by findings that showed as many as 70 children being examined per hour. The idea of "processing" a set number of examinations in a certain amount of time cannot be defended. Examinations, to be worth the time and effort involved, need to be complete from head to toe. Thus a limited number of students should be handled in one year. Thorough examinations every two or three years are becoming more common, with reexaminations of students possessing definite health problems being given whenever necessary.

The American Medical Association, in conjunction with the National Education Association, has suggested a minimum of four medical examinations: one upon entrance to first grade, one in the elementary intermediate school grades, one at the start of adolescence, and one before leaving school. In some places this policy has been quite successful. There is general agreement that all pupils entering school for the first time should have a complete medical examination. This has the support of the American Academy of Pediatrics. Moreover, the examination should be done early enough to permit an adequate follow-up on recommendations. June has been found to be the most satisfactory month for children who plan to enter school in September.

As previously indicated, there is a definite advantage to having the family physician perform the examination. He or she knows the family and background of the child; examination facilities are usually excellent, and there is quick access to laboratory facilities. Moreover a favorable physician-parent-child relationship generally exists. There are a number of communities in the United States that have no school physician for examinations. Everything is effectively handled by local physicians who cooperate fully with the school nurse. In such cases the family physician is completely informed of what the school desires so that there is uniformity in examinations and reporting. Standard examination forms are used. Also, the family physician is advised to use every opportunity to give effective health instruction just as a school physician would do. This kind of program has been working well in Connecticut, where in a recent year over 25 per cent of schoolchildren were examined by personal physicians. There still remains one big disadvantage to using family physicians; there are always some parents who will not take their child to him or her, or they employ delaying tactics while the child's health is in question (see Figure 3-3).

Another very significant item related to physical examinations of schoolchildren is the growth of specialization in medical practice. In many towns the general practitioner has been disappearing. The family doctor—the person who treated all members of a family, provided continuity of care, and showed concern for the general health of the entire family—has been hard to locate. However, there has been a recent upswing in the number of medical school graduates engaging in family practice. Physician-family bonds are stronger when the physician treats the entire family. It seems likely that in the years ahead the health care of the citizen will be a mass cooperative effort in which community physicians and their assistants will work together in group practice and regional medical centers. In the future such centers will service the schools much more than they are doing at present.

It is a good idea to have the parent or parents on hand during the medical examination to consult with the physician. This is particularly true in the case of primary schoolchildren. Often during these formative years, when growth processes are fairly rapid, it is imperative that the physician and parent see eye-to-eye in their efforts to remedy any abnormal situations. The speed with which defects are

DEPARTMENT OF HEALTH, PHYSICAL EDUCATION & RECREATION

Roslyn Public Schools

Roslyn, N.Y.

_____
Date

NOTICE TO PARENTS - HEALTH CERTIFICATES

Dear Parents:

Since _____ has not had an annual health examination
by your own personal physician, he/she will be inspected by Dr._____
our school doctor, on _____.

Please sign and return this slip to the Health Office.

_____
School Nurse

_____
Parent's Signature

_____
School Principal

Figure 3-3. Form used when family physician has not conducted health examination.

remedied has an important bearing on health and happiness in the years ahead. Teeth, for example, do much better when repaired at an early date.

Thoroughly screening preschool children is important. In addition to the discovery of obvious physical handicaps which can limit success in school, there is the opportunity to detect other deficiencies pertaining to the special senses, mental retardation, emotional and behavioral disorders, and physical, social, and cultural deprivation.

The emphasis in school health practice today is to give the physician time to interpret the findings for teachers and parents and to make workable suggestions about current health concerns. This kind of effort sets the stage for teamwork between teachers, parents, nurses, and physicians.

Special Medical Examinations

When the school employs the regular medical examination every three or four years, there will be numerous occasions between examinations when it will be necessary to examine individual youngsters. Children returning to school after an absence due to illness may need a special examination, as will those new to the school system. Those pupils in need of special education may need to be examined from time to time. Since physical education and recreation activities must be adapted to the health condition of pupils, it will be necessary to examine boys and girls who wish to compete on an elementary school team. Also, there will be times in the follow-up and remedial aspects of the program when the physician wants to reexamine a certain pupil. Special examinations have value in that they permit a more careful analysis and diagnosis of the particular child.

Screening Tests

These are measures employed by teachers and health services personnel to select those schoolchildren who appear to be in need of further attention. The most effective screening tests over the years have been tests for vision, hearing, tuberculosis, and the appraisal of physical growth by the weighing and measuring of boys and girls. In recent years a number of school systems have attempted to screen children for dental defects, physical fitness, lateral curvature of the spine (scoliosis), and mental health status. Most of these screening tests can be cooperatively conducted by teachers and nurses. A broader treatment of methods the elementary school classroom teacher can use to screen children for specific weaknesses appears in Chapter 5.

Screening for Vision. As a rule, screening tests are not diagnostic tests. They might well be called processes by which school personnel separate those pupils who are most likely from those who are less likely to need further examination. Therefore, in vision testing the teacher is not an expert, but is simply a careful observer who helps during the screening period. The teacher should be aware that sensory impressions gradually develop from a level of discrimination through a perceptual level to a final conceptual level, and that refractive errors, color blindness, eye muscle imbalances, and more serious conditions such as amblyopia need quick attention. He or she should know that first and second graders tend to be farsighted and that nearsightedness in boys and girls develops at about the fourth grade level.

The pupil old enough to cooperate in a testing situation is ready to be measured. Thus, even a three-year-old child can respond to the symbols on a Snellen E Chart. Proper advance preparation helps improve the response.

The *Snellen Test,* used for a long time in the public schools to test visual acuity, is quite satisfactory as a crude screening instrument when more valid measures are not available[8] (see Figure 3–4).

This test is useful for noting near-to-far-vision. It will tell the classroom teacher whether or not a certain pupil can see the blackboard or wall chart from either the front or back row of seats. The large Snellen Test chart requires reading test objects (letters, numbers, or symbols) on a chart from a 20-foot distance. The E chart is available for children and illiterates, and the mixed-letter chart is for adults and children above the third grade level. The largest letters should be read by the normal eye at 200 feet. Because testing is done at 20 feet, this line of large print is designated the 20/200 line. The normal eye should read the 20/20 line at 20 feet; deviation less than normal is recorded 20/200, 20/100, 20/70, 20/60, 20/40, or 20/30,

---

[8]The necessary testing equipment and detailed instructions can be obtained from the National Society for the Prevention of Blindness, 79 Madison Ave., New York, N.Y., 10016.

Figure 3–4. The Snellen Charts. (National Society for the Prevention of Blindness.)

and any deviation better than normal is recorded as 20/15 or 20/10. In all probability children below the third grade who cannot read the 20/40 line with each eye should be referred for examination by a specialist.

Although the Snellen Test can be given by a person without medical or nursing training, proper attention must be given to the testing procedure and equipment. Some of the more important items to keep in mind to ensure valid results are the following:

Hang the chart so that the 20-foot line of letters is at the level of the child's eyes.

The heels of the child should touch the line marked on the floor 20 feet away.

Children should be at ease and encouraged to do their best.

Both eyes should be open during the test, the eye not being tested covered with a small card or folded paper resting obliquely across the nose.

Test the child who wears glasses first with them and then without them.

Test the right eye first, then the left, and then both eyes together.

Begin with the 30-foot line and follow with the 20-foot line. If the child fails the 30-foot line, start with the 20-foot line.

Move promptly and rhythmically from one symbol to another at a speed with which the child can keep pace.

Consider a line read satisfactorily if three out of four symbols are read correctly.

Record results immediately in fraction form.

Look for eyestrain, signs such as excessive blinking, frowning, scowling, tilting of the head, and watering of the eyes.

Correlate Snellen Test results with classroom observations.

There are several other tests of vision that are recommended when a more complete screening examination is desired. These include tests of far and near binocular vision, depth perception, and color vision. Appropriate vision screening machines include the Keystone View Company Telebinocular, the Massachusetts Vision Test, the Atlantic City Vision Test, the Titmus School Vision Tester, the Ortho-Rater by Bausch and Lomb, and the Sight Screener by American Optical Company.

In recent years considerable attention has been focused on *preschool vision screening* and the importance of visual readiness for learning. Studies show that large numbers of children require professional eye care. In New York City, for example, preschool screening examinations discovered that 7 per cent of the children had visual defects at 20/50 or worse in one eye. In a study carried out in Minneapolis, Minnesota, with a sample of 633 first grade pupils from eight public elementary schools, it was found that over 16 per cent of the pupils required professional eye care. In most communities, therefore, it is advisable to begin the vision screening in nursery schools where the young children are already congregated.[9]

Screening for Hearing. Early and repeated hearing tests are important. Accurate screening is necessary, especially when one considers that an average of two children in every classroom have a hearing problem, that many cases of incorrect speech supposedly due to poor mentality are actually caused by poor hearing, and that there are needless grade repetitions among hard-of-hearing children.[10]

Although whisper tests have been used for years, group audiometers are far more reliable. Six or ten children can be tested together in a pure-tone-audiometer test. Each subject has a set of

---

[9]The booklet *Preschool Vision Screening* and the training film for teachers, *Before We Are Six,* can be most helpful in situations where teachers do the vision screening. They may be obtained from the National Society for the Prevention of Blindness.

[10]In a nationwide study by the National Center for Health Statistics it was found that 16 per cent of 6 to 11 year old children have a hearing abnormality.

earphones. Sound intensity is regulated by a knob up to maximum intensity. Different pitches in tone are given (frequency range) by turning another knob. One hundred pupils a day can be tested and it can be used with children of all ages. Hearing tests for small children are especially important, because of the fact that early discovery of hearing loss and follow-up treatment can frequently prevent permanent loss of hearing (see Figure 3–5).

Screening for Physical Growth.   There is a close relationship between pupil health status, personal growth characteristics, and academic achievement. Learning depends upon sound health. Children who are small or underweight for their age have a higher proportion of communication problems, according to the National Institute of Neurological Diseases and Stroke. Very often a simple sign of retardation in growth, discovered by nurses or teachers, is significant. Yet the growth period of boys and girls cannot be neatly divided and subdivided into set periods. There is too much individual variation in pupil size, shape, and form due to such factors as heredity, constitutional endowment (body build), and physiological maturation.

A number of screening devices to evaluate over-all physical growth have been developed for school use. These involve age-height-weight measures and are usually handled through the health services department. Frequently teachers weigh and measure their own pupils. The children remove hats, coats, jackets, sweaters, and

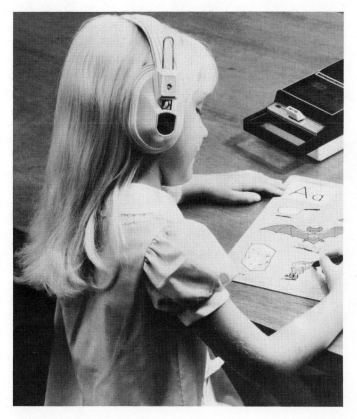

Figure 3–5.   Evaluating hearing at the primary grade level. (Courtesy Avedex, Inc., Skokie, Illinois, 60076.)

shoes. Weight is recorded in pounds and half pounds. Height is recorded in inches and quarter inches.

The child who fails to gain in height and weight in a six-month period frequently has some degree of ill health. This may be due to a physical defect, an organic strain, a prolonged emotional problem, or perhaps a number of unhygienic health habits.

An easy-to-use graph for teachers is the *Meredith Physical Growth Record*. There is a record for each sex, divided into zones (Figures 3–6 and 3–7). For height there are five zones: tall, moderately tall, average, moderately short, and short. For weight the zones are heavy, moderately heavy, average, moderately light, and light. The graphs cover ages four to 18.

Recently, John Spurgem and H. V. Meredith of the University of South Carolina developed *Height and Weight Charts For Black-American Boys and Male Youths of the United States*. The same was done for black girls and female youth.

The child's measurements are plotted on the graph for any one period. Successive measurements permit the observer to note whenever the points do not fall in *like zones* (that is, tall and heavy, short and light). In such instances the pupil is referred to the physician for examination. It may be that the child is perfectly healthy but of a particular body build. On the other hand, he or she may have some infection, need an improved diet, or require changes in daily living habits.

Screening for Scoliosis. Routine school examinations for lateral curvature of the spine (scoliosis) have been established in numerous school systems. Trained nurses and physical education personnel can detect spinal curvature in 30 seconds. Early detection and proper treatment prevent major surgery. In the San Juan Unified School District of California several thousand sixth grade pupils were examined; 17 per cent were reexamined by the orthopedists, and 221 were referred for x-ray studies and further evaluation.[11]

Screening for Mental Health. The need for psychiatric services in grade schools has grown faster than private and public psychiatric services can possibly keep abreast of. Children coming from a background of environmental deprivation frequently are emotionally immature and harbor a negative self-image. All too often disturbed parents raise disturbed children. This is why Abrams and others make a plea for the employment of full-time psychiatrists to work with students, parents, social workers, school psychologists, nurses, and teachers.[12] By observing and talking with individuals and small groups of children, this battery of school personnel will be able to effectively screen out those pupils in need of help and provide early attention.

Screening for Blood Pressure. The American Academy of Pediatrics recommends that children three years old and up have their blood pressure measured annually as part of their continuing

---

[11]Benson, Karen D., et al. "Results of School Screening for Scoliosis," *Journal of School Health, 47*:483–484, October 1977.

[12]Abrams, Richard S., et al. "A Suggested School Mental Health Program," *Journal of School Health, 42*:137–141, March 1972.

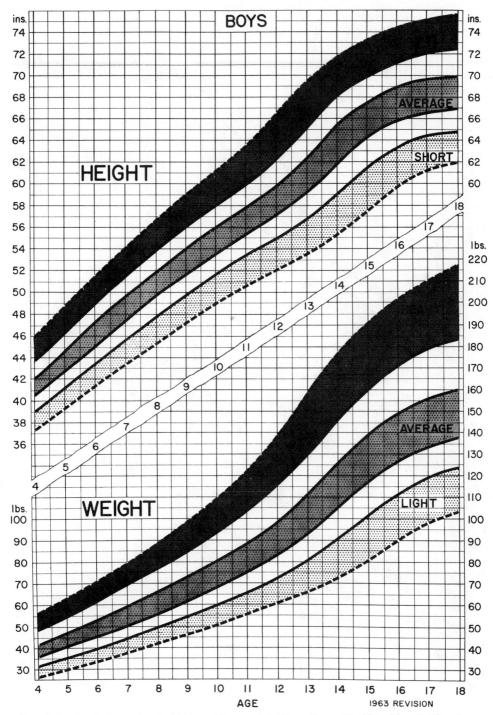

Figure 3–6. Physical growth record for boys. (Courtesy Joint Committee on Health Problems in Education of the NEA and AMA.)

Figure 3-7. Physical growth record for girls. (Courtesy Joint Committee on Health Problems in Education of the NEA and AMA.)

health care.[13] Those individuals with sustained elevated blood pressure should receive a systematic long-term follow-up program, which may include counseling concerning salt intake, weight control, and physical activity. There is great variability in blood pressure readings, so testing is required on several occasions prior to labeling a child as hypertensive and in need of treatment.

Screening for Heart Sounds. When one considers that there are approximately 10 cases of heart problems per 1000 children, the need for mass heart screening programs becomes apparent. As a relatively new technique, heart sound screening shows promise in school use. A highly sensitive microphone placed on the child's chest picks up heart sounds. These are analyzed by a portable computer, which provides information beyond what may be detected with the ordinary stethoscope.

Screening for Lice Infestations. Some four million Americans had lice in 1977, a fourfold increase since 1970. Thousands of schoolchildren may have head lice sometime during the year. The eggs of the tiny insects are transmitted from one person to another on combs, coats hung together, caps, scarves, and upholstered seats in theaters and trains. The lice live by making a small opening in the scalp and sucking the blood. Their feeding can induce intense itching, the most noticeable symptom of infestation. Booklets for distribution written in English and Spanish can be obtained from the Pharmecs Division of Pfizer Inc., New York, N.Y. 10017.

HEALTH MAINTENANCE AND CONTROL

Certainly one of the big tasks of school health services has to do with the everyday prevention of illness. This is accomplished through a program of control of personal and environmental factors. Factors such as communicable disease, emergency care and first aid, accident prevention, and school sanitation are major items.

Communicable disease control involves both the school and the community. The school health services department is generally aware of the prevalence of illness in the area and is prepared to control disease in the school population through widespread use of vaccination, immunization, prophylactic therapy, and isolation of ill pupils. While children are in school, they must be protected from other children who may be ill. The gathering of pupils in the classroom may set the stage for the transmission of disease. Here, the classroom teacher can be most helpful by observing carefully and reporting quickly those pupils who appear to be ill. (For details see Chapter 5.)

Emergency care procedures for children who become ill or injured while attending school are also the responsibility of school personnel. The school administrator and the staff must always act *in loco parentis,* i.e., in place of the parents—not just any parents, but

---

[13]American Academy of Pediatrics. "Report of the Task Force on Blood Pressure Control in Children," *Pediatrics,* 59:799, May 1977.

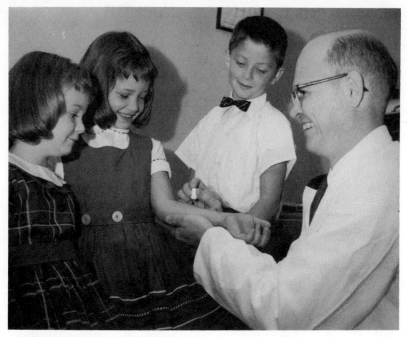

Figure 3-8. Application of TB Tine Test in the screening of schoolchildren. (Courtesy Lederle Laboratories.)

the wisest and most enlightened type of parents. This can be a sizable job because the figures collected by the National Safety Council indicate that some 60 per cent of the accidents to children of school age occur on the school grounds, in the buildings, or going to and from school. It becomes necessary, therefore, for the health services personnel to cooperate with the teacher and school principal in the event of an emergency.

Children who appear to be ill should be segregated immediately. Sometimes an emergency rest room is used. At other times it may be necessary to transport the child back home. In either case the school physician or nurse should make the decision as to how the sick child will be handled. In the absence of either of these people, the principal and teacher will have to use their best judgment. When the child is sent home, the parents should be contacted so that appropriate action may be taken with the family physician. And when the pupil returns to school after an illness, the procedure is to report directly to the health service office for clearance to the classroom. Most local school boards have established a readmissions policy.

Providing effective *first aid* requires careful planning by all school personnel. Ideally, only medical personnel should render emergency care. There will be times, however, when only the classroom teacher is available.[14] What should be done? How far should

---

[14]Practically every major group of educators has recommended that teachers have training in first aid. This includes the American Association of School Administrators, Elementary School Principals, National Education Association, American Public Health Association, and American Association for Health, Physical Education, and Recreation.

one go in giving temporary treatment at the site of the emergency? Each teacher should have some knowledge of first aid procedures. It may be possible to relieve suffering and prevent shock, or prevent a disability, or even save a life. It is effective school health practice, therefore, to have the school physician discuss this topic at the start of each school year in order that all school personnel will be prepared for the emergency when it occurs.

No attempt will be made here to go into the many details relative to the various conditions of illness, injury, and suffering which may require first aid attention. Familiarity with the standard first aid course material of the American Red Cross would be most beneficial. However, there are several points that classroom teachers should keep in mind relative to helping during an emergency:

1. It is important to note whether the child is having trouble breathing or is bleeding profusely.
2. Note also whether the child is in a state of shock. If so, the skin is damp and cold and may be ashen or pale in color. Breathing may be shallow, the pulse rapid and weak, and there may be a vacant, glassy stare in the eyes. The child should be made comfortable and should be wrapped in a blanket with the head lower than the feet. No liquids or stimulants should be given.
3. If the face is flushed, lay the child down on his back with the head raised; if he vomits turn his head to the side.
4. Do not move the child who has had an accident until medical assistance arrives.
5. Always comfort and reassure a child. It is encouraging to know that one will be all right.
6. Do not give food or liquid to ill children. It may cause nausea, vomiting, or strangulation.
7. First aid is always rendered to reduce suffering and discomfort. Remaining with the child until assistance arrives, or until he or she is with his parents, may frequently be quite essential to his or her welfare.

Every elementary school should have a well-stocked first aid cabinet located in the office of the nurse or if necessary in the office of the principal.

Accident prevention is another health control item that requires some organization. It is closely related to the content of the elementary school curriculum, and it is an activity that teachers can discuss at length in the classroom. It is also related to the administrator, for he sees that steps are taken to prevent accidents, engages in research projects to determine the cause of accidents, and prepares plans to use in case of fires, hurricanes, and other disasters.

School sanitation is a responsibility in health maintenance and control that rests primarily with the school physician. The physician cooperates with the local board of health to see that school items such as water supplies, dishwashing facilities, food service areas, and locker and shower rooms are safe and pleasant to use. Occasionally an unsanitary drinking fountain—something that all primary school children seem to like to put their mouths over—will spread a disease.

The design and installation of fountains, therefore, are important to teachers as well as sanitation experts.

SCHOOL ABSENCES

In a number of school systems 15 per cent of all pupils are absent daily. Illness is the major cause. It is also the greatest cause of non-promotion because of the high correlation between illness and poor scholastic achievement.

Respiratory difficulties are by far the largest single group of acute conditions reported nationally. Independent studies in New York and California indicate that close to 50 per cent of all absences are due to respiratory disease, with the common cold heading the list. Accidents also contribute to school absenteeism—about 2,200,000 school days are lost annually owing to accidents.

Good patterns of attendance are cooperatively developed between school, parents, community physicians, and welfare agencies. Both parents and teachers should realize that stressing "perfect attendance" is frequently detrimental to proper school health practice. According to Dr. Carl S. Shultz of the U.S. Public Health Service, the usually healthy child should stay home from school if the child is feverish; if symptoms (headaches, drowsiness, runny nose, nausea, or diarrhea) are sufficiently severe to be disabling; if the child is likely to be disturbing to the class or if it is improbable, due to his general condition, that the child will profit from school. Moreover, the child who is permitted to go to school with a slight fever will probably have more fever later in the day; and the child returning early to school while recovering from an upper respiratory infection may pick up other organisms from classmates that could produce serious secondary complications.

REMEDIAL OR FOLLOW-UP PROGRAM

Healing is a matter of time; it is also a matter of opportunity.

—Hippocrates

To have an effective school health organization, medical and teaching personnel must do much more than carry out a program of detection and discovery. They must have the time, facilities, staff, and know-how to implement effective follow-up procedures.

The efficient follow-up program begins with careful planning. Once a health problem is discovered, one might ask whose job it is to contact the parents. In the small elementary school this may be done by the physician, nurse, or classroom teacher. Notices sent to the parents, telling them of the suspected difficulty, are generally respected when signed by the school physician. There is considerable merit, however, in having the classroom teacher sign the notice. This is especially true at the primary grade level. Here, the judgment and concern of the teacher are appreciated by most parents, perhaps more than at any other period in the school years. If the teacher says, "Your John needs glasses now," there is a very good possibility that something will be done about it right away. Parents, like most people, tend to put off doing what they know should be done soon. Sometimes they fail to realize the seriousness of the situation. They say to themselves, "After all, John isn't blind; he doesn't walk into the side of the barn." As true as this may be, he still could fail to read the printed page.

Formal notices of medical examinations sent to parents are often like report cards. They are easy to send home but difficult to get back with an indication that something has been done. The larger and better organized elementary schools send out notices that provide space for an answer. Parents have the opportunity to check off whether they have taken their child to a physician or dentist, plan to do so, or need help in doing so. Other school systems use a form with a detachable section to permit parents to acknowledge receipt of the notification.

The success of a follow-up system depends upon the kind of contact school personnel have with parents, the availability of needed services, and the seriousness with which parents view the health abnormality. Factors favorably influencing follow-up programs include (1) higher socioeconomic status, (2) small families, (3) parent's national background, (4) education beyond high school, (5) non-working mothers, and (6) parental contact involving personal interaction either by telephone or visits. Also, follow-up is more likely when parents receive more than one notification, and by more than one person.

If the school nurse has some method of suspense date record keeping, such as a suspense file, practically all notifications to parents will be accounted for. It will then be possible to keep in close contact with delinquent parents and see that they proceed with the necessary remedial work for their children. In this way the same children with the same defects will not appear year after year in succeeding classrooms with handicaps that might have been corrected.

DUTIES OF HEALTH SERVICES PERSONNEL

The list of duties and responsibilities of personnel connected with the health services department is an extensive one. Some of the more important functions are as follows:

The School Physician

Ideally he or she is a general practitioner or pediatrician interested in children and their problems and in public health. This individual helps the administrator coordinate the health services with other parts of the school program; diagnoses diseases and defects of children but is not responsible for the medical care of individual children; is familiar with the methods of integrating school health services with health teaching, physical education, special education, guidance, recreation, and lunchroom service; is responsible for control of disease, sanitation, emergency cases, and safety within the school; and practices the techniques of teamwork and directs health service as a cooperative enterprise within the school.

Across the country a large number of school systems are unable to employ a full-time physician. In such instances the part-time physician is concerned primarily with basic health services. The Committee on School Physicians of the American School Health Association formulated a manual outlining the duties of school physicians. The minimum duties set forth for the part-time physician are as follows:[15]

1. Consults and assists in the direction and implementation of health screening programs. Examines all candidates for interscholastic athletics prior to each season and periodically thereafter. Implements state labor laws in those states requiring boards of education to provide medical examinations for employment certificates.

2. Assists in the coordination of the school immunization programs conducted by family physicians and health departments.

3. Advises on the control of communicable disease within the school.

4. Interprets medical information from family physicians pertinent to the appropriate classroom management of the child with a physical or emotional handicap.

5. Assumes responsibility for establishing and supervising school emergency facilities and first aid training programs for school personnel. Arranges for emergency care of pupils injured or ill at school when the parent and family physician cannot be reached.

6. Arranges for meetings with groups of community physicians, at which time procedures and communication are discussed to resolve problems to the mutual satisfaction of the school and the physicians.

7. Assists with the planning of parent-education meetings concerning school health problems.

8. Arranges for medical appraisal of pupils who show signs of health problems and whose parents are unable to pay for such services.

9. Compiles reports of the services rendered by the school medical program and of the health problems identified.

Physicians in the larger school system also handle school employee physical evaluations and school-wide health problems which are staff related. This is part of the total task in which most physicians take a great amount of interest. In fact, in addition to an interest in children (which is strong), most physicians are motivated to enter school health work because of a broad interest in preventive

[15]Report of the Committee on School Physicians of the American School Health Association. *A Manual for School Physicians. Journal of School Health,* 37:395–399, October 1967. (Revised).

CHAPTER 3

medicine which involves people of all ages. Most would give more time to the school system if it could be arranged. Unfortunately, because of economic reasons, and because most school physicians are pediatricians and internal medicine specialists, the demands are great upon them to be somewhere other than in the schools. However, survey findings make it clear that when they are able to be in the schools they do spend their time wisely in the three major task areas: (1) individual evaluations, (2) in-school contacts with nurse, principal, teacher, and parents, and (3) both medical and non-medical contacts in the community.

The School Nurse

The school nurse is a respected member of the teaching faculty, and, as such, participates with other teachers in school affairs. In many places today he or she is a nurse-teacher with special skills in health assessment of schoolchildren, coupled with a background in health education, counseling, and the use of community resources.[16] The school nurse interprets the school health program in the home and assists in the planning of learning experiences in the classroom. He or she cooperates with the health agencies in the community that are interested in child health, assists in first aid and home nursing courses, assists the physician, organizes teacher-nurse conferences, and follows up with parent-nurse conferences. In addition, the school nurse is a consultant to the administrative staff, a participant in curriculum design, a counselor, a member of the team providing for handicapped children, and the facilitator of emergency care for illness and injury occurring in school or school-related activities.[17]

The relationship of the nurse to the classroom teacher is of major importance. The success of a nurse's work in school is directly related to the closeness, continuity, and harmony of his or her association with the teacher.

The clever nurse will involve the children when planning for various screenings. Dorothy Shoobs of Columbia University recalls how the nurse carried out an orientation session for kindergarten children who were to undergo audiometer screening in one school system:

The nurse showed the earphones to the children and asked, "Who wears them?"

The children answered, "astronaut," "pilot," "the man in the police station."

The nurse then had one child try on the earphones. She asked the children to be quiet so he could hear the message she was sending him. The children giggled.

---

[16]In some states, public or county health nurses will be assigned to town and city schools. Some of their duties will be the same as those of the nurse-teacher, yet in many respects experience indicates that they do not become as much a part of the school "team" as nurses employed by and responsible to the school administrator. This is due, in part, to the fact that their loyalties are divided between school needs and the public health needs of the community.

[17]For a more complete and detailed breakdown of nursing activities, see *This Is School Nursing* and *School Nursing for the 70's,* distributed by The Association for The Advancement of Health Education, 1201 16th St., N.W., Washington, D.C., 20036.

She had the child repeat what he heard. He mimicked the sound. The nurse turned up the volume so that all of the children could hear the sound.

Next, she asked the teacher to select a child, and she instructed the child selected to don the earphones and tap with a ruler when he heard the sound. She selected three children to come to the health office with her, and told the class that when each child finished, he would return to class and choose the next child to be screened. The next child would then come to the nurse's office.

As each child came up to be screened, the nurse asked him what he would like to be (astronaut, pilot, policeman, etc.). She repeated her instructions to tap with the ruler when the child received her message (heard a sound). The children generally wore expressions of pleased anticipation as they participated in the screening.

This is a good example of how to make the screening procedure less threatening. By having the children take part in the task they gained some control over what was happening, reduced their anxiety, and set the stage for a more reliable measurement of their hearing.

The School Nurse Practitioner

A large number of schoolchildren in America fail to visit private physicians or utilize the services of neighborhood health centers or hospital out-patient departments. They simply do not get comprehensive care; as a result, numerous conditions affecting the ability to learn go undetected for long periods of time. To help solve this problem, the *school nurse practitioner* program in pediatric health was started in Colorado with Denver Public School personnel.[18]

The school nurse practitioner is prepared to assume an expanded role in providing health care to school-age children. He or she receives extra schooling in order to be able to assess the factors that may operate to produce learning disorders, psychoeducational problems, perceptive-cognitive difficulties, and behavior problems as well as those causing physical disease. Significantly, the school facility serves as the principal setting for comprehensive primary and continuing health care and services since it is the one place where children are regularly and readily accessible.

The School Dentist

Dental health services are under the control of the school dentist. Surveys show, unfortunately, that only about one school in 20 has a dentist that visits the school and participates in the education program.

The effective school dentist likes children well enough to perform dental examinations on each child periodically. He or she supervises preventive dental work and oral prophylaxis done by dental hygienists; may take part in a school-sponsored dental clinic;

---

[18]For details of an early program see Silver, Henry K. "The School Nurse Practitioner Program," *Journal of American Medical Association, 216*:1332–1336, May 24, 1971. See also the later report by Silver, Henry K. "School Nurse Practitioners: A Concise Descriptive Definition of Their Functions and Activities," *Journal of School Health, 47*:598–599, December 1977.

and aids classroom teachers and nurse-teachers in the preparation of curriculum materials in dental hygiene.

The dental health "inspection" includes a cursory observation of the mouth and teeth of each child and clinical observation using a mouth mirror and explorer in good light. This is not a diagnostic examination such as would be carried out in the office of the family dentist. It does, however, have certain benefits: it is a fact-finding process which serves as a basis for the school dental health education effort; it helps build a positive attitude toward the dentist and dental care; and the child and parents are motivated to seek and to accept dental treatment as a part of their total health protection. Such efforts are effective. In Minneapolis, for example, "high dental risk" children were placed in a program that restored them to a state of optimum oral health.[19] The program included dental health education, the topical application of stannous fluoride, decay-reducing diets, and parental reinforcement.

Few school administrators realize that the local dental society, with the blessings of the American Dental Association, will gladly conduct a dental survey to assess dental health. The information obtained may be used as a basis for upgrading dental health education. Societies will also provide teaching materials, sponsor in-service education programs for teachers, and assist with the development of teaching guides.

The Dental Hygienist

Despite the efforts in some of the larger states such as New York and California, the dental hygienist as a member of the school teaching staff is still rare.

The dental hygienist may periodically clean teeth and assist the dentist or school physician in the examination of the teeth. He or she may make topical application of sodium or stannous fluoride where state law permits this. The dental hygienist interprets dental defects for parents and helps them make plans for dental corrections. An increasing number of dental hygienists have a degree in education and are prepared to assist elementary school teachers in the area of health instruction.

COORDINATING PERSONNEL

There are a number of people in the school who have a rather special function pertaining to health services. These specialists are a part of the total school health effort. Their day to day activities may rightly be called health coordinating activities. Moreover, their work comes so close to involving the classroom teacher that brief mention will be made of their duties:

---

[19]Meskin, Lawrence H. et al. "A Preventive Dental Program for 'High Risk' Children," *Journal of School Health,* 47:293–297, May 1977.

The Health Supervisor or Coordinator

The elementary school health supervisor or health coordinator is a trained school health educator who works with teachers to develop an organized health education curriculum. This person coordinates health service activities with classroom activities, is familiar with the techniques of instructional supervision, and meets with the school health council to coordinate all school activities.

The Physical Educator

The physical education teacher is one of the most popular teachers with elementary schoolchildren. He or she is concerned with building health, primarily through large muscle activity. This instructor helps the grade teacher develop physical activitiy programs to meet the needs and interests of children and provides for health safeguards on the playgrounds and in the gymnasium. The instructor cooperates with health services personnel by providing a remedial exercise program for children with postural defects, orthopedic difficulties, and a low level of physical fitness. Total health—physical, mental, and emotional—is promoted through a broad program of individual and group experiences. Identifying physically underdeveloped children is an important task, for unless they are helped they tend not to function effectively. Embarrassed by repeated failure, the underdeveloped child may develop a low opinion of himself or herself, an active dislike of physical activity and sport, and an antisocial attitude. It is quite possible for such a child to become a sedentary, overweight adult with all the health risks that those conditions entail.

The School Nutritionist

Trained in nutrition and home economics, the nutritionist supervises the school lunch program, cooperates with the kitchen staff, and helps in promoting health primarily through nutrition education.

The School Custodian

The unknown hero in many elementary schools is the person responsible for the physical environment—the custodian. He or she is one of the most important health promoters in the school. The custodian is concerned with sanitation, ventilation, heating, cleanliness, and safety conditions in corridors, on floors, along walks and at exits. He or she is one of the best friends a classroom teacher can have. Without the custodian's help the teacher may have a difficult time with young children.

In a study published by the United States Department of Health, Education, and Welfare, it is pointed out that the schools need trained custodians who, by the satisfactory performance of many duties and tasks, can contribute to the educational objectives of the school.

Schools are employing psychologists, social workers, school adjustment counselors, and psychiatrists to provide more specialized help. The psychologist is able to determine individual abilities and personalities. The social worker is the contact between the school and the home and is familiar with community resources. The psychiatrist, in the few school systems fortunate enough to have one, generally does consultative work with school personnel and may do diagnostic and therapeutic work with individual boys and girls. A fairly unique characteristic of the Los Angeles program is the wide use of psychiatrists throughout the school health service departments.

HEALTH COUNSELING

Health counseling follows health appraisals. The child's health needs can often be served best by combining the thoughts of several interested people. Sometimes a person designated as health counselor plans a meeting at which a number of people discuss a particular child. In many places the health coordinator is the logical person to head such a committee or council. This type of group in the elementary school may consist of the school nurse, health supervisor or coordinator, the classroom teacher of the child being discussed, and the parents. Groups such as these are able to make a real contribution to the over-all health program of the school. They solve many difficulties and permit the school to give more than "lip service" to the problem of meeting individual needs.

SCHOOL-COMMUNITY HEALTH COUNCIL

There is also another type of council which is timely, broad in scope, and affords opportunities for widespread discussion of health problems. Serving in addition to teachers, administrators, and parents are medical and dental personnel from the community and representatives of public and private health agencies. This council provides a voice for all kinds of voluntary health groups concerned with heart disease, cancer, drug abuse, mental health, family counseling, and others.

The school is a natural community center, especially for elementary school-age children and their parents. In a number of cities it has been possible to accomplish things using the school health service as a focal point that could not have been done as well elsewhere. The school, therefore, is a fine location from which the school-community health council may operate. In this manner the local problems dealing with economic issues, crowded housing, hazards to safety, malnutrition, and other deterrents of health can be cooperatively aired and pursued. Such activities as publicizing the importance of blood testing to detect sickle cell anemia, securing

Una Guia Para Comer Bien

Consuma Diariamente:

Leche y sus Productos

3 o más vasos de leche—Ninos
vasos más chicos para algunos ninos
menores de 8 anos

4 o más vasos—Jóvenes

2 o más vasos—Adultos

Queso, helado o mantecado y
otros alimentos hechos con leche
pueden suplir parte de la leche

Grupo de Carnes

2 o más porciones

Carnes, ave y pescado,
huevos o queso
—con frijoles secos,
alverjas y nueces, como
suplentes

Vegetales y Frutas

4 o más porciones

Incluya vegetales
verdes o amarillos; frutas
citrosas o tomates

Panes y Cereales

4 o más porciones

Enriquecidos con
vitaminas o de grano
entero. Con la leche
se aumenta su valor
alimenticio

Esta es la base para una buena dieta. Consuma más de éstos y otros alimentos según sea necesario para el crecimiento, actividad y para guardar un peso adecuado.

12 1972, 3ra. Edición—Propiedad Literaria de 1958, 1964, National Dairy Council, Chicago 60606

Figure 3-9. Nutrition information provided for Spanish-speaking families. Comes in leaflet or colored poster. (Courtesy National Dairy Council.)

community action for drug abuse prevention, fostering preschool examinations and immunizations, organizing to alleviate certain social conditions conducive to poor mental health, and many more multiple interest activities can be carried on. Where there are language problems, for example, the council is able to initiate changes and provide help through appropriate written aids (see Figure 3–9).

Where there is a neighborhood health center located apart from the school facility, the school-community health council can provide the necessary bridge between school and center so that the school health program component cannot be separated from its neighborhood context.

The potential for community-action programs seems to be advanced where coordinating councils have been established. In the Des Moines–Polk County area of Iowa a number of health-related projects emerged—a weekly health radio series, health fairs at shopping centers, health cassettes for hospital patients' use, and the organization and use of community resource people for classroom presentations.[20] Similar results occurred in Kokomo, Indiana, where the community organized a school-based project to decrease drug and alcohol abuse, child abuse, venereal disease, promiscuity, teenage pregnancies, and other community-school health problems.[21]

ADDITIONAL FUNCTIONS OF HEALTH SERVICES

In recent years the services to pupils have been extended in a number of ways. Working cooperatively with other school personnel, the physicians and nurses are helpful in two important areas.

Detection of Learning Disabilities

The child with learning disabilities requires some interaction with various concerned groups. This individual is considered to have adequate mental ability, sensory function, and emotional control; his or her problem lies in perceptive, integrative, or expressive processes which severely impair learning efficiency. Some children need careful observation in order to identify central nervous system dysfunction, which is also expressed chiefly in impaired ability to learn. The classroom teacher with the help of a specialist (the team approach) has much to offer. Somewhere between 7 and 10 per cent of schoolchildren need help in this area. Often this help starts with the neurological examination in order to secure objective findings. This includes an appraisal of gait and posture, motor system-muscle tone, coordination, handedness, right-left discrimination, and other motor tasks that may be given fairly quickly (see Figure 3–10). Next comes a thorough look at family history, followed by an appraisal of mental status, vision and hearing, and speech and language.

Administration of Drugs in the Schools

Numerous children need to take medicine while attending school. A policy, therefore, needs to be in effect in each school relative to the procedure to be followed. The principal should delegate the person to administer the pupils' medication. It may be the

[20]Lightner, Melvin D. "The Health Education Coordinating Council," *Health Education*, 7:25–28, November/December 1976.
[21]Seffrin, John D. et al. "A School Based Health Education Project," *Health Education*, 8:31–33, January/February 1977.

Clues to physical health problems may show up in school work. Randy's paper (left) revealed a perceptual problem diagnosed as "minimal cerebral dysfunction." Lynn's rapid decline in writing ability (below) led to a medical diagnosis of St. Vitus' Dance.

Courtesy of Elena Boder, M.D.
Pediatric Neurologist
Parent Teacher School Health Center
Los Angeles City Schools

Courtesy of Wan Ngo Lim, M.D.
Director, Department of Pediatrics
Hospital for Special Surgery
Cornell University Medical School

Figure 3–10. Perceptual problems show up in the classroom. (Courtesy Metropolitan Life Insurance Company.)

teacher in some cases, or the school nurse. Ideally, the school nurse should handle this and be familiar with the proper dosage and method of administration. However, the behavior of the child as observed by the teacher needs to be communicated to the physician prescribing the medication. The nurse is probably the best person to communicate with the physician.

Certain drugs have a promising effect in the treatment of children with learning impediments. Tranquilizing agents as well as anticonvulsant agents are employed in many places. So are central nervous system stimulants such as amphetamines. Hyperactive (hyperkinetic) elementary school children have been helped with amphetamine drugs, and the Office of Child Development (HEW) has sanctioned this kind of treatment after "very careful clinical analysis." There is great concern over the amphetamines because of their abuse throughout society. Out of 12 million standard doses produced in a recent year, an estimated 50 per cent were diverted to the black market. Surveys among student populations show that fifth and sixth grade pupils are involved in amphetamine abuse. However, with proper school control the hyperkinetic children with significant behavior problems are helped to sit still and pay attention to what goes on in the classroom. In this connection, it is especially desirable that there be a regular follow-up program including consultation with school nurses, physicians, parents, and teachers of children who are on behavior-modification drugs.[22]

THE CLASSROOM TEACHER COOPERATES WITH HEALTH SERVICES

Without the help of the sympathetic teacher, the health services personnel would indeed be handicapped. Some significant contributions follow.

Detection and Referral

The limitations of the routine medical examination of schoolchildren make it desirable to use the classroom more fully in the detection of pupil health problems. To the teacher who is trained to observe children carefully will come many significant symptoms of poor health. Although the teacher is in no position to diagnose, he or she can certainly detect changes in behavior and refer those to the health services department.[23] In connection with these detection and referral activities of teachers, it is interesting to note that a great deal of this kind of observation is done across the country in isolated areas where physicians are not plentiful. New York state, for example, is rich in physicians. It has one sixth of all the country's physicians and one fifth of all pediatricians. The figures are quite different in New Mexico or Montana. Yet, even in New York state, the vast majority of the physicians are concentrated in big cities, and upstate counties sometimes have difficulty obtaining one. The health observation role of the classroom teacher is further emphasized by the fact that many small cities have no school nursing service.

Following Up Deviations from Normal Health

The value of an appropriate follow-up program in a school has already been pointed out. The teacher's unique contribution here cannot be overstressed. In this country there are great numbers of children who come from homes where they do not have adequate

---

[22]Recommendations of *NEA Task Force on Drug Education*, Washington, D.C., National Education Association, 1972, p. 16.

[23]Chapter 5 will show more clearly what the teacher may observe and screen out in the way of disease, growth abnormalities, and behavior changes.

preparation for school. They lack the sleep, food, or emotional climate that make for satisfactory schoolwork because of poverty, ignorance, and parental indifference. In the classroom the child falls short of what is expected; he or she may appear listless or lazy, easily discouraged, and show poor scholarship. The alert teacher may be able to notice dry scalp, sallow skin, poor posture, lack of energy in physical activities, restlessness, and general irritability. It is important that something be done quickly. This situation is not different from one in which a boy or girl is in need of glasses because of not being able to see the blackboard. Expert medical judgment is needed. Follow-up to see that something is done is vital. Here, parents and teachers need to cooperate, but it is the teacher who is in a position of *control*. He or she actually controls the situation from the classroom and can do a day by day check on the pupils concerned. Nevertheless, boys and girls still appear year after year with the same defects or difficulties despite the efforts of school personnel.

The following case report from a teacher in upstate New York represents a practical approach to a problem of malnutrition. It is more difficult than most cases, but is the type of case that is present in almost every community. It clearly demonstrates the role of the classroom teacher as a *prime mover* in following up basic health abnormalities. The classroom teacher speaks:

John was an 11 year old boy who lived in a trailer camp. His family consisted of father, stepmother, and two stepbrothers ages one and two years old.

He came to school with dirty clothes and unkempt hair and had been classified for two years as a problem child.

The fourth grade teacher noticed that he was listless, complained of headaches, and was retarded in his schoolwork. Then some of the children who brought lunches to school complained that a sandwich, apple, orange, or cookie was missing from their lunches. On inquiry, it was discovered that John was guilty of the misdemeanor. What was the cause? The teacher took John to the school nurse. A conference of nurse, teacher, and John brought out the fact that he was coming to school without breakfast and going without a noonday lunch.

Since the stepmother couldn't leave her small sons, the nurse arranged for a visit to the trailer. The nurse and stepmother discussed John's physical condition and his meals, but the stepmother displayed disinterest. She said that the milkman didn't come until after John's school bus had gone and that the milk on hand in the trailer had to be used for the babies' cereal. She didn't have time to give John toast or egg or to make him a lunch to take to school.

The nurse contacted the father at the factory where he worked and tried to make an appointment to talk to him. His wife had already mentioned the nurse's visit to the trailer, so his reply to the nurse was, "The wife takes care of the food and the feeding of our family." No satisfaction was gained from him.

The nurse reported the results of the investigations to the principal. The principal, nurse, and school cafeteria manager discussed the case and came to the following decision:

Each morning when John's bus arrived, he went to the cafeteria to perform some little task for the cafeteria manager. In return she offered him juice, a slice of bread and butter, and a glass of milk. He didn't realize that this had previously been decided by the conference.

At noon, tickets were given to the children who purchased school lunches. John had been going without lunch or taking hand-outs from the other children, and was now given a ticket each day with the explanation it was given for doing errands for the principal. This was all arranged without humiliating John.

In June, John had shown a year's growth in achievement over the previous year. This was the greatest achievement he had shown in three years. He was a much happier boy in June than the previous September. Cooperative effort of principal, nurse, teacher, and cafeteria manager improved John's nutritional condition and gave him a new outlook on life.

Assisting in Screening Measures

The grade teacher in most school systems works with the nurse to screen pupils for a number of health problems.

In addition to helping with vision and hearing measures, teachers also screen children to determine rate of growth. Growth is usually steady over a long enough period, so teachers weigh and measure their pupils periodically. Sometimes this is done with the aid of the school nurse so that some kind of further appraisal may be made on the spot.

Children are screened for characteristics of poor mental health in some of the more progressive schools. A program, carried out by the teacher, is set up for administering and scoring selected tests and recording the data obtained. Tests measuring the attitude of the child toward school and toward other children, and tests measuring general behavior are especially useful in combating instances of maladjustment.

It should be pointed out that "screening" tests used by teachers are not intended to diagnose. They serve only to select those pupils who appear in need of a diagnosis by a physician.

Carrying Out a Daily Inspection

The principle of observing hands, fingernails, faces, skin, eyes, hair, teeth, and glands is a good one. The question often asked is whether such a daily inspection should be a formal one or an informal one. Certainly the formal inspection is an orderly approach—one which the pupils soon learn to accept. When teachers are careful not to place *too much* emphasis on health items, the interest of the pupils is just enough to permit valuable learning to take place. Highly competitive morning inspections, however, sometimes force the pupils to be a part of the group "at any cost," even to the extent of being dishonest and reporting that they brushed their teeth when they did not.

Probably the daily inspection can best be carried out on an informal basis. Sometime during the morning activities the teacher moves about the classroom observing the boys and girls. He or she obviously will be more interested in noting the appearance of those pupils who had poor health practices the day before. The teacher can still post a record of his or her observations as a motivation technique for health education. In fact, several companies print daily inspection charts that may be obtained by request. Some teachers, instead of keeping the charts at school, send them home with the children. They are taped to the back of the bathroom door so that the child may keep his or her own record. This can be very effective for it also serves to keep the parents aware of what is going on.

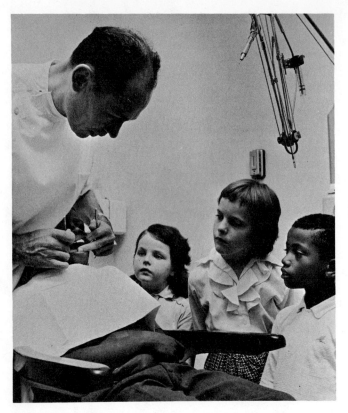

Figure 3–11. Health education is not limited to the classroom. (Courtesy Cincinnati Public Schools.)

Health Counseling

Either individually or as a member of a school health council, the classroom teacher follows up appraisals by discussing the findings with the pupils. This is most generally planned but carried out informally. With younger children the parents are involved right away in the counseling procedure. Some of the finest counseling is done just like good teaching—"as if you taught them not."

Opportunities for Health Teaching

As already suggested in Chapter 2, the classroom teacher has a wonderful chance to educate for health every time the class is scheduled to visit the school physician. If this job is well done, the boys and girls will look forward to going to the physician's office. Furthermore, having a medical examination can be a most rewarding experience for the youngster in the early grades. These children are curious and, as a rule, they need little external motivation to prepare them for the day when they are looked over by the doctor. The teacher with a pleasant and positive outlook can discuss the why, the what, and the how of such a visit.

Why are we going to have the examination? Will it hurt?
What will the doctor find?
How will all this affect me?

These are good questions. If the pupils are allowed to work on this topic a while they will come up with a number of other things that have been bothering them—questions relating to the instruments carried in the black bag, or why doctors do not seem to catch the measles or mumps when they visit sick children.

In some classrooms or nurses' offices children have a chance to handle a real stethoscope before the examination, and listen to the beat of their own hearts. Questions are asked and answered so that by the time of the examination the class is practically bouncing with enthusiasm to get started. This kind of approach almost guarantees a *satisfying experience*.[24] Such positive health teaching may be briefly summarized by referring to a story told by a pioneer in health teaching, Mable Bragg. In a Newton, Massachusetts, school one day, Dr. Emmett Holt stopped a group of children who were skipping merrily down a corridor. "Where are you going?" he asked. "We're going to see the doctor," said a little girl. "Why?" asked Dr. Holt. "Are you sick?" "Oh, no," she replied, "We're going to see how well we are."

THE IN-SERVICE PROGRAM

Orienting teachers and keeping them up to date is the responsibility of the local administration. School health is promoted this way through the in-service program.

A number of school programs have been completely reorganized from time to time because teachers have sat down together to talk about the health of their children. In Indiana, for example, the in-service training of teachers in health education has been successfully carried on for many years. Weekly conferences, under state education department guidance and promotion, have prompted many principals and classroom teachers to modify their existing health efforts. Moreover, in a number of the larger cities, the nurse-teachers speak to all school personnel each year about the health services available in the school and the community. Surveys have indicated that in a number of elementary schools there are numerous teachers who are quite unfamiliar with health centers and the health services available for their immediate use within a few miles or minutes of the school.

QUESTIONS FOR DISCUSSION

1. In a Galveston, Texas study it was found that elementary schoolchildren had considerably more visits for health services than high school children. What do you think is the reason for this finding?

2. What is the current thinking relative to the administration of medication to schoolchildren during school hours? If a pupil must take his pills

---

[24]An expression used by William James to convey the idea of something that gives deep gratification to the individual and will be apt to be repeated again because of this.

regularly should he do it in class under teacher supervision or go to the office of the school nurse?

3. To what extent do teachers of your acquaintance engage in "detection and referral" activities?

4. How would you as a teacher feel about keeping anecdotal records on the health behavior of your children? Would it be a chore or something you believe would be useful to other teachers?

5. Are school psychiatrists necessary ? Is it not possible that a guidance counselor or school psychologist might be a reasonable substitute?

SUGGESTED ACTIVITIES

1. Samuel Braun speaks highly of parents going to school with their young children because they can be helpers in the classroom and health office. (See *Selected References*.) As a teacher, how would this appeal to you? Inquire of several other teachers on the job to sample their opinion relative to strengths and weaknesses.

2. Find out what kind of duties school nurses actually perform. Do they do everything this chapter says they do? How do they relate to handicapped children? To drop outs? To children who may take advantage of illness? To children who miss classes? To the social workers or health center?

3. Read about preschool health screening efforts. (See Belleville article in *Selected References*.) Aside from the positive elements, what are some of the difficulties found in working with these younger children and their parents?

4. Interview a school nurse, preferably one in a large city and another in a small town, in order to discuss factors affecting school health follow-up practices. This may be organized as a committee project to discover some of the difficulties involved in following up and in improving the health conditions of schoolchildren. Write out your comments following the interview.

SELECTED REFERENCES

Anderson, C. L. and Creswell, William H. *School Health Practice,* 6th ed. St. Louis: C. V. Mosby Co., 1977.

Belleville, Marion and Green, Pauline B. "Preschool Multiphasic Screening Programs In Rural Kansas," *American Journal of Public Health, 62*:795–799, June 1972.

Braun, Samuel J. "When Parents and Young Children Go to School," *Health Education, 7*:6–9, May/June 1976.

Cubbage, Mary-Louise. "Jottings of an Early Childhood Consultant," *Health Education, 7*:20–21, May/June 1976.

Dennison, Darwin and Fenimore, Joy A. "A Heart-Sound Screening Program for Elementary Children," *Journal of School Health, 41*:349–351, September 1971.

Diamond, Elliot and LeBendig, Michael. "The School's Role in Preventive Child Foot Care," *Health Education, 8*:36–39, January/February 1977.

Eisner, Victor and Oglesby, Allan. "Health Assessment of Children," *Journal of School Health, 42*:348–350, June 1972.

Greenberg, Jerrold S. "Responding to the Causes of Unhealthy Behavior," *Health Education, 7*:32–33, May/June 1976.

Hoopfer, Leah B. "Awareness Teams in Health Education," *Health Education, 8*:8–11, September/October 1977.

Mayshark, Cyrus, Shaw, Donald B., and Best, Wallace H. *Administration of School Health Programs,* 2nd ed. St. Louis: C. V. Mosby Co., 1977.

McKevitt, Rosemary K., et al. "Reasons for Health Office Visits in an Urban School District," *Journal of School Health,* 47:275–278, May 1977.

Mello, Arthur F. "A School Fluoride Mouthrinse Program," *Journal of School Health,* 47:557–559, November 1977.

Mercer, Cecil D. and Trifiletti, John J. "The Development of Screening Procedures for the Early Detection of Children with Learning Problems," *Journal of School Health,* 47:526–532, November 1977.

National Education Association—American Medical Association Joint Committee. *School Health Services,* 3rd ed. Chicago, AMA, 1973.

Schaller, Warren E. "Positioning School Health Education as a National Priority," *Journal of School Health,* 47:393–394, September 1977.

_____ and Nemir, Alma. *The School Health Program,* 4th ed. Philadelphia: W. B. Saunders Co., 1976.

Schuur, Elizabeth. "School Nurses' Public Relations," *Journal of School Health,* 47:613–614, December 1977.

Silver, Henry K. et al. "School Nurse Practitioners: A Concise Descriptive Definition of Their Functions and Activities," *Journal of School Health,* 47:598–599, December 1977.

Healthful and Safe School Environment

4

Schools can be humane and still educate well. They can be genuinely concerned with gaiety and joy and individual growth and fulfillment without sacrificing concern for intellectual discipline and development.

—Charles Silberman

The environment for learning depends substantially on a variety of physical characteristics and human influences. Yet, schools differ measurably, ranging from those that work very well to those that actually hinder the development of many young students. Silberman's call to create settings where children are respected, where learning is valued, and where equality is pursued is both healthful and humane.

IMPORTANCE OF HEALTHFUL LIVING TO THE SCHOOL PROGRAM

The healthful school environment is one which provides for healthful living throughout the school day. It is not a haphazard setup; there is organization to bring this about. The administrator, the physician, and the custodian work together to provide safe and sanitary facilities and such pupil-teacher relationships as are favorable to the best development, optimum learning, and welfare of all.

Concern for the living conditions of students is not new. Most civilizations have given it some attention. Spartan educators realized the importance of favorable surroundings dominated by teachers with strong personalities. Through the years in American schools there have been numerous distractions such as lack of heat in the winter months, poor lighting, inadequate ventilation, unadjustable desks and chairs, unattractive walls, and poor acoustics. Parents sometimes made their objections known. So did medical doctors who were interested in the schools. At the founding meeting of the American Association for the Advancement of Physical Education, held in Brooklyn, New York, in 1885, Dr. W. L. Savage spoke about "ill ventilated school houses and weary children and of the relief which open windows and physical exercise would bring."[1] Over-crowded classrooms and poor school construction in the late 1800's resulted in several tragic fires which stimulated the populace to look more closely at the school environment. In 1892 William H. Burnham, one of the better known school health pioneers, wrote extensively on "school hygiene" and presented evidence to show the necessity for greater attention to school furniture, cleanliness, growth, schoolhouse architecture, reading, writing, fatigue, and aspects of school health neglected at that time.[2] Gradually, more attention was given to child health, and today educational buildings and programs are continually being modified to provide healthful school living.

No one, however, should be misled into believing that most of the schools are "up to date" just because new buildings are being erected. Teachers still register complaints about inadequate drinking fountains, overcrowded classrooms and playrooms, noisy environment, and insufficient janitorial services. In a great number of schools it is possible to discover inadequacies in basic safety measures. School bus transportation is a good example. Despite an increase in new equipment and improved bus regulations, many states do not forbid pupils to stand in moving buses.

THE INTERNAL ENVIRONMENT—THE SCHOOL BUILDING

Whether or not the elementary school contributes to the over-all purposes of health education depends initially upon the thinking and planning of members of the Board of Education. Where is the building to be located? Is it to be near main highways, busy streets, noisy factories, or active train yards? Of what is it to be constructed? In what direction will it face? Is there play space within the structure? Are the corridors sound-proofed? Are the stairs moderately inclined? What kind of windows does it have? If windows have to be closed, is there air conditioning? Are the classrooms attractive? Is the health examination room adequate in size? Are there locker room and shower facilities? How satisfactory are the lunchroom facilities? These and a dozen more pertinent questions must be discussed by the board members, architects, sanitary engineers, and others before the building is constructed. Moreover, it is not uncommon today for teachers' committees to plan the facilities that to them seem desirable for the maintenance of good health and the promotion of a reasonable degree of individual pupil achievement.

The importance of the internal school environment to the elementary school teacher should not be underestimated. The finest health teaching is done by example. Where there are no facilities for handwashing, for instance, it is difficult to discuss visiting the wash-

---

[1]Proceedings of the Association for the Advancement of Physical Education. Brooklyn: Rome Brothers, 1885.

[2]Means, Richard K. A History of Health Education in the United States. Philadelphia: Lea & Febiger, 1962, p. 62.

room and washing the hands before eating. There are numerous schools that fit this category. Until recent years the city schools were usually better equipped than the rural schools, but with the closing of many old-time rural schoolhouses and the opening of thousands of consolidated and regional schools serving large areas of the population, the trend toward superior facilities is moving away from the large cities.

No matter how poor the facilities are, the classroom teacher owes it to the pupils to strive personally for improvements. He or she should know that:

1. The water supply must meet the minimum standards for chemical bacterial purity established by the state and local health departments.

2. The common drinking cup is prohibited.

3. The sanitary drinking fountain should be installed near the classroom, or at least one on each floor to serve a minimum of 50 pupils; the height of the nozzle should range from 23 inches for kindergarten to 29 inches for intermediate grade school pupils.[3] The fountain should be of the modern, slanting type with self-closing valve and mouth guard. Adequate water pressure must be maintained at all drinking fountains.

4. The drinking fountain water should be cool, less than 75°F.

5. The rural schools without running water should use sanitary privies, either the pit privy or septic privy type, or chemical toilets.

6. In the absence of a garbage grinder, food and refuse from the school cafeteria should be disposed of by local collection, burning, burying, or other methods approved by sanitation authorities.

7. Toilet facilities—clean, well-ventilated, bright, well-kept, and properly lighted—encourage pupils to maintain these conditions. The dark toilet room, without paper towels and liquid soap, poorly kept, encourages a lack of respect for standards of sanitation. There should be a minimum of one urinal for 30 boys and a split-seat toilet for 25 to 30 girls.

8. The handwashing basins should range in height from 20 inches for kindergarten to 25 inches for intermediate grade school pupils. There should be one for every 30 children.

9. School cafeteria sanitation must meet the standards of any public or community eating establishment. The cafeteria should also be an attractive place to eat.

10. The school swimming pools and shower room facilities must meet sanitary standards. The use of pupil footbaths is not recommended; instead, individuals are encouraged to practice proper foot hygiene. This involves drying the foot and using foot powder if necessary. It also includes periodic inspection of the pupils' feet for athlete's foot and other skin infections. Floors should be hosed and washed daily.

11. The teachers' rest rooms should be attractive and functional.

---

[3]National Education Association, American Medical Association. *School Health Services,* revised 1970. Washington: National Education Association.

12. The school custodian is the teacher's friend and needs the help of the teacher and pupils.

13. The gymnasium must be well-lighted and ventilated and have protective wiring over exposed lights.

14. The halls, stairways, classrooms, and auditorium must be checked for accident hazards.

15. The playground should be clean and level and perferably have an asphalt (blacktop) surface.

16. The school area should be relatively free of disturbing noises, obnoxious odors, and other distractions.

17. School personnel must be constantly alert to observe buildings, grounds, and equipment for possible hazardous conditions:

Broken or splintered furniture or playground equipment
Defective stair rails
Broken sidewalks
Protruding objects, such as nails
Holes in blacktop surfaces
Sandboxes not properly maintained
Blocked or obstructed exits
Slippery floors
Gas leaks

18. Fire prevention equipment must be conveniently located and inspected at regular intervals.

ASPECTS OF CLASSROOM ENVIRONMENT

The classroom is the teacher's domain. Here are influences too subtle to measure, and here also are influences of major proportion that may contribute to or detract from learning and pupil achievement. These influences, or environmental elements, may be divided into physical factors and human factors. They touch upon all phases of healthful school living, from physical and emotional climate to classroom safety.

Physical Factors in the Classroom

Children attending school near large airports such as Los Angeles International Airport run the risk of suffering permanent hearing damage and are threatened emotionally because of jet aircraft noise. This kind of stressful situation is exactly what Hippocrates referred to 25 centuries ago when he talked about the state of the organism which results from reactions to noxious stimuli or disturbing situations. Unfortunately, such negative influences are as much a part of the educational process as the favorable ones. Very often something can be done about them.

Other things being equal, if the classroom is a pleasant place to live in, the student will find many opportunities for a satisfying experience. One wonders how "satisfying" the Los Angeles experience referred to earlier can be when decibel readings from airport noise are 80 to 96 in the classroom—far in excess of a reasonably quiet neighborhood of 45 to 50 decibels. Worse still, in this situation the classrooms were neither sound-proofed nor air-conditioned for pupil comfort when windows were closed. At best it is a struggle to learn in such an environment. No wonder Charles Silberman, commissioned by the Carnegie Foundation to study schools near the Los Angeles International Airport, termed the quality of life in the classroom "intolerable."

The teacher should know that the physical aspects of the classroom may have as much to do with success as the motivation techniques and educational methods employed. He or she should know that:

1. An air temperature not in excess of 68°F represents an optimal condition for comfort, with a slightly higher temperature of about 70°F desirable in the primary grades.
2. Items such as humidity, air movement, and children's clothing must also be considered when comfortable room temperatures are being discussed.
3. It is good education for health to have pupils record readings on room thermometers at set intervals.
4. Ventilation is as important to comfort as room temperature; windows should be opened from the bottom to permit incoming cold fresh air to mix with the warm air rising from the radiator, and combined air moves toward the exhaust.
5. Standards of classroom lighting are steadily being revised, both for artificial and natural light. The lighting must be soft, even, properly distributed, and bright enough for eye comfort.
6. The responsibility for checking the operation of window shades and lights is the classroom teacher's.
7. To obtain the best working light from natural sources within the pupil's field of vision and with a minimum of shadows, individual pupil consideration should be given to seating arrangements. The 50° rotation of classroom furniture (in schools with movable desks and chairs) allows for maximum utilization of natural lighting by permitting the light to fall upon the work surface of each child's desk, unobstructed by body shadows.
8. The eyesight of schoolchildren is influenced by differences in brightness. This involves natural lighting, artificial illumination, and the color used to finish the interior surfaces of the classroom. Excessive brightness, which is glare, can be avoided by the type and color of paint used. Upper walls should reflect more light than lower walls and floors. But floors should reflect about 30 per cent of the light; they should not be dark and oiled. Desks should be light enough to reflect 40 per cent of the light, while the chalkboard should not reflect more than 15 per cent. Furniture, chalkboards, and other fixtures should have non-glossy finishes.
9. Uncontrolled sunlight is a fatiguing element that detracts from the total learning process.

10. The classroom should be free from acoustic difficulties.
11. The location and size of desks and chairs should be suited to the pupils using them. Fatigue and tension are often caused by ill-fitting classroom furniture.
12. The writing surface of the desk should be at a height which permits the student to write while squarely seated so that there will be no need to elevate one shoulder when writing.
13. The ability of any one pupil to see or hear should be the major factor in determining where he or she sits in the room.
14. Eyestrain may be relieved by alternating instruction involving close eye work with learning activities that are visually less fatiguing.
15. Clean teaching materials, such as maps and books, are desirable. Too often soiled materials are employed on which there is poor contrast between the paper and the print.

Healthful school living is in itself a health teaching opportunity. All pupils must share the load of keeping the school clean and pleasant. By so doing they gain an understanding of the proper use of school property, the rights and feelings of others, and an appreciation for healthful surroundings. It is of interest to note that on many occasions this kind of pupil appreciation carries over into the home environment rather quickly and is manifested by such actions as cleaning kitchen floors, hanging bright curtains, and helping parents wash windows and paint interior walls.

There are, in addition to the physical factors already referred to, a number of other classroom items that have a bearing upon healthful living. The scheduling of activities and the allotment of time, for example, may be done in such a way that the interest of the class members is kept at a high level throughout the day. This may be ascertained by experimenting with the difficult activities at various hours of the school day. Keeping a rigid time schedule, particularly in the lower grades, does not allow for individual and group variations in capacities and interest. Other classroom environment elements that are of concern here include things such as the length of the school day, the spacing and duration of rest and recess periods, class load, and programs and surroundings adapted to individual needs (see Figure 4–1).

Human Factors in the Classroom

Few laymen have any idea of the complicated juggling of forces and personalities that is the everyday job of the classroom teacher; it is like trying to stage an important show while trying to keep a dozen billiard balls, knives and forks in the air all at once without dropping or forgetting one.

Further complicating classroom success is the myth that student economic inequality is an obstacle. Myths die hard in this country, so negative views get passed around. Rist summarizes them as follows:

Middle-class students can learn, lower-class students cannot . . . control is necessary, freedom is anarchy; . . . Teachers can save a few, but will lose many; the school tries, the home will not; and finally only the naive would

Figure 4–1. A relaxation period fosters healthful school living. (Courtesy Los Angeles Schools.)

dispute these beliefs, as the wise know. *The outcome of this set of attitudes . . . is that the school as an institution sustains, in a myriad of ways, the inequalities with which children first come to school.* The school's response to issues of color, class, and control all mesh together to make two nets—one to catch winners and one to catch losers.[4]

The role of the teacher is to attempt to maintain an environment for good health, which in turn creates the optimum atmosphere for learning. The teacher must be realistic and deal objectively with pupil relationships, must think in terms of individuals while operating in the medium of masses of children, and must exercise leadership and be firm with pupils. At the same time the teacher must demonstrate cooperation and sympathy for children with personal problems of adjustment. And as Mayshark, Shaw, and Best point out, all of this must be accomplished with a genuine enthusiasm for teaching.[5]

Human factors are more difficult to control than physical factors. The elementary schoolteacher is faced at the beginning of each school year with the task of building a mentally healthy environment. He or she must understand child behavior and recognize that the mentally healthy classroom is one where the children have a high level of self-esteem, are relaxed and at ease, are challenged by the situation to want to learn, and are confident that they can succeed. Children should receive a personal satisfaction from such success.

[4]Rist, Ray C. *Urban Schools: A Factory For Failure.* Cambridge, Mass.: M.I.T Press, 1973, p. 330.

[5]Mayshark, Cyrus, Shaw, Donald D. and Best, Wallace H. *Administration of School Health Programs,* 2nd ed. St. Louis: C. V. Mosby Company, 1977, p. 280.

Furthermore, the teacher must recognize that in adjusting to school, children are making three of the fundamental adjustments to life. First of all, they are making a social adjustment, i.e., to classmates. In the second place, they are making an adjustment to authority. This is an adjustment made to teachers and principals, which is just and friendly, and essential for happy group living. In the third place, children learn in school to adjust to their own limitations. This, in itself, places the teacher in a unique position, for every child wants to be the best, the brightest, and the most productive; the teacher must help each child discover his or her own strong points and live with his or her limitations.

In addition to recognizing these factors, the teacher works to create a school environment that promotes mental health. Such activity on his or her part is a first-rate example of proper health education. Some of the more specific tasks the teacher can engage in to foster feelings of acceptance, affection, and achievement include:

1. Making the classroom a friendly place. "Big Brothers" and "Big Sisters" can be assigned to help newcomers feel at home. Look for the child without a friend and see that he or she has a chance to sit with an especially friendly person.
2. Showing concern for each pupil. Celebrate birthdays. Telephone the home of sick children to inquire about them. Welcome them back on their return to class and allow them to talk about their illness to the group.
3. Permitting boys and girls to have a part in planning the class activities.
4. Treating all pupils kindly. Avoid constant nagging, scolding, or correcting. Let children know, without saying in so many words, that you like them, and if they have trouble with something, you will try to see their side of the problem.
5. Accepting children's feelings of the moment. Angry children have their difficulties, but these may be overcome to some extent by directing their attention to some constructive form of expression such as helping the teacher, painting a picture, or talking over the trouble with an older person.
6. Providing for successful experiences. Each pupil needs to feel success in at least one area of effort, whether it be sport skills, music, reading, or in picking up paper from the floor! At the same time it should be noted that children learn by their failures. Thus they should not be protected from their failures but should understand them clearly in terms of their successes.
7. Praising individuals and groups for their fine efforts. Praise, properly administered, acts as an effective tonic which spurs pupils on to greater accomplishments.
8. Making provisions for specific student weaknesses and deficiencies through avenues of adapted instruction and program modification.
9. Helping parents develop a wholesome attitude toward ability and success in the classroom.
10. Recognizing that academic and social pressures may be

somewhat offset by "low pressure" teaching and flexible pupil scheduling.

Liking or disliking school has much to do with classroom atmosphere. Needed are more patient teachers endowed with the kind of sensitivity that makes it possible to see how things look from the other person's point of view. Combs clearly indicates that teachers frequently fail to see children's views, and this accounts for most of the failures in human communication.[6] When children with severe emotional problems are involved, it is even more important to see the child's view and resist reacting to a child's hostility on a personal level. Teacher calmness, objectivity, and warmth tend to rub off on the pupil.

Teacher's Personal Health Status

The most favorable physical and human factors brought to bear in the classroom may mean very little if the teacher's own health status is below par. Yet various surveys of the mental and physical condition of teachers have produced evidence that a good many of them are ill in one way or another.

---

[6]Combs, Arthur W. "The Human Aspect of Administration," *Educational Leadership,* November 1970, p. 197.

Figure 4–2. A healthful environment for learning is a pleasant teacher. (Courtesy National Education Association and Joe DiDio.)

Many communities require periodic health examinations for teachers. Hypertensive individuals showing some irritability and fatigue and teachers with a history of severe mental illness probably should not teach school. Unfortunately a very small number of teachers are prohibited to teach because of poor health. Studies are needed to show more clearly the relationship between classroom-pupil efficiency and teacher health defects and illness. How can a grouchy teacher create happiness? Said Ben Franklin in his *Almanac:*

> If you would have others merry with cheer, be so yourself or so appear.

It is estimated that *ten per cent* of all teachers in the United States have emotional problems deep enough to merit the designation "seriously maladjusted." Withdrawn and depressed teachers are using up their illness days in many localities. In New York there has been a one third increase in teacher absence since 1960. Research is meager in this area, and when teachers exhibit behavior that should keep them out of the classroom, little is done about it, partially because it is difficult to define mental illness clearly enough to permit school authorities to label a person sick without risking a legal suit. Teachers with emotional problems often refuse to admit their inadequacy because they are threatened by it.

The physical health status of the classroom teacher is related largely to personal health practices. Teaching is considered one of the vigorous occupations, on a level with medicine, military life, and police duty, and, as such, demands much of the vigor and enthusiasm of the individual. Practices involving good nutrition, dental care, recreation, moderate exercise, and rest are therefore important if one is to sustain an active constitution for effective teaching.

Every day there are untold circumstances that challenge the strength, ingenuity, and adaptability of the teacher. Some of these exert pressure on conscientious teachers and tend to alter their attitudes so that they are a little less friendly and appear not to enjoy their jobs quite as much as before. Teachers need time for enrichment. Just as other people show signs of psychological stress and fatigue from their efforts to make a living, teachers too need relaxation, diversion, and play. Art, music, golf, fishing, photography, and other hobbies provide "just what the doctor ordered" for harassed teachers. The teacher who understands this point of view is far ahead of the one with great zest who "pushes" himself or herself until he or she becomes unbearable to the class.

ASPECTS OF SCHOOL SAFETY

The topic of safety and safety education is a discipline in itself, but safety programs usually fall within the school health education domain. Safety education cuts across all fields and involves all school personnel. Children learn about safe living through programs of instruction and by well-defined school safety practices that are engaged in by all pupils and teachers.

The school building has its share of hazards to guard against.

There are stairways, corridors, lavatories, classrooms, shower rooms, swimming pools, gymnasiums, cafeterias, auditorium stages, and industrial arts shops to be concerned with. And there are programs associated with these facilities that require constant attention on the part of teachers lest accidents occur that might have been prevented. The same reasoning applies to the external environment. Safety on the playgrounds and playing fields, on the school buses, at the crossings adjacent to the school, and on field trips into the community all relate to healthful school living.

Accidents constitute the major hazard to the lives of children. They account for about half of the deaths among boys and for one fourth among girls. For boys especially, the accident hazard increases rapidly as they reach their late teens. A great many of these accidents occur in the school area.

Research reported by the National Safety Council indicates that 800,000 school injuries occur each year among boys and girls. According to the U.S. Public Health Service, there may be closer to four million accidental injuries per year, half of which are due to falls and bumping. In a Louisiana study it was found that "running when walking was required" and "horseplay" were practices strongly contributing to school accidents. In the first six grades the frequency of accidents is highest in the unorganized activities. Serious accidents, as determined by the average number of days lost from school, occur at the bicycle rack area, stairways, athletic fields, doorways, and school sidewalks, in that order.

Obviously there is a need for safety precautions in every school. Administrators, working with teachers, must formulate school safety procedures and establish local regulations. In numerous large city systems such as Boston, Los Angeles, New York, Cincinnati, and Boulder, special policies on accident prevention and environmental health have been set forth in administrative handbooks.

An appraisal instrument designed to help teachers and administrators improve their school safety efforts is available from the National Commission on Safety.[7] It is a checklist that encourages action on school safety problems related to facilities and other environmental considerations and educational programs.

With over 7200 fires a year in schools, the fire departments carry out inspections, and boards of education are required to implement fire department suggestions with respect to remedying hazardous situations. Police departments frequently study school traffic safety, erect special traffic signals and signs, and order appropriate crosswalk markings. Local civil defense groups also have a genuine interest in school health and safety activities.

Accident Prevention

There are at least four major considerations worth reviewing when an effort is being made to promote school safety. The first of

---

[7]National Commission on Safety Education. *School Safety Education Checklist: Administration, Instruction, Protection,* (revised), Washington, D.C.: National Education Association, 1972.

these, which has already been discussed at some length, is the *determination of pupil health status*. The sick child is a hazard to his or her own safety. Reflexes and responses are slower; the child is less alert; and the physical capacity that contributes to personal safety is missing. Even children convalescing from disease and getting over colds probably should have a modified school program, for it is conceivable that their interaction with children could have some bearing on the safety of others.

The second consideration is *proper maintenance of equipment and facilities*. Activities in the classroom, on the playground, in the gymnasium, and in the shops involve the use of special equipment. It is the teacher's responsibility to see that this equipment is in proper repair and safe to use. Very often when a jungle gym frame is loose, or a sliver of wood breaks off a teeter board, or a stone under the swings works up out of the ground, the classroom teacher will complain that it is the duty of the school custodian to do something about it. But in most instances constructive action will be taken in the way of repair only when the teacher personally discusses the situation with the custodian.

The third program safeguard concerns the *development of activity skills*. In every subject area there are specific skills to be mastered. Proficiency in these skills—in the classrooms and laboratories and on the playgrounds—makes the difference between a low and high accident rate. It would be improper for schools to remove every dangerous piece of equipment or condemn all hazardous activities. Children need the experience of meeting challenging situations by developing satisfactory skills. Electric jig saws are not removed from the shops because they can cut off a wayward finger; playground equipment is not dismantled for fear that some child may fall off; and automobiles are not outlawed because of automobile accidents. We learn to live with these things. There is no substitute for skill. The child, for example, who possesses the skill for operating the jig saw, is far better off than the one who has little ability but is closely supervised.

This leads directly to the fourth and final consideration, *adequate supervision*. The stairways, corridors, halls, playgrounds, and classrooms need constant supervision, not only because teachers are liable but also because youngsters are often too busy to look after their own safety. Satisfactory accident prevention involves a combination of all four considerations, especially personal skills and adequate supervision. For example, children boarding school buses, crossing streets, and taking part in fire drills need to practice well-identified skills in the presence of capable teacher supervision.

The prevention of school accidents has become one of the major interests of board members, teachers, and administrators. A few of the more significant *accident prevention activities* are worth listing, for they have more than a slight influence on school health:

In the classroom:

1. Put sharp objects away.
2. Cover exposed projections such as plant boxes and table corners.

3. Cover exposed lights, radiators, and electric fixtures.
4. Play games that are safe for the particular classroom.
5. Instruct children to move about the classroom in an orderly manner, neither pushing nor running.
6. Use tools at a workbench or desk.
7. Keep furniture in its proper place.
8. Encourage children to keep their feet out of the aisle and under the desk.

In the halls, corridors, and stairways:
1. Do not leave locker doors ajar.
2. Instruct children to avoid running and pushing, especially on stairs.
3. Exercise care at drinking fountains.
4. Use care in passing closed doors; they may be opened suddenly and cause serious injury.
5. Report slippery surfaces and worn or broken stairs.
6. Appraise the hall traffic in terms of congestion; rerouting may be advisable.

In the shops and laboratories:
1. Keep floors clear of litter.
2. Look for "shop sloppies" who wave boards wildly around in the air and leave nails sticking up for others to step on.
3. Check and repair equipment each day.
4. Post and discuss safety rules for using laboratory or shop tools and equipment.
5. Provide adequate first aid supplies, especially for burns and bleeding.

Figure 4–3. Fifth graders study safety in school. (Courtesy National Safety Council and National Education Association.)

6. See that gas, water, and electricity are turned off when no longer needed.
7. Stress the importance of good footing and safe clothing. Sleeves should be rolled and ties removed.
8. Use color to denote parts of machinery or chemicals that are particularly hazardous.

In the gymnasium, locker room, and shower rooms:
1. Encourage safe play through personal example and discussion with pupils.
2. Stress the rules of the game, point out the boundaries, and penalize for infringements.
3. Do not overcrowd the play space. There is danger when groups practice their skills in adjacent areas.
4. Select activities within the physiological and skill limits of the pupils.
5. Seek out the hazards of each game and plan to counteract them.
6. Check exposed projections, gymnasium equipment, lighting, and floor surfaces. Lights should be protected with a heavy wire mesh.
7. Insist that pupils dress in proper uniform with sneakers for all gymnasium activities.
8. Regulate showers from a master control panel.
9. Prohibit pushing, wrestling, and fooling around in locker and shower rooms.

On the playgrounds:
1. Enclose the entire playground area with a fence five or six feet high.
2. Provide adequate space between pieces of equipment.
3. Mark well and properly space all courts for outside games.

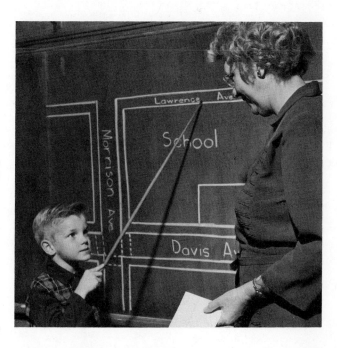

Figure 4–4. City children talk over the best route to school. (Courtesy National Safety Council.)

4. Check apparatus for needed repairs and terrain for objects such as tree roots or stones.
5. Encourage safe play. Teach the correct use of each piece of apparatus.
6. Carry on team games such as soccer, speedball, and softball in an area away from the apparatus and small children.
7. Reserve one section of the playground that is protected and near the school for kindergarten and first graders.
8. Encourage courtesy, patience, and fair play; they breed a degree of respect for the other person and reduce accidents.

Going to and from school:
1. Discuss with children the routes they take home.
2. Encourage parental interest in the safety program, particularly as it concerns going to and from school.
3. Remind children to stay on the walks and in crosswalk lanes, and to obey rules, signs, and the traffic directors.
4. Encourage children to report hazardous obstructions along school routes.
5. Cooperate with school bus drivers in the aspects of bus safety.
6. Provide supervision of school traffic patrols.[8]

QUESTIONS FOR DISCUSSION

1. In this chapter Ray Rist is quoted as saying that a number of myths relative to student inequalities prevail—an attitude and assumption that contributes to unsuccessful school experiences. How do you feel about this? Do you agree or disagree?

2. Does the expression "healthful living" mean more or less to you than "healthful school environment"? Explain.

3. Would parental safety education of school-age children be workable? Could child psychology, child safety, and other environmental topics be taught in such a way that accidental injuries to children could be reduced? Do you have a better idea?

4. Suppose the teacher's personal health influences learning in a negative way. What should be done in a school system to prevent this situation? To remedy it?

5. Discuss the construction of a checklist of items designed to screen the environmental conditions of a school from the viewpoint of health and safety.

---

[8]Standard rules governing the operation of school safety patrols have been adopted by states and on a national level by representatives of the National Safety Council, National Congress of Parents and Teachers, National Education Association, American Automobile Association, National Association of Chiefs of Police, and the U.S. Office of Education. Standard rules have been published by the National Safety Council.

SUGGESTED ACTIVITIES

1. Since students must learn to live with risks by developing appropriate skills, it is the teacher's task to provide opportunities for risk-taking. Look into adventure-challenge activities and assess risk-taking situations suitable for elementary-age pupils. Outdoor education and physical education personnel may be of some assistance.

2. Read what Charles Silberman says about "intolerable" conditions in the classroom (see Selected References). From your experience would you tend to agree or disagree with this Carnegie Foundation writer?

3. Visit several elementary classrooms located in close proximity to a busy airport. Is there evidence that learning is more difficult here than in a quieter environment? Indicate how a study might be arranged in a particular school.

4. Consult the literature of such organizations as the National Safety Council, the National Commission on Safety, and the U.S. Public Health Service, and compare accident statistics for children in the first six grades. Comment on the significance of your findings.

SELECTED REFERENCES

Davis, Charles C. "How to Cope with Stress in the Classroom," *Health Education,* 8:36–37, September/October 1977.

Dithridge, E. H. "Administration of School Health Services," *Nursing Outlook, 14*:50–53, 1966.

Joint Committee on Health Problems in Education of the National Education Association and the American Medical Association, *Healthful School Environment,* Washington: NEA, 1969.

National Commission on Safety Education. *A School Safety Education Program,* (revised): Washington, D.C.: National Education Association.

Mayshark, Cyrus, Shaw, Donald D., and Best, Wallace H. *Administration of School Health Programs.* 2nd ed., Part 3. St. Louis: C. V. Mosby Co., 1977.

Ponder, L. D. and Mayshark, Cyrus. "The Relationship between School Organizational Climate and Selected Teacher Health Status Indicators," *Journal of School Health, 44*:122–125, March 1974.

Rosenthal, Etta M. "Dealing with Emotional Problems," *Instructor, 82*:14, January 1972.

Sellitto, T. J. "There's More to Student Accidents than Offering Insurance Programs," *School Management, 18*:9, 1974.

Silberman, Charles E. *Crisis in the Classroom.* New York: Random House, 1970.

Stone, Donald B., O'Reilly, Lawrence B., and Brown, James D. *Elementary School Health Education.* Chapter 9. Dubuque: William C. Brown Co. Publishers, 1976.

Sugden, John H. "How Effective Are Open Plan Elementary Schools?" *American Schools and Universities, 45*:18–20, January 1973.

Willgoose, Carl E. "Educating for Safety," *Instructor, 81*:62–63, February 1971.

Normal Growth and Deviations from Normal

5

I am a Jew. Hath not a Jew eyes? Hath not a Jew hands, organs, dimensions, senses, affection, passion? . . . fed with the same food, hunt with the same weapons, subject to the same diseases, healed by the same means, warmed and cooled by the same winter and summer, as a Christian is? If you prick us, do we not bleed? If you tickle us, do we not laugh? If you poison us, do we not die? And if you wrong us, shall we not revenge? If we are like you in the rest, we will resemble you in that.

—William Shakespeare
The Merchant of Venice

This quotation is intended to reflect the certain fundamental likenesses of all people. People are never so different that they are not recognizable as human beings, differing only within the limits that human ranges allow. Yet every person differs enough that no two are exactly alike. Tennyson recognized this when he talked of people differing "as heaven and earth." Thus, there is a certain bit of being normal in being different.

THE CONCEPT OF NORMAL

It is sometimes a major task to discriminate between the pupil who acts differently and is really ill, and the one who acts differently but is simply "marching to a different drummer." To ask what is normal at this point is to raise a perplexing question, for in every direction there abounds a multitude of persons and things that are not as they are "supposed to be." A man shuffling along wearing size 13 shoes catches our attention not when he towers well over six feet in height but when he is only five feet tall. His health may be perfectly normal, but his feet are not; they are too long for a man of his height. An appropriate norm table would show this, for a norm is no more than a standard point of reference. It is a kind of average of all extremes of existing characteristics. This may be good or bad, for the norm is in no way an ideal.

A normal characteristic is simply a typical one. It is built around some specific factor or phenomenon and is based solely on generalizations. It considers typical cases and typical behavior and is used for purposes of comparison. If several thousand 12 year old girls have freckles, then freckles are typical. If 1000 12 year old girls, 62 inches tall, generally weigh 90 pounds, then 90 pounds is typical and becomes the norm. We have generalized so that the girls at either extreme, whose weights were part of the several thousand cases, would be below or above normal in weight; they would be labeled "abnormal," "atypical," or "deviant." Yet, there are so many of these deviants in a given sample that they might well represent a large segment of the population. Thus, sociologists, anthropologists, and educators think and speak in terms of individual differences for a very good reason.

To proceed to the question of what is normal health, it must be admitted that it is quite normal to see people with bad teeth, digestive upsets, nearsightedness, baldness, aching feet, advanced obesity, or mental instability. It even seems normal for more than a million people to succumb to heart disease each year, but these items can hardly be accepted as desirable even if they come close to being within the normal range of what might be found in a cross section of the population. It is imperative, therefore, that we do not generalize all health characteristics and behavior and be blind to the distinctions which make each of us an individual. Healthy people are different. Healthy children are different. Sheldon points this out in his monumental work on the study of body build and constitutional behavior.[1] Sheldon's findings have been related to educational practice, and it now seems clear that *if children fail to act as we think they should, it is probably because we have not learned to perceive them as individuals*. Williams illustrates this idea by quoting the Russian novelist Ivan Turgenev.[2] Turgenev pokes fun at scientists and educators by saying that "a man's capable of understanding anything—how the ether vibrates and what's going on in the sun— but how any other man can blow his nose differently from him, that he's incapable of understanding." (See Figure 5–1.)

THE NORMALLY HEALTHY CHILD

Educators usually think of the healthy child as one who is well adjusted to the surroundings, is free from physical defects and organic drains, and demonstrates emotional stability. He or she is not necessarily perfect, but is quite well. There are other children who are almost as well, but they are not quite up to average when it comes to some special function such as heart efficiency or hearing. In this

---

[1]Sheldon, William H. *The Varieties of Human Temperament.* New York: Harper & Brothers, 1942.

[2]Williams, Roger J. *Biochemical Individuality.* New York: John Wiley & Sons, 1957.

respect they are actually atypical or abnormal, but are generally referred to as handicapped. Children with obvious individual differences in body build, physical and mental capacities, behavior, and interests may be completely healthy. But *it will take a teacher who is trained to observe children carefully to be able to select from such a group of individually different children those who deviate too far and appear to need medical or psychiatric help.*

Determining whether a pupil is normally healthy can at times be a most difficult job. Some diseases are carried for a long while and are only slightly noticeable in the early stages. A pupil with a respiratory ailment, for example, may do nothing more serious than cough occasionally for months, thus behaving not too differently from his or her compatriots in the class. Everyday behavior is a complex process and involves an interrelationship of physical, mental, emotional, and social activity. The body operates as a whole; both *psyche* and *soma* are part of the same constitution. A disease or attitude that affects one has a measurable bearing on the other. Thus a malnourished pupil might be irritable and bite his fingernails in class and be mistaken by the teacher for a pupil with an emotional problem. Or a child might have a stomach upset because he or she was unable to recite before the class. This might easily be interpreted to indicate that the child was imagining the pain when in reality it was more likely associated with a defense mechanism resulting in "psychological" or even psychosomatic illness, because the child did not know the lesson and was not prepared to recite before the class.

Figure 5–1. Individual differences. Seventh grade boys of the same age.

THE EXCEPTIONAL CHILD CONCEPT

As far back as 1956, Maslow was saying that no human being is comparable with another.

Therefore his ideals for himself, his path of growth, must also be unique. His goal must arise out of his own nature, and not be chosen by comparison or competition with others.[3]

In recent years an effort has been made to look at children as individuals and to classify them as exceptional when they require special or modified programs of services and instruction in order to make the most of their education. Especially significant in bringing about this thinking has been federal legislation governing the education of the handicapped. Personal and civil rights of the handicapped were guaranteed under Public Law 94–142, The Education of All Handicapped Children Act. By 1980 the curriculum must focus on realistic goals for each learner, according to the law. In addition there must be an "individualized education program" for each handicapped child that supplements instructional activities that are engaged in by all schoolchildren. The objective is to look upon each learner as normal to some extent, and to place him or her in the least restrictive environment.

The variety of exceptional children is extensive. Dunn, in conjunction with the U.S. Office of Education, classifies them into nine areas of exceptionality:[4]

1. *Superior cognitive abilities* (intellectually gifted and creative)
2. *Moderate and severe general learning disabilities* (formerly nonadaptive, noneducable, nontrainable, and severe mental retardation)
3. *Mild general learning disabilities* (formerly adaptive, educable, mental retardation)
4. *Behavioral disabilities* (emotionally disturbed and socially maladjusted)
5. *Oral communication disabilities* (major speech and language problems)
6. *Hearing disabilities* (deaf and partially hearing)
7. *Visual disabilities* (educationally blind and partially sighted)
8. *Neuromotor and other crippling and health disabilities*
9. *Specific learning disabilities* (primarily reading, writing and arithmetic problems)

DEVIATIONS FROM NORMAL HEALTH

Obviously a large number of children do not fit the category of exceptional, yet they vary in health status from time to time. In studying normal health and its many deviations, the beginning

---

[3]Maslow, Abraham. "A Philosophy of Psychology," *Main Currents in Modern Thought,* 13:27–32, 1965.
[4]Dunn, Lloyd M. *Exceptional Children in the Schools: Special Education in Transition,* 2nd ed. New York: Holt, Rinehart and Winston, Inc., 1973, p. 14.

teacher should be familiar with growth and development characteristics of boys and girls. (See Chapter 6.) The extremes of early and late maturation may appear to indicate deviations from normal health when such is not the case. Children do not grow according to a rigid schedule; there is no growth pattern to which every child must conform. One must be aware of the fact that mental and social growth may be retarded due to genuine physical difficulties. Inadequate hearing, for instance, may result in poor speech or a reluctance to speak. And because social growth in children is more abstract than physical growth, it will again be difficult to note behavior deviations from normal.

One can learn the characteristics of optimum child health and can also become familiar with the common deviations. Since most people are more familiar with the marks of good health, this chapter will call attention chiefly to the deviations.[5]

Teachers may see what is often missed by parents who are too close to their children to notice defects, and what would be of interest to physicians and nurses if they had access to the child on a daily basis. They may be puzzled if a hitherto cooperative child becomes inattentive, or the otherwise bright child is unusually slow in learning to read, or the ordinarily happy and enthusiastic youngster becomes extremely docile. They may wonder about pimples around the mouth, swollen glands in the neck, low shoulders, underweight and malnutrition, or excessive sniffling or coughing. It is when teachers *are* this much concerned with what they have seen that pupils may be helped early and at a time when the greatest good can be accomplished in remedying the situation. In this connection, the excellent 32-page booklet, *Looking For Health,* distributed free to teachers by the Metropolitan Life Insurance Company, sets up classroom conditions that make it easy for the alert teacher to observe children.

What are the signs and characteristics of general poor health, specific physical and mental defects, and conditions which can be readily detected in day-to-day contact with boys and girls? Following are some that relate to long-standing defects, chronic illness, neurological disturbances, improper nutrition, and poor health practices.

Important Points for Observation

Height and Weight

Numerous misconceptions exist regarding weight changes and health status. Maturation and growth are influential variables. Bulk weight is not in itself a sign of health. A pupil of normal height and weight may be suffering from some hidden abnormality or disease.

---

[5]The treatment of the topic will be brief, for no attempt is made here to embrace the area of health abnormalities of schoolchildren. Such a topic is broad enough to fill a book. It is referred to here only because observing pupil deviations is a part of the total school health program.

[6]Copies available on request from Metropolitan Life Insurance Company, Health and Welfare Divisions, 1 Madison Ave., New York, N.Y., 10010.

Probably less than 4 per cent of obese or thin children have any glandular disturbances. White and Negro pupils generally are larger than Mexican and Japanese students. Extremes of body build, although somewhat related to nutrition and activity, are quite apt to reflect constitutional patterns passed along from parents or families. The better norm tables allow for individual variations in structure.

Evidence of the wide variation of weight for age was clearly demonstrated by Falkner for white North American children in an extensive study of physical growth. At age 10, for example, boys varied in height (between the 5th and 95th percentiles) by as much as 9 inches and in weight by as much as 40 pounds. Girls at age 10 varied 6.5 inches in height and 47 pounds in weight.[7]

Since there is a relationship between the quality of growth and the rate of learning, it is appropriate to weigh and measure boys and girls. Moreover, this is a first-class health instruction activity.

Children should be weighed wearing as little clothing as practicable and without shoes. Although the frequency of measurement varies in different schools, the most effective screening combines weighing with height measurements two or three times a year. This procedure screens out the approximately 10 per cent of elementary school children who fail to gain weight for three successive months between September and May. Failure to realize a weight gain in three to four months is nearly always a sign that something is wrong, because of either poor health practices, disease, or conditions that call for medical examination.

A simple record for each child is suitable for classroom use. Individual growth records are available for each pupil; the Meredith Tables are useful. (See Chapter 3.) So is the Wetzel Grid for revealing trends in growth.[8]

Deviations in Appearance and Behavior

Failure to gain in height and weight over a three to six month period

Excessive overweight

Small and underweight for age

Fluctuating weight changes

Skin

The skin shows a great deal to the observing teacher. Pale pupils who appear flushed, and rosy-cheeked pupils who appear pale are usually not up to par. Skin eruptions such as impetigo are very contagious. A number of communicable childhood diseases begin with a flushed or spotted skin. Vesicles appear in chickenpox, red rash in measles, and pallor in malnutrition. Skin deviations are often accompanied by fever, chills, headache, and loss of appetite.

From the pupil's viewpoint skin eruptions are serious in terms of personal appearance; social health seems more important than physical health.

---

[7]See report, together with growth tables, in *Obesity and Health*. Washington, D.C.: U.S. Public Health Service, 1966, p. 11.

[8]The Wetzel Grid is published by National Education Association Service Inc., 1200 W. Third Street, Cleveland, Ohio.

Deviations in Appearance and Behavior
Pale or sallow
Flushed appearance
Eczematous condition with rashes, scales and crusts
Persistent sores
Pimples
Acne on face
Boils, warts
Cuts, scratches, bruises, burns
Blueness or pallor of lips
Common skin disease such as ringworm, impetigo, scabies ("itch"), and pinkeye
Sensitivity to several substances; allergy
Easily bruised
Itching or burning skin (with frequent scratching)
Fever
Nits (lice eggs) on hair

Teeth and Mouth

The pupil with a foul odor on the breath day after day probably has a mouth, tooth, nose, or alimentary disorder. Decayed teeth and diseased tonsils are often accompanied by enlarged glands. Total body infection, overall fatigue, and poor appetite may be caused by grossly decayed teeth. Diseased teeth and tonsils set the stage for sore throats, inner ear disturbances, speech disorders, and the more serious viral and bacterial infections. Dental defects occur among children about six times as rapidly as the rate at which they are being corrected.

Deviations in Appearance and Behavior
Bad breath
Cavities in teeth
Excessive tartar at necks of teeth
Toothache
Malocclusion and bad bite
Irregular spacing of teeth
Protruding and broken teeth
Speech difficulty
Inflamed or bleeding gums
Sores in mouth
Cracked lips, especially in corners of mouth

Neck

Swollen lymph glands are visible as lumps on the side of the neck and below the ears. They are readily seen in mumps and other systemic infections. Glands appearing as small lumps may be large when examined by touch. Swollen and tender glands demand immediate attention.

Enlargement of the thyroid gland is usually accompanied by rapid heart rate, more than normal sweating, and irritability and distractibility in the classroom.

Deviations in Appearance and Behavior
Enlarged lymph glands
Enlarged thyroid glands on either side of windpipe
Position of neck out of alignment with spine

Hair and Scalp

Dirty children with dirty underclothes often have unclean hair
and scalp. The white eggs (nits) of head lice (pediculi) cling to hair
while female gray-backs move about. Pubic lice may invade the
pubic hairs in the groin area and cause much scratching. Infections
with microorganisms may follow lice and ringworm; both are highly
communicable.

Brittle hair and dry scalp often accompany cases of malnutrition.
Pride in oneself begins with clean, combed hair.

Deviations in Appearance and Behavior
Uncombed, uncontrolled hair
Dirty, dry scalp
Signs of vermin and ringworm
Brittle, stringy, and lusterless hair
Small bald spots
Crusty sores on scalp
Excessive dandruff
Frequent head scratching

Upper Respiratory Tract (Nose, Throat, Sinuses)

Nasal and throat abnormalities affect the quality of the voice.
Speech improvement comes about when the nasal passage is clear
and mouth breathing ceases.

Sinuses and the middle ear may be acutely infected in colds,
measles, scarlet fever, diphtheria, influenza, typhoid, and infected
teeth. Diseased tonsils and adenoid tissue are deleterious to the
whole upper respiratory tract.

Enlarged mucous membranes (hypersecretion) are present with
severe head colds and hay fever. Mucous membranes are continuous
within eyes, nose, mouth, throat, inner ears, bronchial tubes, and
lungs.

Deviations in Appearance and Behavior
Speech thick or muffled
Mouth breathing
Frequent sore throats
Persistent nasal discharge
Excessive colds
Frequent school absences
Difficulty in swallowing
Sore or scratchy throat
Discharge from ears
Frequent sniffling and coughing
Face or forehead pain (sinusitis)
Fever and bad breath
Sudden sneezing spells associated with allergies

Nutrition

Good nutritional status means much in terms of appearance, vigor, and enthusiasm for school activities. The classroom teacher is more effective here than any other person; behavior is so general that one must notice several of the accompanying signs before suspecting malnutrition.

Deviations in Appearance and Behavior
General fatigue; tires easily
Poor, sloppy postural attitude; postural defects
Frequent and prolonged infections
Restlessness and irritability
Fingernail biting
Difficulty going to sleep
Restlessness during sleep
Lack of ambition
Dark circles or puffiness under eyes
Flabby musculature; possible muscle and joint pain
Poor teeth
Lack of appetite
Dry, scaly scalp, hair, and skin
History of sore mouth, tongue, or gums
Abnormally low tolerance of light

Posture and Body Mechanics

Posture is functional and involves total body movement, especially standing and sitting, and attitude and gait in walking.

Functional difficulties due to weak musculature, uneven length of the legs, or one's temporary mental attitude may be corrected by exercises and activities assigned by the physician and physical educator and reinforced by the encouraging words of the classroom teacher. Structural defects (immobile bumps or enlarged joints) need special medical attention.

Even minor postural defects need to be discovered and remedied early in order to obtain the greatest body efficiency in later years.

Many times postural abnormalities are indicative of poor nutrition, organic strains, hidden disease, low physical fitness, sedentary living, chronic fatigue, hearing defects, emotional disturbance, and asthma.

Other things being equal, the way the schoolchild feels at any one moment is often reflected in the posture.

Deviations in Appearance and Behavior
Flabby musculature
Chronic fatigue
Round shoulders (kyphosis)
Head forward
One shoulder lower than the other
Protruding shoulder blades (winged scapulae)
Pigeon or funnel chest (rickets)
Lateral curvature of spine (scoliosis)

Unequal height of hips
Irregular gait in walking
Arches of feet are flat
Feet toe-out too far in standing and walking
Tendon above heel bone is bowed inward when standing
Heels of shoes wear down on inside borders
Pain in joints of body
Pain in bones of foot

Eyes

The list of deviations is rich in items that the classroom teacher can observe easily, especially in terms of reading difficulties. Some 80 per cent of the work a child does in elementary school is built around visual acuity within arm's reach; it is most important that visual difficulties be corrected as early in the grades as possible.

Seeing is a process of both optics and brain development. Young children are normally far-sighted and see large objects, large print, and pictures quite well. In most schools students are screened for difficulties involving visual accommodation. Three fourths of all study activities in the elementary school require reading ability. Promotion from first to second grade is often based on reading ability. Yet four out of five retarded readers have normal intelligence. The teacher may notice that the retarded reader often achieves considerable success in those activities where reading skills are not of primary importance.

School surveys show that less than half the children who need glasses actually have them. School follow-up programs need more attention and control.

Early and repeated examinations are important. Good lighting, frequent rest periods, and the avoidance of prolonged sewing, drawing, painting, or reading by primary grade pupils are recommended.

Instruction should be given in how to view television and how to protect eyesight in the home and community. Some 20 to 25 per cent of all schoolchildren have eye defects.

Deviations in Appearance and Behavior
Complaints of dizziness, headache, nausea
Crusts on lids among lashes
Red rims on lids
Watery eyes; styes
Swollen eyelids
Reading difficulties:
    Holds book far away from face when reading
    Holds body tense or thrusts head forward at distant objects
    Holds face close to page when reading
    Inattentive in wall chart, blackboard, or map lesson
    Reads for only brief periods without stopping
    Screws up face when reading or looking at distant objects
    Shuts or covers one eye when reading
    Tilts head to one side when reading
    Tends to look cross-eyed when reading

Tends to make frequent changes in distance at which book is held

Confusion in reading and spelling o and a; e and c; n and c; h, n and r; f and t

Apparently guesses from quick recognition of parts of the word in easy reading material

Rubs eyes frequently

Poor alignment in writing

Reversal tendencies in reading

Atempts to brush away a blur

Irritation over work or some emotional display

Strabismus or "squint"

Ear

Children with hearing loss in the classroom account for a sizable proportion of all people with hearing loss. Two children in every classroom have a hearing problem. Early detection through screening tests permits the parent to obtain treatment reasonably quickly for the child. Pure tone audiometer testing permits quick sweep checks up to the 8000 frequency level. Some pupils fail the 4000 to 8000 high range, others fail the range below 500; but it is important for them to hear in the middle range. With middle range loss the child is experiencing much difficulty. Also, 35 per cent of the failures are in both ears.

Hearing loss varies, indicating a need for constant teacher observation and annual screening tests.

Deviations in Appearance and Behavior

Discharge or odor from ears

Earache

Failure to answer and misunderstandings

Habit of saying "what?"

Turning head to one side when spoken to

Facial expressions indicating a lack of awareness of all that is going on

Speaking too softly, too loudly, or with an unusual voice quality

Difficulty in locating the source of sound

Unusual dependence on visual cues

Heart

Children with heart defects total about 1 per cent of the school-age population. Most of these children can take part in the normal classroom program. With some degree of restriction, most of these pupils may engage in modified or adapted physical education activities.

Rheumatic fever is declining in incidence and severity, but there are still many children whose heart valves are impaired due to this disease or other chronic infections such as scarlet fever, pneumonia, *Streptococcus* sore throat, measles, mumps, and tonsillitis.

Heart disease in children is prevented by observing and obtaining medical attention for prolonged infections (sore throats or persistent fatigue) and by making sure the child engages in stimulating physical activity, eats nutritious foods, participates in recreation, and obtains adequate sleep.

Deviations in Appearance and Behavior
Fainting and dizzy spells
Rapid heart beat
Irregular pulse
Frequent complaints of pain in joints, arms, legs
Repeated nose bleeds
Clubbed fingers
Shortness of breath and sudden flushing of the face on exertion
Early fatigue
Failure to gain weight
Blueness of lips (cyanosis)

Social-Emotional Adjustment

All children need from the teacher a degree of love, warmth, praise, and consistency. They need gentle and firm guidance and someone interested in their welfare. When this occurs the child becomes more secure, is more tolerant and creative, possesses an outgoing attitude toward others, profits from mistakes as well as successes, and, above all else, is a happy pupil equipped to live life with zest, enthusiasm, and hope.

The signs indicating deviations from normal social-emotional behavior are all about. To the observing teacher they are as evident as pimples on the face, and, like many physical ailments, they are best controlled or remedied through early detection and treatment.

Deviations in Appearance and Behavior
Infantile speech
Foul language; very low, very high, or very loud voice
Unestablished toilet habits
Restlessness, nail-biting, stammering, or lip-sucking not due to any discoverable physical cause
Frequent accidents or near-accidents
Over-timidity; seclusiveness, withdrawal, shyness, isolation from the group
Over-aggressiveness; constant quarreling with others
Suspicion and fearfulness; expectation of failure
Excessive day dreaming; inattentiveness not due to any discoverable physical cause
Extreme sensitiveness to criticism; feelings hurt easily; cries easily
Failure to advance in school work at a normal rate in spite of adequate physical health and satisfactory intellectual capacity. Or gradual deterioration or sudden drop in educational achievement; disorderly and careless work
Extreme docility or anxiety to please
Excessive boasting, showing off, attracting undue attention
Resistance to authority, constant complaints of being discriminated against or "picked on"

A GUIDE TO CHILDHOOD DISEASES

Disease	Recognition	Prevention	Incubation	Control	General
Common Cold	Sniffles, sneezing. Feels poorly. Coughing common.	General good health helps.	1–2 days.	Isolate fresh cases for 3 days. Encourage parents to keep child home. Teach proper use of tissues.	Most frequent reason for absenteeism. Potentially dangerous because of ear, lung, throat complications.
Influenza	Cold symptoms, but child is sick, feverish, and weak.	Vaccine, particularly effective, protection only 6–12 months.	1–3 days.	Isolate fresh cases for 5 days from onset.	More serious, "grippy" cold with high fever. Occurs sporadically each winter.
Chickenpox (varicella)	Small spots and blisters on body and at hairline. Often fever. Itching.	None.	12–21 days; usually 13–17 days.	Isolate and exclude for 6 days after rash.	Common, minor illness, highly contagious among susceptibles.
Diphtheria	Sore throat with white patches; fever.	Effective with 3 doses of toxoid. Boosters every 3 to 5 years.	2–5 days.	Isolate in hospital. May not return until Health Department approves. Classmates and other close contacts receive immunization.	Very dangerous disease—now almost eradicated through mass immunization.
German Measles (rubella)	Mildly ill, if at all. Pinkish spots on body, arms, *not* on face.	None, for disease.	14–21 days; usually 18 days.	Exclude case 3 days from appearance of rash.	A common, highly contagious but mild disease.
Measles (rubeola)	Cough, red eyes, fever, followed by blotchy rash on face and body.	Measles vaccine.	10 days to first symptoms. 14 days to rash.	Exclude for 7 days following appearance of rash.	A common, highly contagious acute illness. Most common complications: ear infection, pneumonia.
Mumps (infectious parotitis)	Swelling of cheeks or 1 or more salivary glands; fever.	None effective.	12–26 days; usually 18 days.	Exclude until swelling disappears, or 1 week from onset.	A relatively common and usually mild disease in children, not very contagious.

A GUIDE TO CHILDHOOD DISEASES (Continued)

Disease	Recognition	Prevention	Incubation	Control	General
Streptococcal Infections Including Scarlet Fever	Sore throat with fever. Hurts to swallow. Diffuse red rash with tiny spots in scarlet fever.	Antibiotics given promptly.	2–5 days.	Exclude according to pre-arranged school plan. Observe classmates for 1 week.	A common disease which can be complicated by rheumatic fever, heart disease, or nephritis. "Scarlatina" is the same disease.
Whooping Cough	Characteristic cough, with choking, redness of face, and "whoop" on drawing breath.	Vaccine usually given with diphtheria and tetanus to infants. Not desirable for older children.	7–10 days.	Exclude for 3 weeks after onset of typical cough.	An increasingly rare disease, especially among pre-school children.
Athlete's Foot	Peeling, cracking, redness, and occasionally oozing between toes or on sole of foot.	Scrupulous foot hygiene. Rigorous cleaning of locker and shower rooms.	10–14 days.	Exclude from physical education, locker and shower rooms. Check custodial job.	Mild, very common fungus infection of feet, especially feet which perspire easily; occurs wherever people go barefoot frequently.
Impetigo	Moist patches on skin around mouth, on hands with brown yellow crusts.	Good hygiene.	2–5 days.	Exclude until treatment is started and lesions are dry.	Common bacterial infection of skin, mostly in younger children with poor health practices.
Lice	"Nits" seen; itching scalp, "mobile dandruff."	Good hygiene.	1–2 days.	Exclude until treated. Check classmates' heads at discovery and 2 weeks later.	Parasitic infestations of hair, boys and girls, directly related to inadequate brushing and washing.
Ringworm of Scalp	Patchy baldness with stubble left.	Good hygiene.	10–14 days	Exclude until treatment started. Must wear cap and not take physical education.	Hard-to-clear-up fungus infection of scalp. Rare after puberty.

Table continued on the following page

A GUIDE TO CHILDHOOD DISEASES (Continued)

Disease	Recognition	Prevention	Incubation	Control	General
Pinworms	Itching behind, crankiness, vague stomach pains.	Good hygiene.	4–8 days.	No exclusion necessary, little chance of spread in school. Enforce hand washing.	A common, mild, worm infection, with more unrecognized cases than known.
"Pinkeye" (conjunctivitis)	Reddened, irritated, weepy eyes. Often whitish discharge with sticky eyelids.	None.	1–3 days.	Exclude only in grades K–3. Observe classmates 1 week.	May accompany cold; more often a mild viral infection.
Poliomyelitis (infantile paralysis)	Headache, stiff neck, fever.	Oral vaccine. Consult physician.	7–21 days; usually 12 days.	Exclude 2 weeks. Observe classmates and give booster vaccinations.	A potentially crippling disease coming in about 7 year waves.
Tuberculosis	By tuberculin test and x-ray.	Early detection.	6–8 weeks; occasionally 1 month.	Routine mass testing. Test and x-ray of classmates.	Usually very mild and often unrecognized in school age children. Source is an adult.
Meningitis	Fever, violent headache, stiff neck.	None available. Contacts can be protected by drugs.	Variable, but seldom over 10 days.	Isolate in hospital. If meningococcal exclude from family until treatment starts.	A group of diseases, caused by many agents —some serious, others not.
Tetanus (lockjaw)	Stiffness of face muscles, neck and back.	Mass immunization. Booster doses whenever child is cut or wounded.	4–21 days.	Booster dose for child with dirty cuts or wounds.	Poison from germ in dirty wounds affects nervous system; highly fatal. Not contagious.
Infectious Mononucleosis	Persistent fatigue, low grade fever, sore throat.	None known.	4–14 days.	Exclude from school until fever is gone.	A not very contagious virus disease that may take months to get over.
Infectious Hepatitis	Jaundice, fever, vomiting.	Clean water and food. Can be prevented in contacts by gammaglobulin.	10–60 days; usually 25 days.	Exclude 2 weeks or until well.	A viral disease affecting the liver—long recovery period needed.
Cat-scratch Fever	Sore at site of scratch, with swollen glands, accompanied by fever.	Avoid cat scratches.	2–8 days.	Exclude until child feels well.	Viral disease from cats. Mild. Not contagious.

120

Poor sportsmanship, some unwillingness to engage in group activities which might result in losing face; playing unfairly or cheating in group games; suffers from being disliked by classmates

Learning Disabilities

Although health services personnel and the learning disabilities specialist can advise and guide the teacher, referring to known cases in this area, much of the early detection, remediation, and feedback is accomplished by the teacher. Early classroom detection is significant—in the nursery school, kindergarten, and first grade, before formal learning tasks have been assigned. Perceptual-motor difficulties and motor development problems may occur anywhere in the school. If there is no specialist or clinic available, the teacher will probably have to work with the school psychologist and a reading specialist.

Deviations in Appearance and Behavior
Short attention span
Hyperactivity
Emotional outbursts
Erratic body control
Impulsivity
Distractibility
Poor eye-hand coordination
Hearing and speech disorders
Immaturity
One-sided physical development
Sequencing problems
Language difficulties

Drug Abuse

To the observing teacher of intermediate level and middle-school children there is much to notice in the way of schoolwide behavior that helps in the identification of the drug abuser. Any one of the deviations might be misleading, but when several of these appear in one pupil there is good reason to look more closely.

Deviations in Appearance and Behavior
Abrupt changes in school attendance, quality of work, and work output
Withdrawal from responsibility
General changes in overall attitude

The Glue-Sniffer (or User of Other Vapor-Producing Solvents)
Odor of substance on breath and clothes
Excess nasal secretions; watering of eyes
Poor muscular control
Drowsiness or unconsciousness
Plastic or paper bags or rags containing dry plastic cement or other solvent found at home or in locker at school

The Depressant Abuser (Barbiturates, Tranquilizers, "Downs")

Symptoms of alcohol intoxication with one important exception: no odor of alcohol on breath

Staggering or stumbling

Falling asleep unexplainably

Drowsiness; may appear disoriented

Lack of interest in school and family activities

The Stimulant Abuser (Amphetamines, Cocaine, "Speed," "Bennies," "Ups")

Pupils may be dilated (when large amounts have been taken)

Mouth and nose dry; bad breath; user licks lips frequently

Goes long periods without eating or sleeping

Excess activity; user is irritable, argumentative, nervous; has difficulty sitting still

The Marijuana Abuser

In the early stages of intoxication, may appear animated with rapid, loud talking and bursts of laughter

In the later stages, may be sleepy or stuporous

Pupils usually are dilated

Odor (similar to burnt rope) on clothing or breath

Remnants of marijuana, either loose or in partially smoked "joints," in clothing or possessions

Usually user in a group, at least in early habit of smoking

Note: unless under the influence of the drug at the time of observation marijuana users are difficult to recognize; infrequent users may not show any of the general symptoms of drug abusers.

Childhood Cancer

Since cancer kills more school-age children than any other disease (only accidents kill more), the teacher should be alert to symptoms, increasing the possibility of early detection and increased rate of cure. Children with leukemia are most commonly observed with signs relating to blood cell dysfunction. Many are anemic, tire easily, and are irritable, and most always appear pale. Others will have recurrent bacterial infections which are slow to respond to therapy. Still others bruise easily and may suffer prolonged bleeding from a school or home injury.

SUGGESTED ACTIVITIES

1. Starling points out that the malignant process of leukemia could be aggressively treated if only people working with children would be more alert to signs (see Selected References). See if you can determine how practical this is by talking with some teachers and others who have several contacts a day with schoolchildren.

2. Visit a large elementary school and ask the school nurse how many cases there are of serious allergies, heart defects, epilepsy, diabetes, and orthopedic defects. Having determined this, find out how many of these children have restricted programs and to what extent. How do you feel about the adequacies of restricted programs?

3. Arrange for several individuals to solicit from several different school departments copies of health manuals or written instructions to teachers relative to health observations and practices in the school system.

QUESTIONS FOR DISCUSSION

1. What are your comments on the sentence in this chapter which included the following: *If children fail to act as we think they should, it is probably because we have not learned to perceive them as individuals.*

2. From your reading and experience, where does the detection and referral program fail?

3. Samuel Johnson wrote that one should practice ". . . observation with extensive view." He wanted the observer to see many things—even extremes. How might this apply to the teacher in the classroom?

4. Consider the signs of good social-emotional behavior. What are several ways these signs may be developed within the limits of classroom activity? Playground activity?

5. What do you think of the view that practically every human being is a deviate in some respect? Support your answer with remarks relative to elementary-age children.

SELECTED REFERENCES

Bogle, Marion W. "Relationship between Deviant Behavior and Reading Disability," *Journal of School Health, 43*:312–315, May 1973.
Dodge, Philip R. "Neurological Disorders of School-Age Children," *Journal of School Health, 7*:238–243, June 1976.
Dunn, Lloyd M. (ed.) *Exceptional Children in the Schools,* 2d ed. New York: Holt, Rinehart and Winston, Inc., 1973, Chapter 1.
Greenberg, Jerrold S. "Responding to the Causes of Unhealthy Behavior," *Health Education, 7*:32–33, May/June 1976.
───────────. *Student-Centered Health Instruction: A Humanistic Approach.* Boston: Addison-Wesley Publishing Co., 1978, Chapter 1.
McGovern, John P. "Chronic Respiratory Diseases of School-Age Children," *Journal of School Health, 46*:344–348, June 1976.
Nolte, Ann. "The Relevance of Abraham Maslow's Work to Health Education," *Health Education, 7*:25–28, May/June 1976.
Read, Donald A. and Greene, Walter H. *Creative Teaching in Health.* 2d ed. New York: Macmillan Publishing Co., 1975, Chapter 2.
Ritter, Alice M. "Using a Teacher's Health Observation Form to Evaluate School Child Health," *Journal of School Health, 46*:235–238, April 1976.
Schreiber, Clare Adel. "What Is a Healthy Preschool Child?" *Health Education, 7*:10–11, May/June 1976.
Starling, Kenneth A. and Shepherd, Dell A. "Symptoms and Signs of Cancer in the School-Age Child," *Journal of School Health, 47*:144–146, March 1977.
Willgoose, Carl E. "Educational Implications of Constitutional Psychology," *Education, 73*:225–228, December 1952.

The Health
Instruction Program

6

Any teacher who responds to love and is capable of giving love, who is capable of genuine compassion, who finds human relationships challenging and rewarding, who has limitless energy and exquisite sensitivity to human needs—plus the constitution of a professional wrestler—is probably a superman. If so, then let us go about cultivating supermen. There is something in the nature of teaching—especially in today's world—that represents a genuine challenge.

—Norman Cousins[1]

The classroom teacher carries on most of the health instruction in the elementary school. Such instruction is not done haphazardly; rather, it is a planned program in which the teacher has mastered still another subject area. Perhaps he or she is indeed what Cousins would call a "superman." Certainly, being familiar with the complexities of health problems and with how to teach this subject effectively calls for ability. Some help is provided in a number of school systems by an increasing number of coordinating or supervisory personnel who have specialized training in health education.

THE NATURE OF HEALTH INSTRUCTION

Instructional programs are geared to the principles of learning and carried on with individual pupil differences in mind. These programs are good chiefly because of good teachers. When classroom teachers understand the purposes of health instruction, the program becomes a significant part of the total school health effort.

The broad topic of health instruction in the elementary grades is related to a large number of factors which include program objectives, pupil needs, pupil interests, capacities, and other psychological considerations. Also included are teacher qualifications, educational methods, material sources and aids, and evaluation. Thus, instruction becomes a complicated topic, one that must be approached with patience and understanding.

---

[1]From "Norman Cousins Discusses the Human Concept," *Instructor,* 80:58, October 1970.

The general objectives of the health instruction program are about the same for all the elementary grades. But the specific objectives for the primary area will differ from those for the intermediate area. Essentially, this difference is due to the varying capacities and needs associated wtih chronological age and growth.

Health education may be defined as the organization of learning experiences directed toward the development of favorable health knowledge, attitudes, and practices. It is an applied science and an academic field. Facts, principles, and concepts constitute its body of knowledge. It is derived from physiology, sociology, psychology, and the behavioral sciences.[2]

Although the fundamental purpose of instruction is to impart knowledge, there should always be a greater emphasis on the formation of desirable practices and attitudes resulting from instruction. Knowledge of mere facts and mechanical skills is of doubtful long-term value; no knowledge is complete until it is understood enough to be applied.

The desired outcome of health instruction is a change in the behavior of the pupils. This is revealed through daily practices of school and community living, the expression of positive health attitudes, and the grasp of a body of scientific knowledge which provides a basis for intelligent self-direction. To accomplish these goals is quite a difficult task. It is relatively easy to impart knowledge in the classroom. Children, for example, will readily learn the names of the vitamins or the rules of bicycle safety without having this knowledge affect their pattern of living in any way. Moreover, it is even conceivable that the same children may have no particular feeling or attitude toward the previously discussed vitamins or bicycle riding. In such a case the knowledge has been "book knowledge" or "test knowledge." It has not been understood and acted upon.

There are other elements affecting the quality of health instruction that are more organizational than instructional in nature, such as the time element that frequently governs the quality of the instruction. Morton Fine studied a large sample of New York City elementary school teachers in order to discover factors limiting their effectiveness in providing health instruction. Although a sizable number of teachers needed supervisory help and current teaching materials, the highest-ranking limitation was the pressure to produce results in other curriculum areas, thus limiting the time and energy available to provide health instruction.[3] Obviously, more coordinated direction is needed in this area.

CRISIS-ORIENTED HEALTH EDUCATION

When pressure builds in a community, as it so often does, to have the schools "do something" about sex, smoking, drugs, and

---

[2]See the excellent booklet *What Is Health Education?*, distributed by the American Medical Association, 535 North Dearborn St., Chicago, Illinois 60610.

[3]Fine, Morton. *Health Instruction Practices and Problems of Selected New York City Elementary School Teachers,* doctoral dissertation. Teachers College, Columbia University, 1974.

alcohol, the hastily thrown together one-week unit or one-lecture type of activity appears. Frequently it covers only one problem identified this year and forgotten the next. This overemphasis of a health problem resulting in the omission of discussions of a number of other pertinent health problems is inexcusable. To be effective, health instruction cannot be established on the basis of crash programs. This was the position taken by the School Health Division of the American Association for Health, Physical Education, and Recreation in 1970 and given further support five years later by the National Congress of Parents and Teachers. These organizations called for a comprehensive school health program which avoids "band wagon" approaches and piece-meal efforts relative to health topics.

A unified approach to health teaching where there is a planned program throughout the school years is necessary for the formation of positive attitudes and the creation of a healthy lifestyle—the mark of an educated person. Moreover, there is reason to believe that crisis-oriented health programs do not produce immediate results such as a reduction in smoking or drug abuse. Behavioral changes in complex socio-psychological areas are seldom accomplished right away; they evolve over a period of time and are influenced by an improved value system.

SCHOOL-COMMUNITY INTERACTION

If you believe as I do, that schools reflect society and that schools can be no better and no worse than the society they reflect, then you may be skeptical as I am, of any educational program that offers to change the schools without first changing society. . . . Schools are part of society, and society's ulcerations—massive urban hemorrhaging in crime, poverty, population, over-arching permissiveness, and the disnesting of the family—overflow by their nature into the educational system. To separate the problems of the schools from the problems of the city is to engage in sloppy romanticism.[4]

There is more truth in the above lines than in a good deal of the educational theorizing that is so often done today. There is simply no way to *really* make schools accountable—for the health of the children or for anything else—without some soul-searching by the local citizenry designed to find ways of helping the educators. In short, effective school health education is a two-way street between the school personnel and the townfolk. In numerous towns and cities such cooperation exists and there results a warm feeling about what the schools are trying to accomplish. Local groups and individual citizens volunteer their special skills and knowledge so that teachers seeking resource personnel to make their classes more lively know where to go for assistance.

In Rockland, Massachusetts, for example, parents, clergy, law enforcement officials, educators, and health specialists were asked if they would take the bold steps necessary to meet the varied health needs of children. Would they support community planning as the

---

[4]Dan Pinck in "Education Backdate . . ." *Saturday Review,* October 14, 1972.

best alternative available to the problems of illness? The response was enthusiastically positive. A community health council was formed that proceeded to help the schools by conducting open discussion groups, preparing lists of community sources of health information, establishing health education materials sections in the town libraries, arranging workshops for teachers and others of the "father-son" and "mother-daughter" type, investigating youth problems in the community, recommending possible additions to the school curricula, arranging for qualified speakers to lecture on pertinent health topics, and many more similar activities.

Advancing school health education programs by placing them squarely in the community health complex is producing positive results. By involving leaders from the medical, dental, and nursing societies and the voluntary agencies, it has been possible to upgrade instruction in a number of ways. Mayshark, Shaw, and Best illustrate this by referring to the area of mental health:

> The increasing concern for violence, suicide, drugs, and other abusive substances among the school population requires that schools work closely with health, justice, and other authorities to manage community issues that appear symptomatically in the schools, disrupting the educational process. The community mental health centers, half-way houses, and "teenscene" self-organizing programs have been impressive innovations. . . . schools and their communities have sought new methods of reaching those in distress. One approach has been the hotline—a telephone intervention system.[5]

Today, the realistic teacher views health instruction as a *comprehensive effort* that devotes a sizable amount of time to solving health inadequacies through channels outside the classroom. Crase and Hamrick point out that "we must develop more political influence; we must utilize political strategies for the purpose of initiating changes that will improve the quality of life for all; and we must utilize more fully the mass media as a vehicle for dissemination."[6] This is reinforced by Hochbaum in his long-time efforts to get health educators to see beyond the school building and other "ivory towers" and to enter a variety of community arenas so that they may ultimately address themselves to "*all* the factors, *all* the forces, and *all* the conditions that determine people's actions."[7]

THE ESSENCE OF UNDERSTANDING

The term "understanding" is both a psychological process and an educational outcome. To possess it is to have more than a knowledge of particulars. A pupil does not begin to understand until he or she is able to react to factual information by moving, feeling, or thinking intelligently with respect to a given situation. Activity is the key word—the kind of activity discussed at length by educational

---

[5]Mayshark, Cyrus, Shaw, Donald D., and Best, Wallace H. *Administration of School Health Programs,* 2nd ed., St. Louis: C. V. Mosby Co., 1977, p. 306.

[6]Crase, Darrell and Hamrick, Michael H. "Health Education: A Reexamination of Purpose," *Journal of School Health,* 47:470–474, October 1977.

[7]Hochbaum, G. M. "At the Threshold of a New Era," *Health Education,* 7:2–4, January 1976.

philosophers of the John Dewey era, in which "pupils learn by doing" was a predominant theory. The more activity engaged in and the more senses stimulated, the greater will be the retention and recall of information to be learned.

In recent years it has been emphasized that the way to successful instruction and eventual understanding is to take heed of the following:

1. How a child perceives an item is significant. There must be a discovery of meaning in a process that must be a highly personal one. To structure personal experiences in a curriculum is difficult, for the schools are part of the society that has made a fetish of the elements of objectivity—facts, figures, and phenomena.

2. Life in school must be stimulating and rewarding. In the early school years it is more important that pupils develop a liking for learning and for the school environment than that specific subject matter be remembered.

3. Relationships and principles are more important than scattered and rote information. In perceiving what they are learning, children may respond more to specific questions involving personal discovery than to the traditional questions so frequently used to initiate a unit of work. In short, it is not uncommon to ask children the wrong questions.

4. Although verbalization has weaknesses, most understandings should be verbalized.

   Symbols such as words, numbers, or formulas are examples of verbalized understandings. In all areas of instruction they have to be used sooner or later. "Vitamin A" is symbolic of a body of information, but it is meaningless unless it is associated with the realities for which it stands. In health education there may be many empty verbalizations that are recited parrotlike by children in dozens of classrooms around the country. Children are taught too often by rote learning. They sing "My country *tears* of thee" and recite that "the circulatory system is composed of arteries, veins, and *artilleries.*" Why does this happen? It seems that there is too much emphasis on isolated items rather than upon wholes and relationships. Also, there is at times in all classrooms the tendency to make instruction an artificial item by divorcing it from the ordinary activities of life.

5. The student's understanding is inferred from observing what boys and girls say and do with respect to their needs. The child who fails to register any particular attitude is sometimes as much in need of help as the child who takes on a negative attitude.

FACTORS THAT DETERMINE WHAT TO TEACH

Everything cannot be brought to the attention of schoolchildren. There simply is not enough time. How then does one determine what to teach? Where does a teacher begin?

Determining Pupil Needs in General

What children need to receive from the elementary school is pretty much what society wants children to have. Since the child grows up in a particular culture, the culture molds him and influences the nature of his or her needs.

To determine what to teach, Ragan and Shepherd studied the needs of children and set up seven categories of needs:
1. Biological needs
2. Achieving status in changing social groups
3. Growing gradually from dependence to independence
4. Security and satisfaction
5. Getting and giving affection
6. Developing appropriate communication skills
7. Learning to face reality.[8]

Whatever phase of health is taught, it must be done in the light of these needs, for these are bona fide requirements that children have—even if they are not aware of them. The interrelationship of these needs is impressive.

Determining Pupil Health Needs

Prior to setting up the health curriculum, it is advantageous to ascertain the child's characteristics, the health needs, and interests for a certain age. Children vary in constitution, growth and development, health status, and background of experience. Some have health problems that others know relatively little about. If, however, there are enough children with a particular health problem, then

---

[8]Ragan, William B. and Shepherd, Gene D. *Modern Elementary Curriculum,* 4th ed. New York: Holt, Rinehart & Winston, Inc., 1971, pp. 89–93.

A Child Needs:	*Society Wants Every Child:*
1. Interpersonal and inter-group relations.	1. To understand and practice desirable social relationships toward individuals and groups, and within the many varied groups of which he is a member. To be a good neighbor and good citizen of the world.
2. Understanding of the world and people and things.	2. To appreciate and participate in worthwhile activities with others at home and abroad.
3. Self-development.	3. To discover and develop desirable individual aptitudes, interests, and abilities. To develop powers of creative expression. To have sound physical and mental health.
4. Control of the communicative arts and skills.	4. To cultivate the habit of constructive, careful thinking. To gain command of common integrating knowledge and skills.
5. Moral and spiritual values.	5. To develop sound emotional attitudes and habits. To appreciate and accept for himself or herself moral and spiritual values.

there is a need in the curriculum for instruction in this area. Sometimes a problem is school-wide. Hookworm and intestinal parasites, for instance, are always of concern in certain southern states and have to be discussed regularly.

There has been a considerable difference of opinion as to the amount of emphasis that one should place on different types of needs. All are important to some degree, but in the interest of economy, some needs must be considered more vital than others. Furthermore, there is a strong point of view that it is not the school's responsibility to meet all of the needs. There are numerous agencies, institutions, and individuals that share this responsibility. The home, the church, scout organizations, 4-H clubs, libraries, recreation centers, radio, television, and summer camps all play a part in meeting the needs of children. The school must do its share, but not attempt to carry the whole burden by itself. Dispensing health information is an example of a shared responsibility, for other community organizations do it too. Many schools cooperate in 4-H and scout work.

It is quite easy to say that most growing children have about the same health needs. They all need good nutrition and proper eating habits, protection against illness and disease, avoidance of accidents, sleep and rest, regular elimination of body wastes, continuous care of eyes, ears, and teeth, good body mechanics and posture, good emotional adjustment, the right attitude toward the opposite sex, and an understanding of themselves. It is not uncommon to find states and larger cities that have excellent courses of study in health which have been carefully prepared over a long period of time to meet the health needs, interests, and capacities of children. Such courses of study are made available to classroom teachers as a basis on which the program can be planned. But, as good as these courses of study are, they should be used only as guides, for much of the material contained therein will require amplification or adjustment in some way to fit the needs of the local community and the particular pupils.

When one considers the whole child in a society that is continually changing, it is readily seen that needs are something more than psychological, social, intellectual, and emotional; they are also individual, moral, and spiritual. Thus the conscientious teacher has quite a task ahead as each school year begins. It will be necessary to seek the answers to some of the following questions on needs before arranging the course of instruction in final form.

Question 1. What Are the Characteristics of My Children at Specific Age Levels? In short, what are the signs of growth and development in terms of physical, intellectual, social, and emotional behavior? What are the health needs?

Growth is a continuous process—an unfolding as children move toward adulthood. It is difficult to subdivide the growth period into specific age levels, for the child never abruptly completes a particular stage of development and begins the next. Moreover, there is never a time when all children in a class are at the same growth stage. Chronological age and physiological age (maturation level) may be quite a distance apart.

Table 6–1, depicting some of the growth and development characteristics of elementary schoolchildren, is a simple device to help answer the question of what characteristics children display at specific age levels. The subdivisions used serve only as convenient labels for periods of growth.

TABLE 6–1. CHARACTERISTICS AND NEEDS OF THE ELEMENTARY SCHOOL CHILD

General Characteristics	Health Needs
1. *Physical Characteristics* 　　Large muscles are better developed than small ones. Can run, jump, skip, climb; enjoy simple tag games, group singing, and singing games. May frequently be clumsy and awkward, and continuous activity brings on early fatigue. 　　Eye and hand coordination not well established. 　　Farsightedness prevails.	To experience basic body movements involving the arms, legs and trunk, with and without music and rhythms. 　　To participate in games with simple rules and boundaries. 　　To have quiet periods of activity; to have rest periods. 　　To have large pictures and large print to read.
2. *Health Characteristics* 　　Usually healthy except for occasional colds, digestive upsets, and "children's diseases." 　　Accidents are the leading cause of death. 　　Burns off considerable energy in short periods of time.	To be aware of colds and sore throats and how to act with them. 　　To understand how to safely use school equipment indoors and outdoors; to know fire drill procedures; to know about the existence of poisons and neighborhood hazards. 　　To eat mid-morning food, milk or juice.
3. *Mental-Emotional Development* 　　Shows curiosity over a short period of time. 　　Proud of possessions, proud of clothes. 　　Often brags to others, likes to hear stories. 　　Capable of self criticism (Gesell). 　　Active imagination with shifting of ideas as child paints. 　　High interest in dramatizations. Speaks and acts spontaneously. 　　Amazingly ignorant of many facts of life. 　　Very vulnerable and sensitive, quick to feel hurt or humiliated. 　　Naturally "mother-centered" and self-centered.	To have experiences beyond the home. 　　To gain confidence in himself or herself as a person. 　　To have freedom to scrawl and scribble and finger paint. 　　To engage in rich, stimulating activities. 　　To learn what is right and wrong, permitted and forbidden. 　　To love a warm, friendly, reassuring teacher who understands children.

Primary School Age (Early Childhood, Ages 6 to 8 Years)

General Characteristics	Health Needs
1. *Physical Characteristics* 　　Growth is relatively slow during this period as compared with the early period. Large muscles of the trunk, legs and arms are more developed than the smaller muscles. 　　Hand-eye coordinations are incomplete, but developing. Eyes slow to focus and usually far-sighted at start of this period. 　　Bones are hardening. Heart and lungs are small in proportion to body weight and height. 　　The loss of temporary teeth begins at 5 to 6 years and continues up to 11 or 12 years of age.	To experience many kinds of vigorous activities involving many parts of the body. This will increase heart action and respiration and help build endurance. It will also improve skills of body control. 　　To have instruction in habits of personal hygiene, such as using the handkerchief, covering coughs and sneezes, the selection of clothing appropriate to weather, etc. 　　Relaxation periods to follow periods of physical activity. Continued emphasis on posture in all activities.
2. *Health Characteristics* 　　Quite susceptible to infectious diseases at beginning of this age period. Respiratory difficulties common in winter. Toxins and bacteria may damage heart, especially if protection is not afforded during convalescent stages of contagious diseases of childhood.	To be checked regularly for signs of disease and defects.

Table continued on the following page

TABLE 6–1. CHARACTERISTICS AND NEEDS OF THE ELEMENTARY SCHOOL CHILD (*Continued*)

General Characteristics	Health Needs
Alimentary tract difficulties common in summer and fall.	To have twelve hours' sleep a night.
Endurance may be poor. Fatigue is "enemy of childhood," but recuperation from fatigue is usually good.	
Accidents are leading causes of death, especially for boys.	To have constant teacher supervision to reduce risks of accidents and to have proper instruction in the hazards of home and school.
The healthy 5 to 8 year old has bright eyes, color in face, great vitality, is happy and radiates enthusiasm and an exuberance for most activities.	To have the chance to express himself or herself through many activities that stimulate physical, social, and mental-emotional growth.
3. *Mental-Emotional Development*	
Short span of attention.	To engage in a number of health activities all of short duration.
Individualistic and possessive, egocentric after age 6.	To learn to share with others, to play alone and with small groups, and to play as an individual in larger groups. Needs recognition for his or her personal abilities and to shift gradually to more group activities.
Dramatic, imaginative, and highly imitative. Curious about things in general.	To create and explore, and identify himself or herself with persons and things. Primary grade health stories appeal to the imagination.
Wide variety of emotional reactions.	To receive guidance in social development.
Enjoys rhythm and rhythmic sounds.	To respond to rhythmic sounds such as drums, rattles, voice, etc.
Reasoning ability present, but with little experience upon which to base judgment. Concern for sex differences made known by pertinent questions.	To have a chance to discuss and relate personal experiences in classroom health topics. To receive just enough information on sex as is necessary to answer questions of the moment. Best handled at home.
Increase in vocabulary. Language grows with experience.	To visit new places, discuss health implications and stimulate growth in vocabulary of words with a health meaning.
When approaching age 8, the child wants the chance to act on his or her own and is sometimes annoyed at conformity. More sensitive to judgment of peers together with a decrease in concern for adult opinion.	To make own choice in selection of health projects, films, plays, and to help evaluate results of activities.
A group most eager to learn and most eager to please the teacher.	To see own work displayed.
Interests are now, not later; will accept things on "faith," less interested in explanations and reasons.	To cooperate at home and at school in play and other group activities.
Somewhat self-dependent toward end of this period. Brushes own teeth and hair, dresses self and ties shoes; cleans table, dries dishes, empties wastebaskets, sweeps floors, watches younger children for parents.	To taste some success, carefully sprinkled with enough defeats to provide a stimulus for greater effort and sound adjustments.

Intermediate School Age (Middle Childhood, Ages 9 to 11 Years)

General Characteristics	Health Needs
1. *Physical Characteristics*	
A noticeable growth spurt at end of period which continues into adolescence. This differs with individual levels of maturation.	To engage in strenuous activity that taxes the muscles, heart, lungs, and other organs to the limits of healthy fatigue.
Sex differences appear, with girls more mature and taller. Sex antagonism gradually appears. Sexual modesty is seen.	To engage in wholesome corecreation and co-educational relationships both in the classroom and on the playing fields.
Rough and tumble activities highly enjoyed, often by the girls.	To participate in those physical skills which properly utilize elements of roughness to build motor skills and physical fitness.

Intermediate School Age (Middle Childhood, Ages 9 to 11 Years)

General Characteristics	*Health Needs*
A few girls begin menstruation by ages 11 and 12. Muscular strength is behind physical growth, postural habits vary.	To be recognized as different individuals. To have instruction in body mechanics, fatigue, nutrition, and factors influencing growth in height and weight.
Some girls may be more developed in motor skills than some boys. Coordinations are good. Many physical skills are now automatic. Reaction time is improved.	To have chance to appraise self through self-testing activities. To relate success in motor skills to personal health habits.
2. *Health Characteristics* Eyes function well but nearsightedness (myopia) may develop at ages 8 or 9.	To have periodic eye screening tests to determine need for eyeglasses. This should be coupled with health instruction in this area.
Resistance to contagious and infectious diseases is much better than in primary grades. Tuberculosis is a threat. Endurance is improved. More rest is needed for the more mature child.	To learn about personal and community health practices which have direct bearing on their welfare. To get as nearly as possible eleven hours' sleep a night and not to play beyond the point of great fatigue. Girls tire more readily than boys, and because they are usually more mature, they require more rest and food.
Permanent dentition continues with incisors and lower bicuspids appearing. Bad teeth begin to appear in large numbers. Accidents are on the increase for this age group, with injuries from burns, automobiles, and bicycles heading the list. Increased interest in foods together with improved appetite. Fewer food refusals and a wider range of preferences. Girls interested in appearance; boys in developing strong bodies.	To have attention directed to dental care. This is a period when many children's teeth are neglected. To understand the nature of personal accidents at school, en route to school, and in the community. To discuss nutrition and the role of the four basic foods in maintaining optimum health. To talk about personal grooming and nature of physical fitness.
3. *Mental-Emotional Development* Child likes a wide variety of activities, has a longer span of attention and greater interests.	To participate in a wide range of health activities involving several methods of teaching and material aids.
Strong sense of rivalry and noticeable craving for recognition.	To succeed often in a variety of health areas, and to do so through some degree of cooperative effort · which affords individual satisfaction.
An increasing attitude of independence coupled with a desire to help.	To have a chance to formally plan, lead, and execute certain projects and to check the progress made. To assist the teacher in the preparation of health exhibits, specimens, posters, etc.
Strong sense of loyalty to groups, teams, or "gangs." Some children are now in a period to be influenced unfavorably. Greater concern over group approval than teacher approval. Enjoys competition, whether physical or essentially mental, but may become angry when tired, or easily discouraged. Interest in opposite sex indicated by teasing, hitting, chasing, etc. Girls are more interested in older boys.	To participate in those activities in which achievement is recognized in the eyes of the group. To gain respect and approval of others. To compete fairly with others, obtaining an understanding of the place of personal cooperation in the process. To work coeducationally in those health activities which broaden social relationships and obtain answers to questions involving the opposite sex.
Broadening intellectual horizons. Interest shifting from the immediate environment to the wider world. Strong interest in collecting things. Love of pets. More critical, need to be shown why. Adventuresome; interested in all kinds of experimentation. Girls are clearly superior to boys in language development, especially toward end of this period.	To study world health conditions and what they mean in terms of personal, everyday existence. To be given a chance to seek detail in a wide variety of health activities. To stimulate improvement of the health vocabulary, a number of meaningful field trips, projects, or dramatizations may be engaged in.

Question 2. What Am I Able to Observe in the Way of the Health Practices of My Children in Specific Situations? How do the children behave with respect to food handling, play and rest, and handwashing and toilet activities? What do they eat? What kind of lunch do they bring to school? Is the home health teaching in keeping with accepted health practices? The observing teacher can tell a great deal about what children need, and these needs are different. For example, children in rural communities sometimes lack health information that may be quite familiar to city children. The teacher who moves from the city to the rural area will often be surprised at the needs that are evident on the local scene. In one first grade class a teacher found one of the boys drinking from the urinal. The boy came from a part of the town where outside privy toilets were used and water was hauled by bucket from a nearby property. School needs, therefore, relate to home needs.

The statements of classroom teachers who have observed children over the years are very useful in gaining an understanding of health needs, which helps to determine what to teach. Some of the pertinent statements, recorded just as they were made, follow:

"Many children come to school improperly fed. Results in early fatigue and loss of energy."

"Some of my children have been drinking coffee since they were old enough to hold a cup."

"Inadequate lunch. Child brings money for full lunch and buys only soup, saving rest for candy. Hastily made, poorly balanced lunches. Gulping food to get out to play earlier."

"Many of our children lack emotional security because working mothers have no time for them."

"In our school, we have problems of emotional malnutrition such as a child's hunger for affection, status with his peers, and hunger for success."

"Parents send children to school when they are ill . . . parents are working or too busy to have them 'underfoot.' "

"Dripping noses: How to care for the common cold? . . . Certain children will not blow their noses often enough or will not wipe them when necessary. I keep Kleenex available to all, but still some have to be told, 'Blow your nose before we can go on with our work.' "

"Head lice—We have had difficulty in controlling the spread of pediculosis."

"Sleep—television—child acquires spectator attitude—child overstimulated comes to school sleepy."

"Lack of proper sleep and rest at home . . . waiting for mother to come home from working on second shift at the mill, or sleep being interrupted by a parent going to work on the second shift."

"Some of our children live in run-down, rat-infested, cold-water flats. Nothing about this environment in which they live is conducive to good health. This overcrowding often makes it necessary for children to sleep near a kerosene stove, the only source of heat. Such children come to school with a strong odor of oil. . . ."

"Body odor . . . This odor is more evident during the winter months when heavier clothing is not changed when necessary."

". . . older children have to sleep with others who wet the bed. . .

The odor is carried on the clothing of the older children."

"Our greatest cause of absence is toothache. . . . Ninety per cent of the primary children have never been to a dentist."

"General fear of dentists that results in harmful neglect of teeth."

"About 20 per cent of the children in my school did not own toothbrushes at the beginning of the year."

"One teacher in the first grade informed a mother that her child was doing failing work because he was unable to hear, and that he should be given a hearing test. The mother said, 'John is not deaf; he is just naughty, and does not want to listen.' "

"A child in kindergarten was very hard of hearing. Not until an examination by the school nurse was it known that he had infected tonsils. The tonsils were removed and the child's hearing was much improved. The loss of hearing had affected the child's speech so that it was hardly understandable."

It is hard to believe in this day and age that home living conditions can be so different. Unless the teacher actually invades the inner city or tours the countryside, seeks the out-of-way places, gets into the apartment buildings, and sizes up the community health situations, he or she is apt to have little real knowledge of pupil health needs. Where a child in one home has his own room and bed, another child in another home sleeps with three others in the same bed; and it may be in a one room dwelling. Numerous places exist where a family of eight, ten, or more lives under one roof in one room. Here they eat, sleep, play, and exist in unclean surroundings and without respect for personal privacy. Even today, public health workers find it necessary to visit homes on the outskirts of a number of communities from Maine to Georgia, attempting to get the people to provide themselves with better toilets.[9] Attitudes and practices formed in this kind of environment can hardly be modified to change right away in the schoolroom.

Question 3. What Are the Health and Safety Hazards in the Local Community? What are the special health problems? Are there hazardous obstacles such as rivers, waterfalls, open sandpits, or automobile traffic, and are there hazardous activities being carried on nearby?

These questions are partially related to the previous question dealing with the observed health and safety practices of the children in school. The questions go together because local conditions *do* affect classroom behavior and point to the necessity for certain kinds of health instruction to meet existing needs.

Local statistics on the prevalence of certain communicable diseases, the purity of drinking water, the cleanliness of local eating establishments, and the safety of milk are fundamental considerations that should be understood by the teacher. If, for example, a community is bothered by black flies or mosquitoes, this should become one of the health topics covered during the year. Moreover, such a topic is probably somewhat familiar to all pupils in the class,

---

[9]Two thousand years ago in the days of the ancient Hebrews, personal health practices were a concern. The Bible says, "Thou shalt have a place within the camp . . . and it shall be, when thou will ease thyself abroad, thou shalt dig therewith, and shalt turn back and cover that which cometh from thee." (Deut. 23:12–13.)

and very little preliminary motivation work will be required to provoke discussion and get some action. Several years ago in one Georgia community, the sixth grade class became so interested in malaria mosquito breeding that they set out to personally initiate a mosquito control program. They drained small ponds and put oil on stagnant waters. In fact, they became so active with enthusiasm, which blossomed as the job progressed, that the townsfolk appropriated money and joined in to make the mosquito control project one fine example of community cooperation. Health instruction directed along lines such as these becomes a magnificent force, not only for the personal health and welfare of the children and adults but also for the promulgation of worthy objectives such as social efficiency and civic responsibility.

Question 4. What Are the Health Problems and Safety Hazards in the State?   Is the state in question any different from any other state? What do recent statistics, collected and made available by the county health department, reveal? Is it conceivable that Alabama might have problems different from those of Montana?

How does the state compare with the National Health Survey, which indicates that pupil deaths from accidents lead the list, followed by cancer and leukemia, influenza and pneumonia, and congenital malformations? What about disabling difficulties? Usually respiratory disturbances rank first, followed by infections and parasitic disorders, and injuries.

States, as communities of people, differ in many respects. Some are more agricultural; others are more industrialized. Some are reasonably warm all year round, while others are faced with an annual adjustment to cold and inclement weather. There are watery noses, sore throats, and cloudy skies in Cleveland, Ohio and Oswego, New York, while the sunshine blazes overhead in South Carolina. Farm safety is taught in the cornbelt states and industrial safety in Detroit. Water safety is of paramount interest in Minnesota, Wisconsin, and along the shores of the Great Lakes and seacoast states.

In Florida, hookworm is a major health problem of schoolchildren. Many individuals have contact with it some time or other. Children who go barefoot appear to be everywhere—and so are hookworm and other internal parasites. Vast numbers of elementary age children are treated by their county health unit through the schools. They stay free from the worms for only a short while following the cure; then they become infected again. And the chief reason for this is that they and their families will not put into practice certain beneficial health habits that have been brought to their attention by public health and school personnel. *The need, therefore, continues to exist for more effective health instruction. In fact, most of these children have more than enough knowledge on the subject to pass a written test with a high grade. What they lack is an intelligent understanding deep enough to create positive attitudes and changes in health behavior.*

The educational needs of many of the children of Mexican-American descent are greater than in other American communities. The same thing relative to needs could be said for the Puerto Rican–American area of New York City or the Italian-American and

Chinese-American sections of Boston. In fact, health problems are more frequent among people of low economic standing in almost any part of the country.

Socio-economic backgrounds, climate and weather, prejudices and superstitions, and even the terrain of the countryside affect what is taught. In New Hampshire—a rugged state of forests, mountains, lakes, and streams—hunting and fishing are as much a part of one's education as any single subject in the public school curriculum. Every spring, on the first day of the trout season there is a school holiday throughout the state. Practically every boy and girl who can walk or hobble along goes fishing. During the year, and especially in the fall, great numbers of children and youth carry rifles and go hunting. This is not without educational implications. Firearms safety, initiated at the State Education Department level, has spread to almost every city and rural school in the state as a special sixth grade health instruction topic. This is a concrete example of how a particular health and safety need can be met. It not only serves the immediate needs of the elementary age children but also carries over to the older age groups.

Question 5. How Does the Local School Environment Furnish Leads for Health Instruction?   Are there poor physical facilities that may represent a school safety hazard? Do children wonder why they are required to take physical education? What kinds of food do primary grade pupils choose in the school cafeteria? Do food selections differ for intermediate graders?

Opportunities to teach health topics in keeping with health needs and interests abound in the school environment. There are hardly two schools alike in facilities and equipment. Every laboratory, lunchroom, gymnasium, and classroom suggests health items of interest and value to pupils. The cleanliness of corridors, walks, and rooms, the lighting, ventilation, temperature, playground equipment, and space all furnish leads to the observing teacher. And one should not forget the number and types of school accidents. Where do they occur and what can be done about them?

Question 6. What Are the Findings of Medical Examinations and Screening Tests?   Do health histories and cumulative health record cards indicate any special findings which the instructional program may be able to remedy or improve? Do some children show a slow rate of growth?

Children with slight cases of malnutrition, postural defects, and similar deviations from normal need two kinds of attention. Primarily, they need to have remedial work started quickly, and secondly, they need information about themselves and their difficulty. There is no need to keep children in the dark about personal deviations, especially when their attitudes can be improved so much by a little understanding. Also, other elementary schoolchildren are generally very interested in the health problems of their classmates and how these may affect them. Furthermore, the child with a problem may become an effective member of the group and feel quite at home in the class by being singled out as, for example, the teacher's helper for a lesson on posture and body mechanics. In one northern New York

State elementary school the teachers have agreed among themselves to have children returning to school after an absence due to illness speak to their classmates and tell them about their experiences while ill. Very often the pupil who has been absent a few days with something like strep throat will stimulate a real show of interest in the broad area of upper respiratory diseases. Moreover, intermediate grade children want to know what they can do about it.

Question 7. Are There Major Student Interests That Relate to Health Education? Young children are vigorous. Sometimes they are rough and adventuresome. Their play is serious, full of meaning—their way of life. Such children are too often unaware of the things they do that may influence their health and safety. Large muscle activities such as running, jumping, climbing, and wrestling are play activities that are at time hazardous. Climbing out on tree limbs, frolicking in the water in the summer, and testing the ice in the winter are potentially dangerous yet powerfully stimulating forms of recreation. Even interest in becoming Brownies or Cub Scouts presents leads for meaningful health instruction.

Student interests rise and fall according to school and local happenings. A major traffic tragedy, a local epidemic of Asian flu or scarlet fever, and a severe water shortage are current health events that may heighten pupil enthusiasm to the point where the alert teacher can take advantage of it and "make hay while the sun shines."

Current and immediate interests of children can be readily determined in a novel way by providing them with the opportunity to ask questions through a device such as the question box. This makes a bit of a game out of it. The teacher who is observant can determine children's health interests rather well by:

Taking note of what they do before and after school.
Talking with them.
Observing their actions in and about the classroom.
Listening as they talk together.
Watching their activities during leisure moments, unassigned periods, or at play.
Evaluating the stories and materials they bring from home.
Studying their paintings, drawings, crafts, stories, and letters.
Noticing their choices of books, clothing, and other materials.
Studying records of pupils of the same level, such as cumulative records, personal diaries, and class folders of the year's work.
Discussing these records with parents and former teachers.

When young children are carefully observed one finds that they are interested in radio, television, movies, play activities, people of other lands, picture magazines, plants and animals, machines, the care of pets, their own bodies, and many other factual and creative items.

Health interests may also be checked through the use of a teacher-constructed questionnaire or pupil check list. Questions pertaining to medical and dental care, food habits, cleanliness, rest, and posture indicate a great deal in terms of pupil behavior and needs but also in terms of health guidance. In the primary grades, direct ques-

K–2	3–4	5–6
How does my body get made?	What shape are my bones?	Why do we have hair?
How does my heart beat?	Why are people so different?	How does a baby grow?
How does God get your heart in there?	How does your mind think?	Why was I born male, not female?
What makes people cry?	What makes you sweat?	How do you get a cold, measles, chickenpox, etc.?
How can I tell if I have a fever?	If a nerve were cut in your arm, could you feel?	What else besides smoking causes cancer?
How can you tell which is a cow or bull?	What goes on inside my body?	Why do people take drugs?
What makes your finger move?	What are the right games to play?	Why don't people stop killing and start loving?
	Where does a baby come from?	What makes it a boy or a girl?

tions which may be asked by the teacher will indicate and stimulate interest in health. For example:

1. Do you wash your hands after going to the toilet?
2. What foods do you eat between meals?
3. Do you stay home when you have a cold?
4. When were you to the dentist last?
5. At what time do you usually go to bed at night?
6. How do you sit in your chair? Do you lean over or slide down in the seat?

Perhaps the most impressive study of children's health interests was *Teach Us What We Want To Know,* completed by the Connecticut State Board of Education.[10] Techniques were used to *get at* the true concerns of students by asking them for advice and suggestions as to what should be taught about health in schools. Through such means as discussions, role-playing, observation, and tape recordings it was possible to gather authentic information. The 180-page paperback book has to be read to be fully appreciated, but a few sample pupil responses relative to interests and picked at random are as shown.

Question 8. Have the Pupils Had Experiences in Other Areas of Learning Which Provide Leads for Needed Health Instruction? It takes many ideas from several study areas to educate for health. Experiences from one subject area carry over into another and enrich health instruction. The teacher plans for this in advance by correlating teaching materials with the content of other areas and the activities of other teachers.

Physical education games, dances, and stunts can be directly related to health instruction topics such as strength, vigor, nutrition, rest, and social health. In fact, for children to have physical education activities and fail to learn why they are important to their health and welfare is indeed a shortsighted kind of education. Yet many opportunities are overlooked to explain why exercise, physical skills, and social contacts are necessary. The same may be said for the special

---

[10]Byler, Ruth, Lewis, Gertrude and Totman, Ruth, *Teach Us What We Want To Know.* Hartford, Connecticut: Connecticut State Board of Education, 1969. Available from Mental Health Materials Center, 419 Park Avenue, New York, New York 10016.

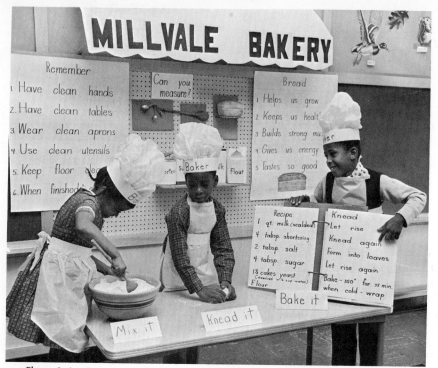

Figure 6–1. Permanent attitudes are formed through interesting activities. (Courtesy Cincinnati Public Schools.)

areas of music and art. Do children know that healthy people, free from worry and organic problems, sing and paint better because they are happy?

TEACHING FOR ATTITUDES AND PRACTICES

From an instructional viewpoint, what can be done with the rank and file of elementary school students to develop a proper attitude toward managing oneself and one's environment? And even more important is the question of how this attitude can be extended to decision-making and actions. This, of course, is the very meat of this whole book. It has never been an easy topic to resolve, despite much research and extensive literature. Gordon Allport spent a lifetime struggling with questions in this area. He made it clear, however, that personal feelings are so ingrained, so carefully protected, and even hidden from the holder that a valid appraisal of attitudes following a certain period of instruction is most difficult. To further complicate the matter is the fact that attitudes are frequently more than a feeling—they represent a predisposition to act or a potential behavior—which makes it even more difficult to consider them accurately.

Combining medical and psychological expertise, Palmer and Lewis researched the health attitudes and behaviors of California children in grades 1, 3, and 6 toward concepts of personal health and illness. They found that the higher the grade, the greater was the increase in discrimination between ill and injured states and the greater was the awareness of the need to seek care. Moreover, the younger children followed the more unrealistic thinking mentioned by Piaget in his *Growth of Logical Thinking* and attributed illness to items such as eating too much candy or going outside without a jacket on. Older children attributed the illness to contact with ill people and germs. Palmer and Lewis concluded that attitudes and behaviors are best advanced when health interventions are appropriate for the developmental level of the child.[11] Teaching children in third grade and older how to become involved in their own health care has their support. It can be done directly, whereas with younger children it requires a more indirect approach, frequently with parental assistance.

What has been said about teaching attitudes applies as well to behavior change. For decades teachers have taught useful health information, yet the world is full of people who failed to apply what they apparently learned. Often the pupil who receives an "A" in the topic of dental health grows to adulthood harboring a mouth full of decaying teeth greatly in need of care. The sixth grader who creates the finest project depicting the relationship of diet to overweight sometimes grows up to be a heavyweight with an attitude of complete indifference toward avoiding certain foods. And every social misfit in our country has been exposed to the influence of a number of reasonably good teachers. Add to this the millions of cases of people involved in vocational failure, chronic unemployment, marital unhappiness, emotional instability, and other expressions of failure, and it becomes quite evident that working to create attitudes and behavior change is a most difficult task requiring the best in curriculum, methodology, and teaching.

One way to assess behavior change is to seek the cooperation of the students. An anonymous questionnaire can be employed to find out what action students have taken following the teaching of a number of health topics. For example, one might respond to these three considerations in terms of decision making:

1. Having studied this topic, my *attitude* toward the improvement of health practices is (—better, —worse, —unchanged).
2. Having studied this topic, my *actions and/or activities* in this area are (—better, —worse, —unchanged).
3. Having studied this topic, I (—have, —have not) helped someone else improve a personal health practice.

When this kind of analysis of decision making is made, it is possible to discover a number of individuals with improved attitudes and practices. Also, there are many students who will admit having tried to help someone else improve a practice. This happens more often with the older and more mature students who, for example, speak up in favor of automobile seat belts and encourage others not to start to smoke.

---

[11]Palmer, Beverly B. and Lewis, Charles E. "Development of Health Attitudes and Behaviors," *Journal of School Health*, 46:401–406, September 1976.

Health Teaching

Instructional programs become effective in promoting pupil achievement when they have good teachers behind them. The finest fashioned course of study, carefully modified at the local level to consider immediate needs, is but words on a sheet of paper to the incompetent and unsympathetic teacher. Fortunately, however, most elementary schoolteachers like children and make an effort to understand and work with them.

Teaching has been defined in many ways, but in general it may be considered a procedure involving leadership. If education may be defined as a process of changing behavior toward certain preconceived goals, then teaching is the act of exercising leadership in this process. Good teaching can be so effective that children are taught numerous things without even being aware of it. "We are," wrote Lord Chesterfield, "more than half what we are by imitation. The great point is, to choose good models and to study them with care." This has a profound meaning for educators. Someone has said that "teaching is a process of making little images of the teacher in the minds of pupils." If such is so, and it appears to be, then teachers of impressionable youth and eager-to-learn children might well tremble at the thought of how much power they wield for good or evil.

The Competent Teacher

A writer once asked Dr. Albert Schweitzer if he did not think that personally setting a good example was one of the best ways of influencing people. Dr. Schweitzer replied, "No! It's the *only* way." The implication is clear that in order to really influence others in developing good health, teachers must be fit themselves.

"Each honest calling, each walk of life," says Conant, "has its own elite, its own aristocracy based on excellence of performance."[12]

There is little question that the teacher must be much more than an ordinary person. Needed are the characteristics, vision, and understanding of the clergy, the zeal and devotion of the medical worker, and the earthly human qualities of the missionary. The teacher must be an idealist and aim high with enthusiasm for teaching that might well exemplify the immortal words of Robert Browning: "Ah, but a man's reach should exceed his grasp, or what's a heaven for?" In short the *real* teacher has everything. This is demonstrated time and time again by the testimony of successful men and women who pay tribute to their teachers of earlier years.

Competency as a teacher is not something which automatically accompanies being hired to teach school. Almost anyone can get a job teaching. The question is, what constitutes a competent teacher?

It has been said that the competent teacher is neither a poem nor a paragon. Assets overcompensate for liabilities, and liabilities do not occur in crucial areas.

---

[12]Conant, James B. *The Education of American Teachers.* New York: McGraw-Hill Book Company, 1961, p. 183.

There are many excellent characteristics that might well describe the competent teacher. Certainly this individual should possess a number of superior traits—personally and professionally. Here are six earmarks or minimum essentials of the competent teacher:

1. A Person with a Personality. Certainly the personality of a classroom teacher who is aiming toward the successful teaching of health must be one capable of registering a deep personal concern for the welfare of every pupil in the class. Children influenced by the attitudes and practices of the teacher's warm, unflagging interest in them receive a lesson in what can be done by the teacher who really cares about the mental, physical, emotional, and social well-being of his or her students. Several years ago a Harvard University graduate study indicated that this *feeling* of warmth and understanding (empathy) was the quality more instrumental in good teaching than anything else. Yet, one cannot legislate or command this quality. Given a little help, it may be developed, especially among teachers who profess to like children.

Not all teachers have the personality that is desirable for school teaching. It has been stated that the chances are seven to one that in the course of 12 years of school a child will come under the thumb of at least two teachers with personality maladjustments. They may be unstable and neurotic or even seriously psychopathic. This is a most serious problem, not only for the health of the teachers but also for the children they teach. Inappropriate emotional response, faulty personality reactions, and devastating character maladjustments can develop and be spread under bad classroom as well as bad home conditions.

2. A Person with a Significant Store of Useful Knowledge. A limited knowledge of the science of health cannot be offset by a broad understanding of educational philosophy and method. A balance of both is required.

Teachers of health need increasing knowledge. New medical discoveries and changes in public health practices are occurring all the time. The well-informed teacher is one who has sought extended instruction.

3. A Person Who Has Considerable Success in Selecting Important and Strategic Things to Be Learned. The key word here is "select." Competent teachers, through study and training, know what they should select to teach, but because there is so much variety to choose from today, the selective function becomes an art.

4. A Person with Decided Skill in Arranging What Pupils Do in Order That Learning Will Take Place. The key word here is "arranging." The ability to arrange the teaching situation so that children get the most out of it is high-level skill. Today, with the many teaching instruments available—movies, field trips, libraries, and outside speakers—it takes a competent teacher to move from one to another so that all children receive maximum benefits. This holds true whether one teaches health or English.

5. A Person Who Succeeds in Establishing Constructive, Stimulating Relationships with Individual Pupils. Although most personal contacts with children are made on a mass basis, the competent teacher knows how to go beyond the mass approach and reach individuals.

6. A Person with at Least One Well-Developed, Useful Specialty. It is good for a teacher to be well-rounded, with many abilities useful in education. At the same time, however, excellence in some phase of educational endeavor seems to be a common characteristic of the competent teacher.

Faith in the Worth of Teaching

No discussion of the competencies of teachers of health would be complete without mention of the teacher's personal attitude toward teaching. This attitude may have more to do with successful health teaching than any other single factor. The teacher who likes the work and approaches the lesson with a pleasant and enthusiastic manner demonstrates a positive approach to the topic that sets the stage for optimum learning. The great New England pioneer in health teaching, Mabel Caroline Bragg, taught her teachers-to-be that the teaching of health—perhaps more than any other subject—calls for a teacher with dynamic vitality, an inspired interest in the welfare of children, and a faith in the worth of teaching. Miss Bragg herself was the magnificent example of this faith, for wherever she went, in college or grade school classrooms, she created an atmosphere of radiant, positive health. One must, therefore, possess a profound conviction of the worth of his or her work. There must be a sense of greatness in one's profession.

Finally, this faith in the worth of teaching is expressed through service. Through the basic concept of service the individual teacher establishes a place in the group. And through service the group takes on more significance. Unless humanity can be guided by a motive of service, selfishness and materialism eat at the roots of individuals and nations. Antoine de St. Exupéry attributes the fall of France to this lack of the concept of service. In his *Flight to Arras* he says that if man insists upon giving only to himself, he will receive nothing, for he is not a part of anything. Later when he is asked to die for something he will refuse to die, for his own interests will command him to live. There will be no deep love for something else strong enough to compensate for his death. Men do not die for tables and walls; they die for a home. They die for something bigger than themselves. Says St. Exupéry, "Men die only for that for which they live."

HEALTH GUIDANCE: TEACHERS AND PARENTS

The number of schoolchildren who need health guidance is increasing. There have always been a number of children with minor physical deviations needing attention, but in recent years more and more children have problems of adjustment on the mental-emotional plane. Although there are school psychologists, guidance counselors, and in some places school psychiatrists, there are nevertheless far too few dedicated teachers who are both interested and capable of sitting down and talking at length with children in need of special consideration. Yet, this is necessary and it needs to be done with measurable parental cooperation. As Don Davies has indicated, there are indeed schools where parents make a difference.[13] And they are everywhere from Boston to Los Angeles to the Indian reservations. The involved parents help operate and shape their schools to meet the special needs of their own communities and children.

SUGGESTED ACTIVITIES

1. The challenge of the late 1970's and early 1980's rests with the approach health education takes in responding to health education concerns. Russell (see *Selected References*) wants the focus to be on communication and motivation and less on knowledge per se. Is there any danger here that essential information will be overlooked? Talk with others in professional preparation to see if they agree or disagree.

2. In their book, Ryan and Cooper describe the "New Teacher" (see *Selected References*). They feel that elementary teachers have been prepared as universal superteachers with all the skills, whereas in the future teaching should consist of teams of people with differential skills. Survey a number of teachers and see if they subscribe to this view, even to the extent of having a health specialist come to the classroom.

3. Discover whether research carried on in a school health services department is used in some way by teachers. Some cities, for example, survey tooth decay and relate it to a number of school variables. How is this accomplished? Are those who teach children involved in any significant way?

4. Read several sources pertaining to the objectives of elementary education. What are the objectives held in common? Is there any indication that health education goals at the elementary level are incompatible with the overall elementary education objectives?

QUESTIONS FOR DISCUSSION

1. High-level conferences frequently recommend better health services, a higher quality of health care, and a more equitable distribution of health manpower. Very often missing is a solid recommendation for more meaningful health teaching. Why does this happen? Is the obvious overlooked, or is there a lack of faith in what education can provide?

2. What evidence is there that we are bridging the gap between health knowledge and health behavior? How can we better apply what the psychologists have learned about human motivations?

3. To what extent do you believe parents receive health education through the health instruction program in schools?

4. What health instructional activities are suggested by the prepubescent growth spurt?

5. As civilization becomes more complex, is there a tendency for education to become somewhat divorced from life? Is this true for health education as contrasted with other subject areas?

---

[13]Davies, Don. *Schools Where Parents Make A Difference*. Boston: The Institute for Responsive Education (Boston University), 1976.

SELECTED REFERENCES

Anderson, C. L. and Creswell, W. H., Jr. *School Health Practice*. 6th ed. St. Louis: C. V. Mosby Co., 1976.

Mallan, John T. and Hersh, Richard. *No G.O.D.s in the Classroom: Inquiry into Inquiry*. Philadelphia: W. B. Saunders Co., 1972.

Parcel, Guy A. "Skills Approach to Health Education: A Framework for Integrating Cognitive and Affective Learning," *Journal of School Health,* 46:403–406, September 1976.

Russell, Robert D. *Health Education,* 6th ed. Washington: National Education Association, 1975.

Ryan, Kevin and Cooper, James M. *Those Who Can Teach*. Boston: Houghton Mifflin Co., 1972.

Schaller, Warren E. "Positioning School Health as a National Policy," *Journal of School Health,* 47:393–394, September 1977.

_____. "Communication and the School Health Program," *Journal of School Health,* 47:413–417, September 1977.

Shane, H. G. "The Seven Cardinal Principles Revisited," *Today's Education, 65:57–72,* January 1976.

Willgoose, Carl E. "Sequential K–12 Courses Replace Old Style Health,"*Nation's Schools, 85:78,* March 1970.

Designing the Health Curriculum

7

If I had my choice now, in terms of a curriculum project for the seventies, it would be to find the means whereby we could bring society back to its sense of values and priorities in life.

—Jerome S. Bruner[1]

Organizing the curriculum around the activities of mankind will not only bring about a needed unification of knowledge but will also permit such a curriculum to be of maximum value to students' day-by-day life, as well as to prepare them for participation in a culture.

—Hilda Taba[2]

In his day, Thoreau was critical of those who would "build castles in the air" as philosophers far removed from reality, but he did not take serious issue with them if they would follow his urging and "put the foundations under them."

Designing the health curriculum needs a solid foundation of program particulars that represents a logical outgrowth of the viewpoints and aspirations of school personnel regarding health instruction. This calls for conscientious planning and the development of a *reasonable design* that translates remote goals and near-at-hand objectives into a workable program which can be started gradually, subjected to pilot studies, and evaluated with comment from school and community groups.

THE NATURE OF THE CURRICULUM

Curriculum is a word derived from the Latin *currere,* which means "to run." Whereas it was earlier associated with race courses and the running of races, it is now commonly defined as a "work schedule" or a "particular body of courses." It is generally linked with an orderly plan and progression.

---

[1]Bruner, Jerome S. "The Process of Education Reconsidered," in Haas, Glen. *Curriculum Planning: A New Approach,* 2d ed. Boston: Allyn and Bacon, Inc., 1977.
[2]Taba, Hilda. *Curriculum Development: Theory and Practice,* New York: Harcourt Brace Jovanovich, 1962.

In recent years the word curriculum has taken on an all-inclusive meaning which refers to the total school program of planned or intended learning experiences. It is anticipatory and "prescribes the results of instruction."[3] It has emerged from the time when educational offerings were conceived in terms of the "trained mind" and isolated teacher goals, to the present-day child-centered curriculum.[4]

In any subject area, it is important to note where curriculum stands in relation to other educational influences. As a body of experiences, it commands a central position between one's philosophy and objectives on the one hand and teaching methods and evaluation practices on the other. The degree to which it is implemented, therefore, depends not only upon how it is put together but also on how well it is taught and appraised.

Types of Elementary School Curricula

Curricula are designated in a number of ways. The *separate-subjects curriculum* is regarded as the traditional curriculum. It is often called by such other names as the subject-matter curriculum and the scientific-subjects curriculum. Students study each subject that the school has to offer for a certain amount of time each day. Little attempt is made to relate one school subject to another. For example, physical education is taught without reference to health or social living. Health is taught as a subject by itself. Critics point out that the artificial separation of subjects and the extreme fragmentation of the curriculum are inconsistent with the integration of knowledge and full intellectual development. A multi-disciplinary approach to education is needed.

Since 1925 the trend has been to employ the *broad-fields curriculum* in which closely related subject-matter areas are grouped together. Subject matter is organized, but the emphasis is on large fields or areas rather than on separate subjects. This type of curriculum may group such items as spelling, writing, reading, language-grammar-oral communication, and literature under the broad topic (field) of language arts. Health, safety, and physical education are often grouped together, for they possess several things in common. Health may also be taught in the broad areas of science and social studies. This curriculum helps students to see relationships between several things learned in one general area. For example,

---

[3]Zais, Robert S. *Curriculum Principles and Foundations.* New York: Thomas Y. Crowell Co., 1976, p. 9.

[4]Curriculum and course of study are not the same. Curriculum applies to a larger web of influences, whereas a course of study is more specific—performing the function of a guide to help teachers in planning and carrying out activities.

| Educational Philosophy | Aims and Objectives | Curriculum | Teaching Methods | Evaluation Practices |

students learn from the broad field of health and social living that vitamins are more than something to be concerned about for personal health at the moment; they learn that they are related to historical accomplishments. The sailors who manned the ancient ships in the days of Columbus, Magellan, and Sir Francis Drake were somewhat limited in their capacities by vitamin deficiencies in the form of beriberi and pellagra.

Other types of elementary curricula include the *life situations curriculum* based on the problems of everyday living in the home, school, and community, a program established on needs of the moment; the *emerging curriculum* in which no preplanned program is arranged; and the *correlated-subjects curriculum* in which two or more subjects are articulated and relationships between and among them are made without destroying subject boundaries. More recently Goodlad has pleaded for a greater concentration on human values and interests. Because it involves the requirement for a warm, human approach to learning, it is called the *humanistic curriculum.*[5]

There is much agreement that the contemporary elementary school curriculum should stress the relationship of experiences to the learning process. The key word is *experiences.* The curriculum is organized for living and learning. These two words go together. No longer do we educate just for "later life." Education *is* life. It is concerned with the improvement of living—a better life for children and adults at the very moment—because of the *kind* of living that goes on in the school.

More and more curriculum theorists are calling for a curriculum which is organized into a planned series of encounters between the pupil, the teacher, and the wide community of persons and things outside the school.

CURRICULUM DEVELOPMENT

Leadership in curriculum development has gone from the subject specialists and university and college professors to the "grass roots" of the community—to the teachers, supervisors, psychologists, specialists, and parents working together. The curriculum, in a sense, is part and parcel of the society, the local community, the classroom, and the pupils and teachers. All of these persons enter into the planning of the program so that the curriculum is viewed in the light of total influences. Materials and topics are carefully selected and developed cooperatively; supervisors and classroom teachers work together to rethink the curriculum periodically in terms of current problems which confront teachers in the school, the classroom, and the community. Where there is a need to make a change, an effort is made to implement the findings rapidly.

---

[5]Goodlad, John L. "The Educational Program to 1980 and Beyond," in Morphet, E. L. and Ryan, C. D. (eds.), *Designing Education for the Future*, No. 2. New York: Citation Press, 1967.

Too often in the past, programs have not been properly updated to reflect a changing emphasis on health needs. Sometimes they have not been properly field-tested or subjected to quality control (examining the quality of implementation). More recently, it has been popular to be associated with change—even to the extent of believing that change is automatically equated with a seldom-defined "progress." Change = Progress = Benefit represents a concept of change that becomes regarded as an unqualified good. Certainly there is merit in the expression, "We must adapt to a changing world," but it frequently gives rise to a doctrine of over-enthusiastic adaptability which advances the assertion of "change for change's sake." When this happens, it raises the question as to whether the traditional or existing curriculum has been fully evaluated in terms of its usefulness in modifying health behavior, or if it is being discarded simply because it is "old" and not subject to the seemingly new charm of "innovation" and "creativity." Although local research is frequently given a low priority, there should be some sincere effort to appraise existing programs before entirely new organizations for learning are explored. In short, it is good curriculum development practice to inquire and explore both the new and the old, with comments solicited from many sources. For example, it is possible that a more appropriate health program can be planned in a particular school if new information is available, such as the three findings from the Connecticut study, *Teach Us What We Want To Know:*

1. Children have acquired a large amount of accurate information about health and are more mature in thought and judgment, and at an earlier age, than adults generally think.
2. Young people wish they had been taught about health and often recommend that such information should be given to younger children.
3. Children are capable of making valid suggestions about how and when health topics should be taught.

Most of the larger schools have committees that are responsible for improving the program of studies and articulating it so that all elements of the school's offerings complement each other. This kind of planning guards against unnecessary duplication or gaps in the child's learning experiences. A good amount of preplanning is necessary.

This can be accomplished if the following points are kept in mind.

1. If a program is to succeed, it must have the commitment and support of the community, administration, and staff.
2. The personnel involved are important for success.
3. Basic considerations in developing a curriculum need to be outlined. See *Elements That Affect the Teacher's Planning for Health* (Figure 7–1).
4. A philosophy must be developed in order that value judgments may be made and educational objectives selected.
5. Controversial areas must be considered carefully; methods, materials, and content must be reviewed in reference to their legality, educational validity, and social acceptability.

Health Needs
   Health Knowledge
   Health Habits
   Health Attitudes
   Health Status
Health Interests
Individual Capacities
Characteristics of Growth
   and Development

Significant Curriculum Trends
Time Allotments
Scheduling of Activities
Organization of Health Curriculum
Health of Teacher

PUPIL IN THE CLASSROOM

State Education Department
Elementary Education Objectives
School Department Policies
   School Committee
   School's Objectives
Health Education Objectives

Course of Study and Bulletins
School Environment
Parents and Community
Special Resource Personnel
Available Textbooks and the
   Teaching Materials

Figure 7-1. Elements that affect the teacher's planning for health.

6. A work schedule should be developed early with target dates for assignment completion.

Curriculum Research Studies

New programs in health education are best developed by studying the shortcomings of the existing curriculum. This was done several years ago throughout the state of Rhode Island. More recently, three other states have made a serious attempt to appraise existing programs by analyzing student understandings.

Georgia Health Education Study[6]

In an effort to upgrade elementary and secondary school health instruction, the 1976 Georgia Health Education Study set out to determine the health knowledge of young adults throughout the state. Several thousand students from 29 colleges and universities, all of whom were products of the Georgia schools, were given the Fast-Tyson Health Knowledge Test. It was apparent from the results that subject matter knowledge was not strong in any health content area, and it was especially weak in the areas of exercise, relaxation, sleep, nutrition, tobacco, alcohol, mental health, and human sexuality. Because so many students scored below projected norms, state officials initiated a planned health instruction program for all young people in Georgia.

Kansas School Health Education Study[7]

This 1977 study of 1700 students in 22 colleges and universities who had been educated in Kansas schools was modeled somewhat

[6]For details contact R. Morgan Pigg, Jr., Georgia Health Education Study, The University of Georgia, Athens, Georgia 30602.

[7]For copies contact Parren R. Watts at Emporia State University, Emporia, Kansas 66801.

after the Georgia study. The Fast-Tyson Health Knowledge Test was employed and most students did poorly on it. In fact, health content weaknesses were practically identical with those found in the Georgia study, with the greatest weaknesses appearing in the areas of nutrition and drugs. Also disturbing was the fact that those students who had had health instruction performed only marginally better than those who had not. Especially disappointing was the evidence that the students who participated in a college health course failed to score higher than students who had never completed a formal health course. The result of this study was a forthright call for a critical review of what was being taught in the Kansas health education program. The development of statewide legislation called for several curriculum improvements. Significant among these is the provision for "every elementary child to have daily instruction in health education as a separate subject." Also, elementary classroom teachers are to receive preparation in health education through graduate courses and in-service programs.

South Carolina Health Education Study[8]

Concerned with the quality of health instruction in the grades, a selected population of twelfth grade students attending the public schools of Aiken County was tested for understanding with the revised Kilander-Leach Health Knowledge Test. The average percentage of correct responses was below 50; the areas of greatest weakness were community health, stimulants and depressants, personal health, and communicable diseases. The obvious conclusion was that Aiken County needed a thorough evaluation of its health education program with corresponding improvements in the implementation of the state law, which mandates teaching only about drugs and tobacco and fails to focus on comprehensive health education.

The School Health Education Study

The inadequacy of health education has been the concern of many groups and individuals for a number of years. In 1960 the NEA-AMA Joint Committee on Health Problems in Education recommended a survey of the nation's schoolchildren to determine the status of health education in the schools. Under a grant from the Samuel Bronfman Foundation in 1961, the School Health Education Study (SHES) was begun. Its purpose was to discover the status of health instruction and gain public support for reform measures.[9]

Large, medium, and small school systems were studied. Health behavior questionnaires were submitted to the students in the sixth, ninth, and twelfth grades in order to secure information which would reflect the accumulation of health experience in the years prior to graduation.

---

[8]Further information available from John A. Conley, Chairman, Department of Health and Safety, The University of Georgia, Athens, Georgia 30602.

[9]Sliepcevich, Elena M. *School Health Education Study: A Summary Report.* Washington, D.C.: SHES, 1964.

The findings at all grade levels indicated serious misconceptions about health. Only one in five sixth graders brushed his teeth or rinsed his mouth regularly after eating. Sixth graders also scored poorly in safety education. This was not a strange finding, for it was discovered that health instruction practices were of poor quality throughout the country.

The School Health Education Study undertook a project to bring together health education specialists, supervisors, and classroom teachers to develop sample experimental curriculum materials based on a concept approach. These were carefully prepared and tested during the 1964–1965 school year in test centers in Alhambra, California; Evanston, Illinois; Great Neck–Garden City, New York; and Tacoma, Washington.

In 1967, packets of materials pertaining to the concepts were available commercially.[10] The ten curriculum concepts developed by the project are:

1. Growth and development influences, and is influenced by, the structure and functioning of the individual.
2. Growth and development follows a predictable sequence, yet is unique for each individual.
3. Protection and promotion of health is an individual, community, and international responsibility.
4. The potential for hazards and accidents exists whatever the environment.
5. There are reciprocal relationships involving man, disease, and environment.
6. The family serves to perpetuate humanity and to fulfill certain health needs.
7. Personal health practices are affected by a complexity of forces, often conflicting.
8. Utilization of health information, products, and services is guided by values and perceptions.
9. Use of substances that modify mood and behavior arises from a variety of motivations.
10. Food selection and eating patterns are determined by physical, social, mental, economic, and cultural factors.

THE HEALTH CONCEPT APPROACH IN CURRICULUM DEVELOPMENT

It is appropriate at this stage of curriculum planning to consider outcomes of learning. In recent years, the two terms frequently employed to denote learning outcomes are *concepts* and *competencies*. Although they share a common ground, they are not the same. The concept is a point of view or idea held about something, whereas a competency is a solid ability or proficiency. Both are necessary in

---

[10]Teaching-learning guides, together with the basic document *(Health Education: A Conceptual Approach to Curriculum Design, Grades K–12)* and printed originals for preparing overhead projection transparencies are available from Visual Products, 3M Co., Box 1300, St. Paul, Minn. 55101.

health education. Ultimate health behavior starts with one or more health concepts and culminates in a skillful and appropriate action—a health competency.

The concept approach offers the program planner a realistic pattern for the development of curriculum materials in health education. This topic has been well explored. (See especially the references to Bruner, Darrow, Phenix, and Woodruff at the end of this chapter.) Also, there have been several national curriculum studies that have used this approach quite successfully.[11]

A concept is a generalization about something. It is usually built from a number of related sensations, precepts, and images. Concepts range from ideas about very simple things to high-level abstractions.

To the individual pupil, a concept is a personal organization of a number of interpretations of things. In this respect concepts cannot be taught as such. However, teaching is directed *toward* concepts. This means that the instructor is working with pupils in terms of whole ideas, even though pieces and bits of knowledge are being employed along the way. More specifically, the concept approach to learning is one in which all the facts, skills, and techniques are interdependent and interrelated. For too many years teachers of health have taught isolated facts about vitamins in about the same fashion as history teachers have taught places and dates. The pupil learned facts by memorization or repetition without seeing them as a part of a whole—a part of life. They did not become a part of a value system. The dates, places, and vitamins were soon forgotten.

Therefore, the writers of the School Health Education Study materials realized that all health instruction activities must ultimately be related not only to the individual but also to the family and community at large. Health education attempts to unify humanity physically, mentally, and socially by developing health education behavior in the form of knowledge, attitudes, and practices with a dynamic focus on the individual, family, and community.

In a conceptual framework there are broad key concepts which represent the highest conceptual level of the health curriculum. In the School Health Education Study the three overriding concepts or processes affecting health behavior are:

Growing and Developing: a dynamic life process in which the individual is in some ways like all other individuals, in some ways like some other individuals, and in some ways like no other individuals.
Interacting: an ongoing process in which the individual is affected by and in turn affects certain biological, social, psychological, economic, cultural, and physical forces in the environment.
Decision Making: a process unique to man of consciously deciding to take an action, or of choosing one alternative rather than another.[12]

Practically all health education experiences can be fitted to the pattern of growing and developing, interacting, and decision making. In the SHES project these key concepts were established as the three

[11]See especially Pa. Department of Education, *Conceptual Guidelines for School Health Programs in Pennsylvania,* Harrisburg, Pennsylvania: Department of Education, 1970.
[12]School Health Education Study. *Health Education: A Conceptual Approach to Curriculum Design.* St. Paul, Minnesota: 3M Education Press, 1967, p. 20.

Cognitive Domain	Affective Domain	Action Domain

Understanding
Comprehending
Realizing
(Knowledge, intellectual
  abilities, skills)
	Awareness
	Appreciation
	Consciousness
	(Interests, attitudes,
	  values)
		Improving
		Modifying
		Developing
		(Application of knowledge
		  and attitudes)

unifying threads of the health program from which the ten major curriculum concepts emerge. There are also subconcepts which were developed by elaborating on the basic ten concepts. These subconcepts were set up in terms of physical, mental, and social dimensions. From this the long-range goals were formulated in three domains. (See table.)

Finally, the progression and sequence for the teaching-learning experience were developed. These were set up as four levels of progression rather than by the more traditional grade level approach.

Since teaching can be directed toward concepts, this fosters a striving for goals that are pupil-oriented instead of teacher-oriented. It also gets away from the segregation of factual information from practical knowledge and improves the chances of building larger generalizations. There is nothing automatic about this; it requires work to help students conceptualize. Marion Pollock speaks well to the point when she says, "Conceptualization is a natural process, and the difficulty is not in arranging for it to take place, but in arranging for the kinds of perceptions that lead to positive, constructive concepts."[13] In this connection there is some research to indicate that the concept approach to learning is not sufficient to produce a substantial number of significant changes in student-reported health behavior patterns.[14] It would seem that the approach is only as effective as the teacher's ability to use it.

[13]Pollock, Marion B. "Speaking of Concepts," *Journal of School Health, 41*:283–285, June 1971.
[14]Allen, Robert E. and Holyoak, Owen J. "Evaluating the Conceptual Approach to Teaching Health Education," *Journal of School Health, 42*:118–119, February 1972.

Environmental and Public Health (Grades 4–6)	
Outline of Content	*Major Understandings and Fundamental Concepts*
1. The Environment and Health Status	Man is in constant interaction with his environment which is capable of improving his health or harming it.
A. History of Environmental Control	Man improves his health status when he understands his environment and uses it wisely. We must constantly adapt to environmental conditions because our environment constantly changes. Many of the devices we have created to improve our way of life have resulted in environmental destruction.

An example of how concepts may be set up so that they influence curriculum planning and implementation appears on page 155. Note the clarity of the concepts.[15]

BEHAVIORAL OBJECTIVES AND DECISION MAKING

Currently a fair amount of discussion is being done about behavioral objectives. These are student objectives at the instructional level, as opposed to the general objectives of an institution or a society. Moreover, the behavioral objectives are stated in such precise fashion that they describe a behavior. If they are realistic, they can be achieved and measured. They are noticeably different from the usually stated goals and concepts in that they are written not in terms of understanding and feelings, but in terms of action. It is as if someone took the verb *to do* and applied it generally. Thus words such as the following usually preface the objective:

identified	distinguishes
analyzes	relates
evaluates	modifies
describes	improves
applies	performs
gives	makes

By stating educational aspirations in terms of behavioral objectives, the focus is on action and behavior change from the beginning. Note the difference:

Grade 3

Example 1 *Traditional objective:* To understand that certain foods build strong teeth and bones.
Concept: Certain foods build strong teeth and bones.
Behavioral objective: Identifies foods that build strong teeth and bones.

Example 2 *Traditional objective:* To know that a program of physical activity and rest contributes to well-being.
Concept: Physical activity and rest contribute to well-being.
Behavioral objective: Describes how physical activity and rest contribute to well-being.

An example of how behavioral objectives can be arranged for elementary school health education is shown for the topic of dental health. Note the gradual progression toward the more difficult material. Turn to the Appendix for a graduated list of suggested student behavioral objectives for each of the major health topics, grades one to six. This may be employed as a guide in building a course of study.

---

[15]From the State Education Department Strand IV *Environmental and Community Health,* Albany, N.Y.: State Education Dept., 1970 (Grades 4–6).

DENTAL HEALTH
STUDENT BEHAVIORAL OBJECTIVES

Grade One

Brushes teeth in proper fashion
Describes loss of first teeth and appearance of first 6-year molar

Grade Two

Uses toothpaste or powder correctly
Practices proper care and brushing of first teeth and can explain why
Distinguishes between proper care and improper care of toothbrush
Describes and shows how raw foods help keep teeth clean
Relates how sweets affect teeth
Expresses self clearly on the value of regular dental care

Grade Three

Demonstrates ways the teeth may be cleaned without brushing
Identifies foods that build strong teeth
Relates in detail what the dentist does for children
Improves his or her appearance through cleaning own teeth and
    appreciates the reason why
Analyzes the causes of toothache

Grade Four

Presents a clear description of the structure of the tooth
Identifies the several harmful effects of decayed teeth
Plays and works so as not to injure the teeth
Evaluates the importance of teeth for talking and digestion
Examines own teeth for cavities and appearance

Grade Five

Describes tooth structure and relates it to function
Identifies malocclusion and tries to have something done about it
Distinguishes good dental health practices from poor practices
Is familiar with dental office instruments and their use
Makes a point to interest others in orthodontia when it appears to be
    necessary

Grade Six

Figures when self and other sixth graders are apt to have a full set of
    second teeth
Appraises dentifrice advertisements in newspapers and other media
Assists the dental hygiene teacher or other health services personnel
    with younger children
Describes how decayed teeth may cause illness and a disturbance in
    other bodily processes

	CONCEPT 1	CONCEPT 2	CONCEPT 3	CONCEPT 4	CONCEPT 5
	GROWTH AND DEVELOPMENT INFLUENCES AND IS INFLUENCED BY THE STRUCTURE AND FUNCTIONING OF THE INDIVIDUAL.	GROWING AND DEVELOPING FOLLOWS A PREDICTABLE SEQUENCE, YET IS UNIQUE FOR EACH INDIVIDUAL.	PROTECTION AND PROMOTION OF HEALTH IS AN INDIVIDUAL, COMMUNITY, AND INTERNATIONAL RESPONSIBILITY.	THE POTENTIAL FOR HAZARDS AND ACCIDENTS EXISTS, WHATEVER THE ENVIRONMENT.	THERE ARE RECIPROCAL RELATIONSHIPS INVOLVING MAN, DISEASE, AND ENVIRONMENT.
LEVEL I APPROXIMATE GRADE LEVELS K-3	**A** Relates good nutrition, adequate sleep, and physical activity to optimal growth and development. **B** Names major body parts and organs and their related functions. **C** Explains how body types and other factors determine differences in height and weight. **D** Defines the meanings of heredity and environment. **E** Identifies ways in which plants, animals, and children resemble their parents.	**A** Cites examples showing how people of the same age differ and yet are similar while growing and developing. **B** Explains why differences in the rate of growing and developing among children of the same age are to be expected. **C** Identifies ways in which one grows over a given period of time. **D** Describes how each person becomes unique.	**A** Defines the meanings of health and of community. **B** Describes the relationships of health and community. **C** Identifies familiar health problems which are the joint responsibility of individuals and groups. **D** Recognizes local community efforts designed to meet common health needs. **E** Is aware of the variety of health personnel involved in solution of community problems.	**A** Describes what accidents are and the need for their prevention and control. **B** Detects environmental factors which affect health and safety. **C** Indicates hazards existing in the home, school, and community. **D** Identifies procedures which help protect personal health and safety and that of others. **E** Is aware that groups exist to help prevent accidents and eliminate or control hazards.	**A** Distinguishes between being ill and being well. **B** Identifies factors which affect wellness. **C** Discusses ways in which disease-causing organisms can be transmitted from person to person. **D** Identifies ways in which a person can protect himself and others from disease.
LEVEL II APPROXIMATE GRADE LEVELS 4-6	**A** Describes the basic structure and function of the human organism as it relates to growing and developing. **B** Concludes that although each organ and system has a special task, each is dependent on the other in meeting body needs. **C** Identifies ways in which girls are both physiologically ahead of boys and different in behavior and interests at some stages of growth. **D** Explains the importance of certain personal health practices as they relate to the process of growing and developing. **E** Illustrates the effects of heredity and environment on growth and development.	**A** Describes how growing and developing occurs unevenly for body parts, systems and functions. **B** Identifies different ways children grow physically, mentally, and socially. **C** Differentiates among the variety of influences which continually affect growing and developing. **D** Predicts the kinds of changes that may occur during adolescence.	**A** Explains why some health-related efforts are common to all communities while others are unique to certain communities. **B** Identifies factors that influence the nature of community health activities. **C** Compares health programs, facilities, and services provided by organized segments of society. **D** Describes skills and techniques required to meet existing and emerging community health needs. **E** Explores functions of and the range of career opportunities in health-service professions and allied fields.	**A** Cites authoritative data related to the occurrence of accidents. **B** Illustrates relationships between accidents and human behavior. **C** Reports the effects of environmental factors on the health and safety of individuals and groups. **D** Relates precautions to the reduction of hazards and accidents.	**A** Names various methods by which disease can be prevented, controlled, or cured. **B** Identifies various sources of disease. **C** Concludes that immunization prevents and controls some diseases. **D** Cites examples of the effects of disease upon individuals, families, communities, countries. **E** Recognizes that a concern for wellness motivates individuals and organizations.

CONCEPT 6 — THE FAMILY SERVES TO PERPETUATE MAN AND TO FULFILL CERTAIN HEALTH NEEDS.	CONCEPT 7 — PERSONAL HEALTH PRACTICES ARE AFFECTED BY A COMPLEXITY OF FORCES, OFTEN CONFLICTING.	CONCEPT 8 — UTILIZATION OF HEALTH INFORMATION, PRODUCTS, AND SERVICES IS GUIDED BY VALUES AND PERCEPTIONS.	CONCEPT 9 — USE OF SUBSTANCES THAT MODIFY MOOD AND BEHAVIOR ARISES FROM A VARIETY OF MOTIVATIONS.	CONCEPT 10 — FOOD SELECTION AND EATING PATTERNS ARE DETERMINED BY PHYSICAL, SOCIAL, MENTAL, ECONOMIC, AND CULTURAL FACTORS.
A Describes the role and responsibilities of individuals within the family.	**A** Tells **why** personal health practices affect participation in life activities.	**A** Names familiar people who promote, protect, and maintain health.	**A** Identifies substances commonly used by many individuals in society that modify mood and behavior.	**A** Distinguishes among a wide range of foods.
B Describes how family members contribute to the health of each other.	**B** Identifies practices which affect oral health.	**B** Is aware that there are differences among health products and among health services.	**B** Names ways common mood and behavior modifying substances are used in homes and community.	**B** States reasons for eating a variety of foods.
C Lists similarities and differences between boys and girls in appearance, interests, and activities.	**C** Is aware of the influence of growing and developing on personal health practices.	**C** Identifies various sources of health information.	**C** Is aware that there are differences between alcoholic beverages and other beverages.	**C** Is aware of factors that detract from or enhance eating certain foods.
D Discovers that all living things come from other living things.	**D** Discovers that decision making is involved in personal health practices.	**D** Recognizes that laws and regulations exist to protect the consumer.	**D** Realizes there are differences in family practices and feelings about use of tobacco and of alcoholic beverages.	**D** Identifies ways that types of foods and patterns of eating may be related to different cultures.
A Illustrates relationships within a family that influence the degree of health and happiness of all members.	**A** Discusses **why** guidance is necessary in determining a balance of sleep, rest and activity.	**A** Is aware that emotions, family patterns, and values influence selection and use of health information, products, and services.	**A** Describes the range of substances used by man to modify mood and behavior.	**A** Describes food nutrients and their functions as they relate to health.
B Is aware that families in present day society display a wide range of characteristics.	**B** Distinguishes between practices that promote and those that hinder development of the oral structures.	**B** Compares and contrasts health information, products, and services.	**B** Differentiates among controls on purchase, possession, and use of substances that modify mood and behavior.	**B** Develops acceptable criteria for food selection and patterns for eating.
C Describes personal qualities which affect peer group relationships.	**C** Illustrates ways in which personal choices affect health practices.	**C** Identifies different kinds of medical, dental, and health related specialists and their role in health services.	**C** Illustrates how, when, and where certain mood and behavior modifying substances are used for dietary, ceremonial, social, pain relieving, and other reasons.	**C** Cites examples of social and emotional influences on nutritional behavior.
D Explains body changes which occur during puberty.	**D** Identifies conflicting forces affecting personal health practices.	**D** Cites examples of agencies, groups, laws, and standards that protect the health consumer.	**D** Discusses why certain mood and behavior modifying substances are used rather commonly and others only under special circumstances.	**D** Relates different eating patterns to circumstances of living.
E Is aware of the reproductive process and how life begins.	**E** Illustrates relationships between personal health practices and well-being.	**E** Applies the knowledge that harm can result from self-diagnosis, self-medication, and the unwise use of drugs, medicines, devices, cosmetics, and dietary supplements.		
F Defines heredity and is aware of inherited and acquired characteristics.				

Figure 7–2. Behavioral objectives with concepts. School Health Education Study. (Courtesy of Minnesota Mining and Manufacturing Co., copyright 1970.)

In the State of California guide, *Framework for Health Instruction,* both grade level concepts and behavioral objectives are a part of each of the major health units.

In the School Health Education Study, behavioral objectives were developed for each of the ten concepts. This permits the teacher to focus on certain behaviors during daily classroom activities. Progression in behavioral objectives in the K–3 and 4–6 levels is nicely illustrated in Figure 7–2.*

A careful look at the wording of these traditional objectives, concepts, and behavioral objectives indicates considerable similarity. The real difference, therefore, must lie in *how* the teaching is accomplished. If one does not teach for *decision making,* the usual knowledge will be obtained and little action beyond that will occur. This is exactly why the relevance of utilizing behavioral objectives in the classroom has been a source of debate among educators since 1918 (see Ebel's research in *Selected References*).

Interestingly enough, pupils seem to enjoy focusing on objectives and learning activities that provide a choice of one alternative rather than another. Inquiring and making a decision rather than simply accepting information on a health topic tends to keep one alert. Inquiring about a topic, seeking answers to a problem, and experimenting boosts specific values which are instrumental in decision making. The emphasis is on teaching the valuing process and not specific values. Without such involvement any action would be impulsive.

Competency-Based Programs

In competency-based instruction (CBI), specific skills, knowledge, and behaviors are identified in each major health area in advance of instruction. There is a progression in competencies that the learner must follow. As proficiency is demonstrated, the learner moves ahead and the teacher is free to be a resource person, to observe, and to check, among other things, with a student's peers about his or her advancement in competencies. This is more a method of teaching than a program. However, the establishing of competencies to be achieved is an appropriate curriculum development activity.

Curriculum Scope and Sequence

Curriculum development deals specifically with the scope and sequence of the total program.

The word "scope" is used to define the breadth of the health curriculum. It tells *what* should be taught at all grade levels. The scope is either wide or limited, according to the persistent and identifiable wants and desires of boys and girls. "Sequence," on the other hand, refers to the *when* of the curriculum and determines the grade placement of the health learning experiences. It defines the curriculum vertically, whereas scope defines it horizontally.

---

*Some materials on these pages reproduced by permission of Minnesota Mining and Manufacturing Company, copyright 1970.

Determination of Scope. The basis for the scope of a health course is found in the necessities of life as revealed by close analysis, not by peremptory judgment. *The scope should present as great and as rich a selection of ideas as possible. Teachers then do their own organizing. This is the modern elementary approach of stressing experience rather than subjects.* The better school systems are steadily moving in a direction beyond and above a static course of study and to a wealth of documentary materials based upon the needs of the group.

One who understands children will select, eliminate, and adapt experiences and materials to meet all their needs. The scope of the health curriculum, therefore, is made effective by greatly improving existing courses of study, by following guides to child development, and by using source units or course of study units. The last factor, the unit, is by far the most effective curriculum item. For example, in the health curriculum a very wide variety of learning and materials is organized into areas of experience or in broad fields or within single subjects from which selections may be made. Health may be taught in the broad field of social studies or science, or it may be taught as a separate subject, or both. (It is most effective when taught as a separate subject.) Physical, mental, emotional, and social health embraces so much in the realm of human welfare and behavior that the scope of the health curriculum cannot easily be contained. There are limits, however, to the number and kind of topics that children should be introduced to at any one grade level. And there are obvious limits to the amount of emphasis or concentration afforded a particular topic at a certain grade level.

Determination of Sequence. Sequence is defined in most elementary schools today, but it is not fixed with a rigid order of required topics for each school year. The trend is away from the fixed sequence to the more flexible one.

It cannot be stressed too emphatically that the need for a planned course of instruction is essential for effective health teaching in the elementary school. The chief problem which faces most teachers is not what to teach in the major topical areas, but *how far one should go in the area at specific grade levels.* Answering this question would help eliminate or minimize unnecessary repetition. Unfortunately, in many schools today health teaching is simply a "do-gooder" activity. The teacher, feeling sympathetic to the need for health instruction, decides to do "her bit" for the cause. She frequently teaches a little about the teeth, foods, and how to keep clean. This she does all too often with no knowledge of what her pupils have already received in the way of knowledge from the year before or what they will be getting in the year ahead. Both scope and sequence are foreign terms in such a haphazard setup. A business run in this manner would go bankrupt in six months.

The only sound way to insure proper scope and sequence in health teaching is to set up the essential topical areas of instruction, under which are listed the pupil objectives that should be achieved at each grade level. Until this is done in every elementary school, health teaching will be at best only a "busy work" activity. An excellent way for the new teacher to appreciate the sequential development of health topics is to carefully examine curriculum guides and courses of study. This may be accomplished in a curriculum library of a teacher preparation institution. In this fashion, progressions within an area are observed along with appropriate content, materials, and teaching ideas.

Time Allotment and Scheduling

Health instruction has to become a part of the total elementary school program by being scheduled; any program takes time to carry out. How much time should be spent on the health activities? Should a health curriculum, because of its wide scope, justify a rather large part of the school day? Is it conceivable that some teachers, extremely interested in a topic, might spend 30 to 40 per cent of a week's time on it? Who is to say whether this is right or wrong? Of course the classroom teacher must have a fair sense of value and use good judgment when allotting time to health instruction. Time ratios vary because of pupil factors relating to interests, experiences, and maturity; environmental factors involving facilities and materials; and the overall curriculum plans of the particular school.

Many schools have a planned health curriculum which represents the results of long-term study and research. This curriculum, coupled with state recommendations, may suggest a time allotment. For example, in New York City 10 per cent of the time allotted to primary grades and 15 per cent in the intermediate grades is to be devoted to science and health teaching. The amount of time spent in any one exposure should be flexible, in keeping with the nature of the lesson, and depending on whether it is taught by an individual or a team. In most schools the teaching is carried on by the regular classroom teacher, as indicated in the requirement for the State of New York (see Figure 7-3). However, assigning suitable time for health teaching is still a problem. In a Massachusetts study, for instance, a high percentage of teachers recognized this lack of time as their first problem.

HEALTH EDUCATION IN THE ELEMENTARY SCHOOLS

2. *Health education in the elementary schools.* The elementary school curriculum shall include health education for all pupils. In the kindergarten and primary grades, the health teaching shall be largely done by guiding the children in developing desirable health behavior, attitudes and knowledge through their everyday experiences in a healthful environment. This guidance shall include systematic practice of health habits as needed. In addition to continued health guidance, provision shall be made in the school program of grades 4, 5 and 6 for planned units of teaching which shall include health instruction through which pupils may become increasingly self-reliant in solving their own health problems and those of the group. Health education in the elementary school grades shall be carried on by the regular classroom teachers.

Figure 7-3. Regulations pertaining to health education, State of New York.

Although primary graders have a short span of attention, they do not learn too effectively in very short periods day after day. Periods should be of sufficient length to have meaning, perhaps 15 minutes to half an hour. Several authorities prefer a set daily period for direct health teaching.

Daily classroom programs should also be planned so that different types of activity are scheduled for alternate periods; for example, active work following quiet work, such as project construction following reading, or physical education following arithmetic. There is little reason why classroom topics cannot be shifted around from week to week. Children like variety and innovations and respond very well to them. A health topic may be taught in the middle of the morning one day and just before lunch another day.

HEALTH TEACHING IN THE KINDERGARTEN

The health curriculum for kindergarten children may be quite informal. It is integrated with all other areas of instruction. Health topics are taught "as though you taught them not." The children are physically active, extremely individualistic, very imitative, dramatic, and imaginative. What they use in the way of material is largely manipulative and experimental. What they understand is generally developed through active participation and first-hand experience. Fantasy and reality appear to be the same to many children. The time-space concept is slow to develop.

Kindergarten boys and girls show interest in a number of items related to health. They are:

Gaining confidence in themselves as persons.
Developing better motor coordination.
Speaking and acting spontaneously.
Assuming some responsibilities.
Learning to clean up and put things away.
Becoming observant of sights and sounds.
Becoming aware of the natural environment.
Gaining a number of specific health interests, such as:
Acting quickly and orderly in fire drills.
Practicing safe ways of going to and from school.
Visiting the school physician.
Carrying a clean handkerchief and covering the cough or sneeze.
Eating midmorning food and having a warm noon meal.
Resting between periods.
Having a relaxed atmosphere for classroom work and playground recreation.
Having proper toilet habits and practicing cleanliness.
Eating the right foods and caring for the teeth.

The observant kindergarten teacher will find numerous opportunities for health instruction every hour of the day. There will be times when it seems desirable to create situations which will appear to the pupils quite natural and unplanned. Daily health experiences in a healthful environment do much to build lasting impressions. Moreover, the kindergarten is a period of acculturation for children who have been neglected, "spoiled," or overprotected at home. It is a place for socialization and for getting to know people of one's age and what they are like.

The overall kindergarten curriculum in health varies somewhat the country over. Generally, what happens is pretty much up to the individual teacher. Some of the kindergarten teaching opportunities common to most school situations today follow:

1. Health examinations and tests, including examination of teeth by dental hygiene teacher.
   a. Opportunity to make friends with the physician, nurse, and dental hygiene teachers and other members of the school health services staff.
   b. Opportunity to learn that everyone should have periodic health examinations by physician and dentist to help in keeping well.
2. Early morning checking time.
   a. Opportunity to inspect children, to recognize achievements, and to care for health needs.
3. Weighing and measuring.
   a. Opportunity to arouse interest in growing and gaining weight and in doing things which will maximize children's growth.
4. Mid-session lunch, noon lunch, real and play parties, preparation and tasting of real foods.
   a. Opportunity for practicing washing hands before touching food; sitting down to eat, relaxing, eating slowly, and enjoying lunchtime; eating and liking certain foods; taking small bites, chewing food thoroughly and enjoying its flavor; touching only one's own food; washing and preparing food so that it is clean; discarding food which has been dropped to the floor or ground; table manners.
5. Playground activities.
   a. Opportunity to arouse interest in activities in the sunshine and open air.
   b. Opportunity for fun, getting along happily with playmates, promoting physical development, increasing appetite and enjoyment of food, and maintaining or improving posture.
6. Rest periods.
   a. Opportunity to improve ability to relax and rest.
7. Cleanliness and health protection.
   a. Opportunity to learn desirable practices related to cleanliness of body and clothing, food and eating, use of handkerchief, and protection of self and others when ill.
   b. Opportunity to learn to use toilet, handwashing, and drinking facilities properly.
8. Reading and other close eye work.
   a. Opportunity for learning proper position of books and other materials and adjustments of lights and shades.
9. Cooperation in keeping air in classroom fresh.
   a. Opportunity to help regulate air conditions by notifying cus-

todian or by other appropriate means; to enjoy the feeling of a well-ventilated room; to become aware of the teacher's attention to the thermometer and air conditions.

10. Seating.
    a. Opportunity to learn to select seats, desks, and tables so that the child may work and play in comfort and to change position to meet changing needs.
11. Clothing.
    a. Opportunity to learn to put on and take off outdoor clothing and to care for it properly.
12. The total program.
    a. Opportunity to enjoy and be reasonably successful in work and play, to get along happily with children and adults, and to become increasingly self-reliant in caring for own needs and in helping others.
    b. Opportunity to participate fully in the daily program with decreasing need for adult guidance to the end that the child's own safety and the safety of others will be an important outcome of the program.

Research indicates that normal children of kindergarten age, though young in years, are quite receptive to ideas and are capable of learning many presumably difficult things. Because of the interest span and time factor, selecting what to teach is a necessary consideration. Many studies indicate that information on foods and safety is important. Other research indicates a need for emphasis in health instruction to be greatest in the following health areas:

Rest and sleep (correct bedtime and habit of taking a nap during the day)

Grooming (habit of hanging up clothes)

Growth and development (habit of sitting quietly and listening when others speak)

Prevention and control of disease (acceptance of immunization shots and habits of keeping hands out of mouth, and covering mouth and nose when coughing and sneezing)

The new teacher, with the help of the children, will find it wise to build a series of teaching units covering the several areas of emphasis at the kindergarten level. These may be in skeleton form so that they can easily be amended from year to year with appropriate modification.

Kindergarten Health Charts

One of the most effective health teaching items for the kindergarten-age child is a series of 36 full-color charts (17 inches × 20 inches size).[16] Each chart presents a basic health concept in pictures—a method of learning most appealing to and effective with youngsters of this age level. People, young and old, are portrayed in familiar situations stressing fundamental health and safety practices *with which children can identify.*

---

[16]Gallagher, J. Roswell, Spencer, Mary E., and Willgoose, Carl E. *Health Charts for Kindergarten (How About You?).* Boston: Ginn and Co., 1965. A *Teachers' Manual,* offering detailed suggestions for presenting the pictures, is included with the charts.

Figure 7–4. Kindergarten health chart. (With the permission of Ginn and Co., Boston, Mass. 02217.)

Teachers show these large charts (with spiral binding and easel-back for convenient viewing) to their class in order to provoke discussion relative to personal health practices. Figure 7–4 is a greatly reduced picture of chart No. 11 entitled *Warm and Dry?* In this particular illustration, the teacher might begin the lesson by showing the chart and asking: "How do you know that it is a rainy, cold day? Do you think the children in the picture are wet or cold? Why not? Do you think the dog is cold? He certainly is wet. Why do you think this picture is called *Warm and Dry?*"

HEALTH TEACHING IN THE PRIMARY GRADES

The health curriculum for the first three grades is one in which the pupil is not held responsible for a great amount of specific health knowledge. Children may engage in a large number of experiences, but informality continues as it did in the kindergarten. The approach is one of definite exploration of the important health practices. There will be opportunities for integration of the health instructional program with social studies, science, and physical education.

Since growth is a continuous process, there will be varying degrees of maturity, capacities, and interests among primary grade pupils. Where first graders are beginning to differentiate between fancy and reality, third graders will have pretty much established this differentiation. As children mature during the primary years, they gain in ability to present their own ideas and problems orally and in writing. They gradually begin to appreciate cause and effect relationships, project their feelings more and more toward others, become less individualistic and possessive, and are more cognizant of adult opinion. Growth is slow and steady; they continue to tire less as they approach eight years of age, and show an increase in physical strength and dexterity.

Primary children show interest in a number of items related to health. They are:

Beginning to show some muscle growth

Advancing to a state of full visual fusion

Watching the first permanent teeth appear

Accepting greater responsibility for personal safety and appearance

Talking about nourishing food, going to bed early, playing out of doors, and brushing teeth

Choosing lunch foods wisely

Practicing good sportsmanship

Aware of defective sight and hearing

Concerned with minor cuts and bruises

Curious about disease prevention

Beginning to develop some group responsibility, and are adjusting quite well to school.

The primary grade curriculum in health is designed to help children solve a number of health problems of the moment. This curriculum is presented not in great detail but in the manner of an orientation so that a firm foundation may be laid for the more ad-

Figure 7–5. A "surprise" activity stimulates everyone. (Courtesy National Education Association and Joe Di Dio.)

vanced curriculum content in the intermediate grades. The big teaching task is to arouse curiosity, promote questions, and lead pupils to express their thoughts (see Figure 7–5).

The teaching areas common to most primary school situations may be seen by reviewing current courses of study. Opinions of health curriculum specialists are also valuable. In the Massachusetts health education study it was found that the popular primary level topics were accident prevention, cleanliness and grooming, dental health, and rest and sleep.[17] Two additional examples of content areas follow:

ANDERSON AND CRESWELL[18]
Physical Health
- Personal and school cleanliness
- Rest and sleep
- Eating practices
- Posture
- Play practices
- Dental health
- Lighting
- Common cold
- Safety to and from school
- Schoolroom safety
- Playground safety
- Home safety
- Body growth

Mental Health
- Sharing
- Working together
- Kindness
- Being friendly
- Orderliness

- Depending on ourselves
- Attaining goals
Community Health
- Home life
- Sources of water and milk
- Sunshine and health

STATE OF ILLINOIS[19]
- Consumer health education
- Dental health education
- Drug use and abuse*
- Human ecology and health
- Human growth and development†
- Mental health and illness†
- Nutrition†
- Personal health
- Prevention and control of disease
- Public and environmental health
- Safety education and disaster survival*
- Smoking and disease

*Mandated instruction for primary and intermediate grades.
†Third grade emphasis.

HEALTH TEACHING IN THE INTERMEDIATE GRADES

The health curriculum for fourth, fifth, and sixth grade pupils is one that builds on what has already been taught in the first three grades. There is greater depth in subject matter and a little more formality than in the primary grades. *The sole reason for this change is that the pupils are ready for more detail.* Now their curiosity is

[17]Massachusetts Department of Education. *Health Education in Massachusetts Public Schools: A Summary Report.* Boston: Department of Education, 182 Tremont Street. August 1971, p. 20.

[18]Anderson, C. L. and Creswell, William H., Jr. *School Health Practice.* 5th ed., St. Louis: C. V. Mosby Co., 1976.

[19]Part of a comprehensive health education program for Illinois elementary schools. Developed in part by Thomas M. Janeway and W. H. Creswell, Jr. (1973).

aroused and they ask searching questions having more to do with the exception rather than the rule. They want to know, for example, why some man or woman of their acquaintance who never uses a toothbrush and eats haphazardly has such fine white teeth.

This is the age when the questions asked are often a real challenge to the teacher. It is a period in the growth of the 9, 10, and 11 year olds when there is a magnetic "awakening" to all that goes on around them. There is an adventurous spirit demonstrated by a willingness to try anything once, to look here and there, and to explore eagerly. There is a heightened interest in science and machines—how bugs walk, what germs look like under the microscope, how the skeletal muscles hold up the body, and the effect a trip to the craters of the moon has on a person in a rocket. Here is a time when dreamers begin to look ahead and imaginative minds are literally "on fire." Health stories of adventure, mystery, travel, science, sports, animal life, and nature go over big.

In addition to placing greater emphasis on the fundamental topics of the primary grade curriculum, there is a need for special instruction in alcohol and narcotics. By the fifth and sixth grade period a number of pupils, boys in particular, have a desire to try a cigarette or taste alcoholic beverages. Both of these items are readily available in many homes today. This is the age when the "gang" develops, and boys and girls begin to conform to the wishes of the group. The ten or eleven year old shows an increase in self-direction and responsibility. The "wise guy" has a cocky walk and the rounded shoulders of the "man about town." He is seen all too often a block from school flicking the ashes from his cigarette as he heads for home. He is ready for a realistic picture of smoking directly from a classroom discussion.

Antagonism between the sexes grows and becomes acute by the sixth grade. Boys are interested in boys; girls in girls. Both profit from instruction pertaining to family relationships. Although sex education really begins at home, little is said about it in most cases. It should be integrated with the total health education program at all grade levels. It should not be singled out for separate or undue emphasis. In back of the 11 year old pupil's sex antagonism is a smoldering interest in the subject. This is evidenced by the previously referred to Connecticut report, *Teach Us What We Want To Know*. Sex education should be taught without apology by showing its positive aspects in terms of creative drive and family happiness.

A list of major health topics for the intermediate grades can be compiled by viewing the listings of local schools and state education departments. Reports of professional organizations and independent research studies are sometimes helpful. A notable state that has developed and updated health curriculum guidelines and courses of study is New York. It shares top honors with Pennsylvania, Oregon, Washington, and California. The New York curriculum was thoroughly researched and set up for grade levels in five strands (see Figure 7–6): physical health, sociological health problems, mental health, environmental and community health, and education for survival. An examination of the strands indicates where the major

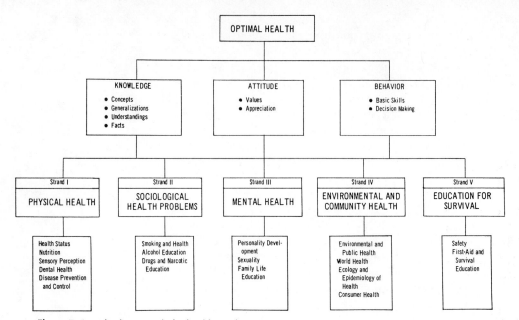

Figure 7-6. The five strands for health teaching. (Courtesy New York State Education Department.)

subtopics fall. It may be seen that when there is planning for a full program there is opportunity for wide coverage of health problems and concerns. This does not occur in all states. For instance, in the previously mentioned report, *Health Education in Massachusetts Public Schools,* it was pointed out that there were omissions in the elementary grades in such areas as sex education and family living, venereal diseases, foot care, alcohol education, and noncommunicable diseases. It was concluded that the updating of present health education programs had not kept pace with revisions in other subject matter areas. Moreover, there was too much emphasis on cleanliness and grooming from kindergarten through grade eight, with too much repetition relative to dental health, sleep, and rest. It was also found that topics such as smoking, alcohol, drugs, and family living were being held off until grade eight instead of being started by grade five at the latest. The Massachusetts guide is similar to New York's.

MASSACHUSETTS DEPARTMENT OF EDUCATION
Area I *Physical Health*
    Body Structure and Function
    Cleanliness and Appearance
    Dental Health
    Fitness and Body Dynamics
    Nutrition
    Diseases and Disorders
    Sensory Perception
    Sleep, Rest, Relaxation
Area II *Mental and Social Health*
    Drugs, Alcohol, and Tobacco

    Emotional Development
    Sexuality and Family Life
Area III *Consumer and Environmental Health*
    Ecology
    Health Careers
    Community and World Health
    Consumer Health
Area IV *Safe Living*
    First Aid and Emergencies
    Safety and Accident Prevention

What makes the scope-establishing task so difficult at any grade level is the great increase in the number of health topics over the years. Twenty years ago Oliver Byrd listed 20 major topics with a number of significant subtopics. Since that time topical emphasis has changed. Recently, Hardt came up with 370 subtopics under Byrd's original 20 major health topics.[20] The task of providing responsible coverage for each of these in the school program could be overwhelming.

THE GRADUATED PROGRAM OF MAJOR HEALTH TOPICS

In view of recent curriculum research, it seems that the most appropriate health instruction curriculum for elementary school children is one that is spelled out in much more detail than were the usual programs of the past. This means that teachers must work together and carefully plan for both scope and sequence in health teaching. The major health topics or health areas for each grade level have to be established along with a *graduated* list of knowledge and understandings (or concepts and competencies) to be achieved by pupils. This task requires the combined deliberations of several top teachers, frequently under the leadership of the elementary curriculum specialist and the health education coordinator for the school system.

In order to insure a graduated program under each major health topic, *all of the desirable knowledge, understandings, and behaviors should be recorded for all six elementary grades.* This extensive list is then reviewed and arranged in such a manner as to place the easier-to-learn items first and the difficult-to-learn items last. It is then carefully divided into six divisions according to grade level with the more detailed knowledge and understandings falling at the fourth, fifth, and sixth grades. This kind of order prevents important topics from being omitted and other topics from being taught at an inappropriate time.

The *major health topics* for the elementary school as determined for this text are as follows: (P-Primary Grades; I-Intermediate Grades)
1. Personal cleanliness and appearance (P, I)
2. Physical activity, sleep, rest, and relaxation (P, I)
3. Nutrition and growth (P, I)
4. Dental health (P, I)
5. Body structure and operation (P, I)
6. Prevention and control of disease (P, I)
7. Safety and first aid (P, I)
8. Mental health (P, I)
9. Sex and family living education (P, I)
10. Environmental health (P, I)
11. Tobacco, alcohol, and drugs (I)
12. Consumer health (I)

---

[20]Hardt, Dale V. "Health Curriculum: 370 topics," *Journal of School Health, 48*: 656–660, January 1978.

Notice that the topics of Tobacco, alcohol, and drugs (No. 11) and Consumer health (No. 12) are introduced at the intermediate level. Notice also that health careers and international health are not included. They are reserved for the early secondary period.

It should be pointed out that planning for the first six grades must be done in terms of future junior and senior high school programming. In the earlier dental health example, it is obvious that more technical knowledge and understanding is not called for here, but with this foundation the student is prepared for more detailed study in grade seven or eight. Moreover, a detailed structuring of knowledge, understandings, or competencies should be included in the finished curriculum guide or course of study.

ORGANIZING MAJOR HEALTH TOPICS

How does one organize the major health topics in the instructional program from grades one to six? Is each topic referred to each year? Is there a danger of too much repetition on a yearly basis? Is there merit in a cycle plan in which certain topics are omitted or simply reviewed every other year?

Certainly it has been the custom to have a considerable spread of information through the grades rather than a concentration at certain grade levels. Each major health topic has been taught at each grade level rather than being omitted at any grade level. Sometimes this insures healthy repetition and frequently acquaints the pupil with something that may have been missed the year before, especially in schools that do not follow a planned health instruction curriculum.

It is common knowledge that it is extremely difficult to keep from repeating too often what is said in the second grade to the children in the third grade. Health teaching may be more effective when there is a concentration of instruction on certain health topics on an every-other-year basis instead of spreading a limited amount through each of six or eight grades. Where the *total* elementary school health instruction program has been carefully planned there may be value in such a cycle plan.

In the Brookline, Massachusetts schools, health programs are maximized at certain key grade levels—kindergarten, four, five, and eight. Although other grades are partially ignored, there appears to be a "spin off" and spread effect from one grade to another. Also, the feeling is that it is better to do an outstanding job at key developmental points in a child's life than to offer a number of shallow programs every year over the years.

The cycle chosen may vary slightly for each major health topic. Almost all topics should be introduced in the first grade. It may be wise to introduce "nutrition and growth" to first and second grades, skip the third, and continue in four and six. The same thing may be true of "safety." Obviously, there is much safety teaching to accomplish right away in the first three grades. Here, one might skip the fifth grade and proceed to the sixth. There is so much to cover in

Summary of Topics by Grades

	1	2	3	4	5	6
Nutrition and growth	x	x	R*	x	R	x
Personal cleanliness and appearance	x	R	x	R	x	R
Dental health	x	x	R	x	R	x
Accidents and safety	x	x	x	x	R	x
Mental health	x	R	x	R	x	R
Sex and family living education	x	R	x	R	x	R
Body structure and function	x	x	x	x	x	x
Disease control	x	R	x	R	x	R
Environmental health	x	x	R	x	R	x
Physical activity, sleep, rest, relaxation	x	x	x	x	R	x
Tobacco, alcohol, and drugs					x	x
Consumer health			x	R	x	R

*R = Review year (brief treatment of topic).

"body structure and function" that the topic might be spread through all six grades. In the planning stage, a chart would be constructed to reflect the organization.

This cycle plan seeks to get away from needless repetition, which all too often is deadly, because it smothers curiosity and kills the interest of boys and girls. Frequently children are bored with lessons on such subjects as brushing the teeth, or standing tall, or something similar; they see nothing new, fresh, and stimulating. Much of this may be prevented when the major health topics are thoroughly covered on the "on" year and very simply reviewed on the "off" year.

UNIT TEACHING IN HEALTH

One of the most popular and often misused terms in education circles today is the "unit." Teachers loosely use the word *unit* to refer to a topic, an outline, a block of subject matter, a project, and even a chapter in a textbook. They divide and subdivide units at random and according to their own particular system of classification of instructional materials.

Most writers agree that a unit, whether for the teacher or the student, represents an organization of activities and information designed to develop useful understandings, appreciations, and practices which will contribute favorably to educational goals. Ragan and Shepherd say:

"When this method is used, learning takes place through a great variety of activities; activities are unified around a central theme, problem or purpose . . .; and the teacher serves as a leader rather than as a task-master."[21]

[21]Ragan, William B. and Shepherd, Gene D. *Modern Elementary Curriculum.* New York: Holt, Rinehart & Winston, Inc., 1971, p. 190.

If a health unit stays within these definitions, one can hardly question its value. It begins with the health needs and interests of children who, with the help of the teacher, create and arrange an environment out of which will grow the purpose and enthusiasm for the work to be undertaken. Health units cut across subject matter lines, thereby providing for integration. They furnish "grassroot" or first-hand experiences, and satisfy a number of innate drives to be active, to create, to dramatize, to communicate, and to construct. Lifelike opportunities in which the pupil may build something, experiment, read, share, interview, and express ideas in various media are important parts of the units. The health unit centers on the present but stimulates an interest in future living. Early in its progression, it encourages pupil discovery. Meaning is given to factual material when a unit requires problem solving. Democratic group living is encouraged as desirable social habits are developed while children work on committees and in groups. Moreover, unit teaching stimulates critical thinking. It is rich in opportunities for children with varying degrees of ability and capacity to work along with others toward the success of the unit.

The Teacher's Resource Unit

A resource unit is simply a collection of suggested learning activities and materials organized around some central theme or given topic to be used by the teacher in preplanning. Often a resource unit in health is the product of a committee of teachers pooling their best ideas and then assigning to one teacher the responsibility of organizing the materials and to another the final writing. School nurses, dental hygienists, and even physicians may sit in and help with the unit. These units need not be complex or involved. They may be developed locally or at the state level. In either case they are not units of instruction but are chiefly collections of ideas and materials which may be helpful to an individual teacher in planning work for the class.

It is worth repeating that the resource unit, no matter how complete, is not a teaching unit; it is strictly an aid to help the teacher and students in planning a teaching unit. It usually is organized with a title and grade level designation, an introductory statement, a statement of proposed objectives, a content guide, suggested pupil activities, a list of teaching aids—books, pamphlets, music records, and films—and suggested evaluation procedures.

Resource units in health may be built for a separate health course. Sometimes they are built to fit a broad-fields or core curriculum. They contribute to the core of a curriculum built around social living or science, and are sometimes thought of as units where there is a fusion of subject matter as part of the *integrating* experience which the unit provides. Certainly integration is desirable in health teaching. Children do not put knowledge in categories and classify it the way scholars do; life situations seldom fall within these artificial boundaries. The specialist in health education can be very helpful here in assisting core teachers. A number of classroom teachers will want to turn to the health educator for professional help in setting up units complete with problems to be studied, bibliographies for both pupils and teachers, and suggestions for school and community activities.

The Health Teaching Unit

The essential difference between a teacher's resource unit and a teaching unit involves purposes. The purpose of a resource unit is to give the teacher a well fortified background in a particular area of study. In the teaching unit the organization is in terms of a given class. It is not nearly as broad and inclusive as the resource unit; it includes only those activities, materials, and evaluation techniques that will actually be used. Thus it is quite realistic and practical in both terms of time available and the nature of the learner. Where a number of stories, films, and suggested activities appear in the resource unit, in the teaching unit the second grade teacher might read only one story, carry out two projects, and show one film.

Some planning of a teaching unit has to be done by the teacher in advance of meeting the class. Then the pupils are given a chance to select activities. They may examine or be given a choice of activities that appear in the resource unit. Those that seem to arouse enthusiasm may be selected for the teaching unit. This unit is then ready to implement. When pupils share in the planning of their own work in health, they have greater retention of what they learn. Activities tend to be vital and are more apt to promote new health habits and appreciations. This is modern education at its best.

There is a difference in emphasis in health teaching between the primary and intermediate grades which influences the building of the teaching unit. Health education in the primary grades is centered on helping children to live healthfully at home and at school. Much health is taught incidentally, indirectly, and informally in an effort to convey elementary health concepts and simple health practices. It would be very easy, therefore, for the teacher to "overorganize" the teaching unit in the kindergarten and first three grades. A few "tried and proven" ideas or activities may well make up the major part of the unit. Obviously, during the planning stages of a unit, children come up with suggestions that are both excellent and impracticable. Through proper manipulation of the planning session, the teacher guides the boys and girls into agreeing on the better suggestions. Evidence abounds in the primary grades to show that young, creative, and dramatic minds have imaginations that at times run wild. Gently curbing this wonderful quality, without at the same time reducing enthusiasm, is what makes teaching an art as well as a challenging profession.

Health teaching in the intermediate grades tends to be more specific, more formal, and generally planned in relation to broad areas of experience. Teaching units, therefore, are often constructed as subunits or integrated units of the broader field. Although they should not attempt to cover too much material in any one health area, nevertheless it is difficult sometimes to strictly limit them. This is because health, in its fullest meaning, relates to physical, mental, emotional and social welfare. Practically everything that affects humans may in some large or small way be connected to health teaching.

Organization of Health Teaching Units

There are a number of ways to organize the teaching unit. Basically it needs some kind of introduction followed by objectives, a main body of activities, source materials, and finally some reference to evaluation.

Teaching units are generally organized along specific lines. This crystallizes the thinking of teachers and pupils. Klausmeier and Dresden use the same form that was employed in the resource unit. Various writers and educational groups have their differences and similarities in unit arrangements, but the similarities seem to outweigh the differences.

As a rule, the following outline is satisfactory for the development of teaching units for the major health topics:

1. Title
2. Introductory statement
3. Concepts and behavioral objectives
4. Outline of content (primary level) (intermediate level)
5. Suggested learning activities
6. Resource aids and materials
7. Evaluation techniques
8. Student and teacher references

An example of an especially detailed presentation dealing with a major health topic is taken from the guide of the New York State Education Department.[22] The strands and topics have already been mentioned (see Figure 7–6).

| Strand V |
| Education for Survival |
| Safety First Aid and Survival Education |
| GRADES 4–6 |

[22]The State Education Department Strand V *Education For Survival (First Aid and Survival Education)*, Grades 4–6, Albany, New York: The State Education Department, 1971.

Some 250 school districts in 30 states, as well as schools in England and Israel, have been involved in preparing teachers to work with their students by employing an *in-depth unit approach* to the health curriculum. What began in 1967 as the Berkeley model, under the administration of the National Clearinghouse for Smoking and Health, is now referred to as the School Health Curriculum Project and is under the leadership of the Bureau of Health Education at the Center for Disease Control in Atlanta.

Each grade unit extends over eight to ten weeks' time and is organized around the structure, functioning, interactions, and care of a *body system*. Energy, nutrition, and the digestive system are covered in the fourth grade, the lungs and the respiratory system in the fifth grade, the heart and the circulatory system in the sixth, and the brain and nervous system in the seventh.

Each unit follows the same pattern of phases:

1. An *introduction* to pique curiosity, acquaint pupils with the methods, and assure that they are aware of the importance of the study to be undertaken.
2. An *overview* of body systems and their relationships to the function of the whole being.
   a. structure and functions of the particular system under study
   b. diseases and conditions to which the system is subject
   c. what the individual, community, and society can do to prevent problems
3. A *culminating* phase that reviews and gives the students an opportunity to realign their thinking and share with parents and others what they have learned.

The objectives of the model are reached by multi-level, multi-media, and multi-methodological approaches. By employing a variety of teaching methods and aids to learning, the approach to health education is refreshing to both teachers and children. Longitudinal studies are needed to determine the effectiveness of this model over a period of time. Heit finds, however, that a number of positive attitudes have emerged.[23]

The success of the program depends upon the special training of teachers. An intensive 60-hour workshop is conducted over a three-year period to acquaint three different grade-level teams from the same school or district with the model. Besides an introduction and culmination preparatory program, the teachers study each unit in terms of five distinct phases. Phase 1 focuses on *awareness,* phase 2 on *appreciation,* phase 3 on *structure and function,* phase 4 on *diseases and disorders,* and phase 5 on *prevention.* The presence of both financial and administrative support has much to do with the effectiveness of this unique health instruction program. At least one appraisal instrument, Cook's Sixth Grade Knowledge Test for the cardiovascular system, has resulted from the project.[24]

---

[23]Heit, Phil. "The Berkeley Model," *Health Education,* 8:2–5, January/February 1977.

[24]Cook, Ron J. *Sixth Grade Knowledge Test (Cardiovascular),* University of Wisconsin, Quant Gymnasium, Stevens Point, Wisconsin 54481.

Outline of Content	Major Understandings and Fundamental Concepts	Suggested Teaching Aids and Learning Activities	Supplementary Information for Teachers
I. Introduction to First Aid	First aid involves immediate temporary care and not treatment.	What is first aid? What is the difference between first aid and treatment?	
A. Definition	First aid is the immediate and temporary care given to an injured or sick person until the services of a physician can be obtained.		
B. Values of first aid training	Having knowledge of first aid will give students a feeling of some competency to care for themselves and others and will serve to make them aware of preventable safety problems.		Pupils can care for their own injuries and the injuries of others. They are helped to improve their safety consciousness which aids in the prevention of accidents. First aid can be extremely valuable during catastrophes such as wars, floods, hurricanes, earthquakes, and tornadoes.
C. General procedures to follow in first aid emergencies	The first aider should function in a logical and systematized way rather than in a state of panic and disorganization. Learn the meaning of panic.	Describe several accident situations and discuss with pupils the general first aid procedures that should be followed in each case. Example: A man has just been hit by a car. He is lying in the street and a large crowd is beginning to form around him. As a first aider, what would you do to help this man? Point out that securing necessary help is vital. Call for professional help as soon as possible. Show McGraw-Hill film *Your Responsibilities in First Aid*. An introductory film also may be shown, such as the American Red Cross films *Checking for Injuries* and *The How and Why of First Aid*.	Factors that should be considered include: determining the victim's injuries; determining what injuries should be dealt with first; getting the victim's name and address; carrying out the determined procedures; securing necessary help; protecting victim from further harm; psychological reassurance for the victim; dealing with external factors of weather, traffic, crowds, etc. The following bibliographical sources may be checked for further information: Cole, pp. 1–16, and Henderson, pp. 34–56

SIGNIFICANT HEALTH CURRICULUM TRENDS

If there is any one overall trend in health curriculum planning, it is to teach health through a variety of experiences in a broad and flexible program. A list of other trends follows.

1. The health curriculum is not limited to the activity and four walls of the classroom. It moves about the building. Primary grade children discuss playground accidents out where

Outline of Content	Major Understandings and Fundamental Concepts	Suggested Teaching Aids and Learning Activities	Supplementary Information for Teachers
		Discuss the consequences that might occur if it were proven that a first aider did something that further injured the victim.	It is best to summon medical help immediately and keep the victim comfortable.
		Panic can be worse than or as bad as an injury. Keep yourself and the injured person calm. Encourage others to do the same. Discuss possible injurious results of panic. Act out in simple skits.	A first aider might find himself in a lawsuit if he negligently and carelessly administered first aid which resulted in injuries or aggravation of the original injury.
		If an injured person is found unconscious keep him lying on his side so that his tongue does not fall back in his mouth to choke him.	See bibliography: Gold and Gold: "First Aid and Legal Responsibility."
D. First aid kits and materials	First aid kits *should* be available in situations where accidents are likely to occur. Very often the first aider must improvise with available materials.	Have several kits available to show to pupils. Show and discuss the contents of each kit. Have pupils report on first aid supplies they have in their homes. Have the pupils make first aid kits for the home and car, and one for camping trips. Wooden boxes 8″ × 5″ × 2″ may be constructed to house these kits. Make a list of possible kit items and discuss this list with your school's nurse-teacher. Discuss materials that might be available when there is no first aid kit for supplies.	Contents of kits usually include adhesive compresses, bandage compresses, plain gauze pads, gauze roller bandages, eye dressing packets, plain absorbent cotton, triangular bandages, tweezers, scissors, antiseptic soap, aspirin, elastic bandage 3″ wide, and safety pins.
II. Wounds and the Control of Minor Bleeding		It is vital to keep wounds clean. Wash with soap and water if possible.	First aid for wounds varies according to the nature and possible results of each.

(This is only the first part of the guide—pages 1–3, out of 39 pages.)

they might occur. Sixth graders visit the local sanitation department and talk with restaurant owners about food handling and dishwashing practices. The health curriculum is practical.

2. There is increasing emphasis on the manner in which principles and objectives influence the curriculum.
3. The health curriculum is being revised continually by classroom teachers working together with health services per-

sonnel, supervisors, and parents. Health needs change, and teachers are becoming more flexible in their teaching. They are more alert to the values of cooperative planning for health.

4. Health in the school is integrated with health in the community through the curriculum and teaching methods. Elementary teachers are learning more about their community health programs and agencies that can enrich their own health instruction.

5. Provision is being made in more schools for formal, direct teaching of health in the elementary curriculum.

6. Health curriculum aids, such as bulletins, courses of study, and the state syllabus, are considered only as suggested guides for the teacher. The teacher must be sufficiently oriented to the modern elementary school purposes and instructional methods to be able to choose wisely those activities best adapted to the health learning situation in his or her classroom.

7. Because of the impact of advertising and quackery, a sharper evaluation is being made of health services and products.

8. The school nurse is more than ever an important member of the school health teaching team.

9. Sex and Family Living Education is being introduced in more elementary school health education programs.

10. There is slowly emerging a unified approach to health teaching in which all major health topics are properly considered instead of singling out one or two urgent topics (such as drugs and smoking) for special attention. There are fewer "one shot" assembly programs as token gestures of a health education program.

As indicated in a national committee report, elementary schools desperately need a school health coordinator, a designated, interested, and well-qualified faculty member who is responsible for the efficient operation of the health education program.

Team Teaching

A number of approaches are being tried to define the functions of the elementary school teacher. One of these which has had an early success in Davidson County, Tennessee, and Lexington, Massachusetts, is *team teaching*. Here, an instructional team, free from the record-keeping clerical duties, teaches children in large or small groups or individually according to the nature of the subject matter. This arrangement, for example, makes it possible for all sections of an entire third grade to assemble for one type of lesson such as a superb film, a special lecture, or a speech by an outstanding resource person. Classroom teachers especially interested and talented in a phase of health may handle certain parts of the instructional program while others are free to develop new teaching materials or work with individual pupils.

The health curriculum lends itself to this kind of teaching. Although the large group will meet, often to introduce a unit of work, it is the medium-size group in which the bulk of the teaching is regularly done, so that teachers can have a continuing relationship with the same children over a period of time. The small group is especially valuable for carrying out vital discussions of health problems of interest to the age group. Also, there is ample room for individual tutoring within the school.

Non-graded Classes

A number of large school systems are currently using a non-graded sequence in at least some elementary schools. In this arrangement grade levels are removed from some or all classes, and the children who would normally be in these classes are placed in the non-graded sequence. This occurs mostly in the primary grades. Each pupil works according to his or her ability—beginning the new school year where he or she left off the year before.

Those who favor this organization point out that the pressure is off the pupils and material is better understood. There is also an opportunity for more continuity in learning experiences. One of the limitations of non-graded plans is the burden on the teacher to follow individual pupil progress. Another limitation has to do with parents who need much help to understand and work with the plan.

Because of the built-in flexibility, the non-graded class seems to be a good place to try new ideas that may make health education more dynamic. Micro-unit work is an example. This is a technique of weaving (integrating) health education content into a topic the students are already studying. For example, disease rates can be integrated with arithmetic, and nutrition can be worked into the social studies unit dealing with cultures in other lands. The micro-unit has been very well received in the Novato, California elementary schools. Four units: "The Waves Rolled and the Ship Creaked—Health Conditions on the Mayflower"; "Puritan Land of Plenty—Food and Medicine in Colonial America"; "Sugar and Spice and the F.D.A."; and "Into the Valley of Death—The State of Medicine at Valley Forge" were highly successful.[25]

Alternative Schools

In an effort to get away from the stultifying climate of so many public schools, close to 1000 "alternative" schools have been born. In addition to these, many alternative programs and alternative paths have been established in traditional schools. Founders of such alternative programs, influenced greatly by the writings of Kozol, Holt, Glasser and others, seek an education for children that is unregimented, alive with flexible teachers, and a fertile climate for learning because of sympathetic administrators. Teaching groups are small,

---

[25]Feldstein, M. and Swabb, L. "The Use of the Micro-Unit in Health Education," *Journal of School Health*, 42:105–107, February 1972.

and what is taught appears unconventional only because it does not take the usual subject matter form.

The key element in the alternatives concept is process rather than product. The specific activities and outlets are secondary. Of primary importance is the process that takes place within the individual of exploring and searching for ways to satisfy inner needs. The secret of success in such programs is in providing multiple options. Numerous educators feel that the well-managed public school should provide these options—and in each school building at every educational level. In short, alternative ways to educate should be available everywhere in public education—programmed learning, Montessori classrooms, community-oriented projects, non-graded sections, multi-cultural arrangements, etc.—to supplement and complement traditional models. Especially important is the need to evaluate alternative efforts to determine how effective learner-controlled activities really are. Do certain students cope with their society any better than they might have in the traditional program? Fantini believes they do.[26]

Compensatory Education

The health problems of the disadvantaged are such that education for them should be different—not so much in terms of subject content, but in terms of teaching emphasis. In their writings, Gentry, Jones, and others make it clear that because there are disadvantaged and culturally handicapped children, a variety of misdirected programs have been created to get at the problem, based primarily on the proposition that ghetto children need "compensatory," "special," "catch-up," "head start" programs.[27] The authors claim that the assumption that compensatory education will clear up the difficulties is a myth. This thinking leads to *lowered expectations* and thereby results in lower educational successes. Children of blacks and other minority groups and the poor are shortchanged because less is expected of them as "disadvantaged" people. What is really needed is a teaching approach that is as vigorous as it would be with so-called normal children and void of defeatist attitudes. There would be no need for compensatory types of education if health and other learning experiences would be personalized and individualized and middle class values would not be applied somewhat abruptly to lower class children and youth.

Differentiated Staffing

Instead of having groups of children assigned to a teacher in a traditional way, a "differentiated staff" is formed where there might be 160 children in a class with two senior teachers, two staff teachers,

[26]Fantini, Mario. "Alternatives in the Public School," in L. Golubchick and B. Persky, *Innovations in Education*. Dubuque: Kendall/Hunt Publishing Co., 1975, pp. 90–93.

[27]Gentry, Altron, Jones, Byrd, et al. *Urban Education: The Hope Factor.* Philadelphia: W. B. Saunders Company, 1972, pp. 12–14.

and four teaching assistants or aides. It is a team teaching effort which attempts to accommodate the many learning styles of children with different instructional approaches. The teacher becomes an "instructional manager" and resource person, and not a "giver of directions." From a health curriculum viewpoint, there is hardly a limit to what might be planned for pupils of various backgrounds and needs. Differentiated staffing anticipates the introduction of new personnel into the instructional process. Resource people from the health professions and health-related areas of the community are worked into programs in a meaningful way. Currently, there is little to report relative to the successes of differentiated staffing in advancing understandings and practices relating to health education. However, if this type of teaching offers pupils a chance to become less bored, less frustrated, and less turned off to school, then it is contributing to sound mental health and deserves more attention.

THE SCHOOL LUNCH PROGRAM

In many schools today a special and somewhat formal effort is made to improve the nutritional status of children, while at the same time increasing their knowledge and appreciation of foods, through the school lunch program.

In 1946 Congress enacted the National School Lunch Program as a "measure for national security, to safeguard the health and well-being of the nation's children, and to encourage the domestic consumption of nutritious agricultural commodities and other foods." The program was amended in late 1970 to put more emphasis on school feeding of children from identified poor families. This program is carried on today on a nonprofit basis without physical segregation or other discriminations by the school against any child because of inability to pay the full cost or any part of the cost of the meals.

A school plan with such worthy objectives as these certainly cannot go unnoticed as a means of further implementing the health instruction program. One cannot dismiss the educational implications of an activity that serves over two billion lunches to millions of children. Surveys, however, indicate that school personnel are not capitalizing on the opportunities inherent in the school lunch program and little is said about the school lunchroom as a learning laboratory.

The school lunchroom offers a place to teach diet and food practices in their natural setting, making the lunch program an educational operation rather than a business function. Here, boys and girls may learn to be self-sufficient, to make decisions, and to spend their money wisely. There are meals to plan and serve, sanitation to be considered, and numerous chances to promote climates favorable to appetite, to growth, and to mental-emotional health. There are few total school activities so conducive to a practical, down-to-earth kind of teaching as that afforded by the school lunch operation. This is a real-life situation where the teacher can find in a single lunchroom an assortment of eating patterns—from the plate lunch to the à la carte lunch; from the home lunch supplemented with school lunch items to the all too typical lunch with the weak combination of a jelly sandwich and a piece of cake.

Beginning in the primary grade classroom with the study of foods, the teacher encourages the class to share their thoughts relative to school lunch menu planning. The planning, especially in the third grade and above, may begin with a school survey of current dietary practices or a study of the components of a well-balanced lunch as a part of the total daily diet. Other ideas include the following:

Discussions may be directed toward overcoming food dislikes. Foods left on the trays may provide a basis for such a study.

New foods may be accompanied by a class discussion on the values of the foods and ways of acquiring a taste for them.

Assisting with the serving of lunches gives pupils a first-hand opportunity to learn about proper sanitary practices.

Help in the preparation of food and cleaning up the lunchroom after the meal may be arranged. Where this is done, pupils should be rotated so that all have an equal chance.

Survey the school lunch facilities and consider ways of improving them.

Observe the social graces. Take turns as hosts and hostesses. This is a social hour for pupils and teachers. It is pleasant and enjoyable—a tonic to learning.

Where proper studies have been conducted, the school lunch has proved to be an effective medium for developing good eating practices which have been sustained throughout the school year. However, the nutritional status of children on school feeding programs does not always improve. This lack of success is attributed to high rates of absenteeism among nutritionally disadvantaged children, incomplete consumption of lunch, and poor nutritional reinforcement at home.

Perhaps the biggest difficulty in the school lunch program has been with the children who bring lunches from home. Many schools and homes have cooperated to improve the home-packed lunch. In Petaluma, California, for example, the school health council and local PTA established the nature of the problem through a city-wide survey, cooperatively prepared a *Guide to Home-Packed School Lunches*, and took steps to revise the health curriculum to integrate this nutrition work into the classroom situation.

In Long Beach, New York, a very complete booklet entitled *For Your Children at Lunchtime* was developed by the PTA for parents. The school health council and classroom teachers assisted.

QUESTIONS FOR DISCUSSION

1. In discussing curriculum development and curriculum reform, Lewy calls for field try-outs following the planning stage (see *Selected References*). Does this time-consuming practice seem practical to you?

2. Bloom, Hastings, and Madaus have written at length on the structuring of objectives in education so that adequate evaluations can be made after learning activities have taken place (see *Selected References*). How might this kind of information be used wisely in planning a new elementary school health curriculum?

3. Because of its high drop-out rate, teaching has been called a profession of low commitment. Many people undergo training for teaching, but few make a career of it. Cooper feels that this may be due to personal disappointment with the first teaching experiences (see Cooper in *Selected References*). Differentiated staffing may have an answer to this concern. What are your comments?

4. As a humanist, Joseph Wood Krutch felt that the school curriculum should provide more opportunities for social intercourse that would foster mental health. Comment on how this can be planned for in the local elementary school.

5. List several ways of achieving both scope and sequence in planning a health education curriculum. Also list the references on curriculum development that you consulted.

SUGGESTED ACTIVITIES

1. John Goodlad points out that "health has never been a clearly defined study in our schools." Ask two or three elementary classroom teachers how they feel about this statement. Is it generally true or generally false? And what is the reasoning behind the answer?

2. Recently curriculum changes have been more widespread and intensive than at any time in the history of American schools. One should ask if the curriculum changes are really significant. Do children learn better in the new programs than they did in the old? Suggest several means of finding out how valuable certain curriculum changes are in a school.

3. Read some of the material that has been written about the advantages of differentiated staffing. From the point of view of health instruction, does it seem to be more or less practical to teach by this method or the method frequently employed in the self-contained classroom unit? Support your answer with appropriate references to the literature on the topic.

4. Formulate your own list of behavioral objectives or competencies suitable for a grade of your choice which pertains to one of the major health topics. Examine several curriculum guides before putting your list in final form.

5. Select one of the following topics and prepare a resource unit for use in a primary grade of your choice:
   a. Safety
   b. Dental health
   c. Sleep, rest, and relaxation
   d. Communicable disease control

6. Visit the college library and look over a number of curriculum guides in health education. List some of the ways in which they differ and some of the ways in which they are similar.

SELECTED REFERENCES

Bloom, Benjamin S., Hastings, J. Thomas, and Madaus, George F. *Handbook on Formative and Summative Evaluation of Student Learning.* New York: McGraw-Hill Book Company, 1971.

Bruner, Jerome A. *Toward a Theory of Instruction.* Cambridge, Mass.: Belknap Press of Harvard University, 1966.

_____. *The Relevance of Education.* New York: W. W. Norton & Co., Inc., 1971.

Cooper, James A. *Differentiated Staffing.* Philadelphia: W. B. Saunders Co., 1972.

Darrow, Helen F. "Conceptual Learning," *Childhood Education,* 287–288, February 1965.

Davies, Ivor K. *Objectives in Curriculum Design.* New York: McGraw-Hill Book Co., 1977.

Ebel, R. L. "Behavioral Objectives: A Close Look," *Phi Delta Kappan,* 52:171–173, November 1970.

Glatthorn, Allan A. *Alternatives in Education: Schools and Programs.* New York: Dodd, Mead & Co., 1975.

Golubchick, Leonard H. and Persky, Barry. *Innovation in Education.* Dubuque: Kendall/Hunt Publishing Co., 1975.

Haas, Glen. *Curriculum Planning: A New Approach,* 2d ed. Boston: Allyn and Bacon, Inc., 1977.

Lewy, Arieh (ed.) *Handbook of Curriculum Evaluation.* New York: Longman, Inc., 1977, Parts 1 and 2.

Macdonald, J. B. and Wolfson, B. J. "A Case Against Behavioral Objectives," *Elementary School Journal,* December 1970, 119–128.

Mager, Robert F. *Preparing Instructional Objectives.* Belmont, California: Fearon Publishers, Inc., 1972.

McNeil, John D. *Designing Curriculum: Self-Instruction Modules.* Boston: Little, Brown & Co., 1976.

Oberteuffer, Delbert, Harrelson, Orvis A., and Pollock, Marion B. *School Health Education,* 5th ed. New York: Harper & Row, 1972, Chapters 2 and 4.

Olsen, Larry K., Stone, Donald B. and Saunders, Jane A. "In-Service Training for Elementary School Health Education," *Health Education, 7*:27–29, March/April 1976.

Phenix, Phillip H. *Realms of Meaning.* New York: McGraw-Hill Book Co., 1964.

Pigg, R. Morgan, Jr., "A National Study of Competency-Based Health Education Programs," *Health Education, 7*:15–16, July/August 1976.

Shuster, Albert and Plughoff, Milton E. *The Emerging Elementary Curriculum,* 3rd ed. Columbus: Charles E. Merrill Publishing Co., 1978.

Sutherland, Mary and Hemmer, William B. "Competency-Based Health Education," *Health Education, 8*:24–28, September/October 1977.

Willgoose, Carl E. "Saving the Curriculum in Health Education," *Journal of School Health, 42*:108–112, March 1973.

Woodruff, Asahel D. "The Use of Concepts in Teaching and Learning," *Journal of Teacher Education, 20*:81–99, March 1964.

Zais, Robert S. *Curriculum Principles and Foundations.* New York: Thomas Y. Crowell Co., 1976.

Implementing the
Health Curriculum

8

What is needed is not only the art and science of healing of disease, important as that is, but the art and science of health enhancement, in which the individual himself becomes his own practitioner.

—Jonas Salk[1]

If an individual is to become his or her "own practitioner," there will have to be a new learning environment offering a wide variety of learning experiences that will do justice to the diversity of the students. It is easy to acknowledge the need to nourish the dissimilarities, variations, and pluralism of modern life. It is much more difficult, however, to put into practice the health understandings that contribute to survival in a multi-dimensional society. The best of instructional programs require a personal dimension—a dimension that Combs highlighted very well when he said that "knowledge is likely to have little effect upon our behavior until such time as we discover the personal meaning of the ideas for ourselves."[2]

IMPLEMENTATION—THE POWER WORD

If indeed the educational need *is* to increase "health enhancement" in order to prepare youth for our diversified culture, then the process of implementation takes on greater meaning.

Coming from the Latin *implere,* the word implementation means to fill up or finish. It is associated with such words as fulfill, accomplish, carry out, and complete. It relates to getting somewhere by putting plans into action through the careful selection of learning activities (the variety of student experiences which include things to think about and try) together with pertinent resources and aids. The word implementation is an all-encompassing term which ultimately gets at the roots of the curriculum by answering the old question of *"how to do"* in education. It is a term which makes methodology practical; and in this chapter it is spelled out by a wide variety of school-community tested learning activities designed to challenge

---

[1]Salk, Jonas. "What Do We Mean by Health," *Health Education,* 9:14–16, January/February 1978.

[2]Combs, Arthur. *Educational Accountability,* Washington, D.C.: Association for Curriculum and Instruction, 1972.

the diversity of learners by providing something that should capture the imagination.*

The view that the program of health activities at any grade level should be a broad and varied one can be supported not only on the basis of a pluralistic society but also on the firm understanding that children differ widely in their personal interests and need to be able to make choices in a school setting. In such a fashion, sooner or later everyone will discover something that he or she likes very much.

As teachers and health coordinators work together to prepare interesting content for a major health topic, they have to keep in mind that the selection of learning activities to be engaged in has to be carefully chosen from an ever-growing list of ideas and activities embracing a great many facts and concepts. With such a wide variety of possibilities and a limited amount of teaching time, *selection* becomes the essence of planning. The learning activities selected must be so succinct and reasonably complete that they will serve to generate the kinds of student practices that relate to total instructional content instead of isolated views and bits and pieces of information.

Although a number of research studies have been conducted about pupil interests, major health problems, the nature of the elementary school health curriculum, the major topics for elementary school study, and the particular knowledge and understandings for each grade, very little research has been done regarding specific *teaching activities* in the major topical area of instruction. This has resulted in a conglomeration of activities and experiences under a particular topic, with or without reference to properly stated outcomes. Every activity employed to teach a health topic, whether it be an experiment, a story play, a poster drawing, or an independent project, should contribute to the pre-determined objectives and be subject to periodic reappraisal.

SUGGESTED ACTIVITIES FOR MAJOR HEALTH TOPICS

A number of special health topics for elementary schoolchildren follow. These topics are the ones that make up the health curriculum and were set forth in some detail in Chapter 7. In order to do justice to current courses of study and at the same time be complete, a total of 12 categories or topics are covered. They are (1) Personal Cleanliness and Appearance; (2) Physical Activity, Sleep, Rest, and Relaxation; (3) Nutrition and Growth; (4) Dental Health; (5) Body Structure and Operation; (6) Prevention and Control of Disease; (7) Safety and First Aid; (8) Mental Health; (9) Sex and Family Living Education; (10) Environmental Health; (11) Tobacco, Alcohol, and Drugs; and (12) Consumer Health. These topics have been set up separately as follows: *Behavioral Objectives* for primary level and intermediate level students; *Comments* relating to instruction; and *Suggested Activities*

---

*Chapter 9 will provide a more thorough discussion of methodology, in terms of both student behaviors and teaching techniques.

for each elementary school level. The *Behavioral Objectives* are samples of what might be developed at the local level. They are reasonably appropriate for the grade level. They tend to be more realistic in any community when developed by teachers themselves. The same can be said in part for the *Suggested Activities*. The teacher should find them useful when considering how far to go with any one particular grade. Although primary grade children are quite different from intermediate graders as a group, there will be times when there is considerable overlapping of interest between children of different grades. More specifically, a precocious third grade child may be ready for a suggested experience or project suitable for the typical fifth grade class.

The activities suggested for the primary and intermediate grades are not all-inclusive nor are they offered as ideals or "musts" in any way. They are simply a collection of appropriate experiences for a particular category of health instruction. No teacher will carry out all of the suggestions, but he or she may use those most applicable to a particular grade. Practically all of the activities have been tried in one school or another and found to be worthwhile in promoting a greater understanding of health. Many of them are suitable for initiating a unit of study. When employed with appropriate questions, they contribute to the discovery method of instruction. Obviously, depending on local circumstances or local teachers, some of the activities are better than others in their tendency to change behavior and promote acceptable health practices and attitudes.

In using this suggested material, *keep these points in mind:* (1) the effectiveness of the activities will be increased after a review of the chapters on methods and materials; (2) evaluation techniques (Chapter 11) will help measure the worth of the activities selected; and (3) sources of materials to accompany these activities (films, filmstrips, charts, posters, pamphlets, and stories for children) should be used. These are listed in detail in Chapter 10.

---

1. PERSONAL CLEANLINESS AND APPEARANCE

Behavioral Objectives* (Primary Level)

Explains why cleanliness and grooming are important to personal health and appearance.

Demonstrates ability to wash the hands when necessary, use toilet facilities properly, brush teeth, keep clean, use the handkerchief, care for the clothing, comb the hair.

Dresses appropriately for the climate and weather.

Behavioral Objectives (Intermediate Level)

Relates why clothing needs to be changed frequently and in keeping with weather conditions.

---

*For a finer breakdown of behavioral objectives grade by grade, see the Appendix. All of these are attainable pupil objectives which lend themselves to appraisal by the teacher.

Distinguishes proper from improper practices of cleanliness related to food and eating.

Explains the structure and function of the skin and the elimination of wastes through the skin.

Describes the relationship between appearance and daily living, social success, and self-respect.

Analyzes the ways to assume personal responsibility for the maintenance of good health.

Comments

The child entering school is faced with the somewhat new idea of being responsible, more than ever before, for personal cleanliness and appearance. As he or she progresses through the grades there is a growing understanding of the reason why cleanliness and grooming are important to personal health and appearance. The student becomes aware of how cleanliness helps to prevent the spread of disease and how it makes one more acceptable to classmates.

Although standards of cleanliness vary, most homes are equipped with the basic facilities for helping children keep clean. When children through no fault of their own fail to meet accepted standards of cleanliness or appearance, care should be taken not to humiliate them unintentionally.

In the intermediate grades, cleanliness may be related to the prevention and control of disease. (Merely keeping clean for esthetic reasons will no longer hold attention.) After learning the characteristics of bacteria and their relationship to disease, the practice of keeping clean becomes more closely related to a desire to preserve health. Cleanliness then becomes a social asset.

With the active aid of the students, cleanliness and neatness in the classroom can be achieved. With a little encouragement, children take pride in the condition of their books, desks, and materials. The alert teacher recognizes that it is only a step from such individual accomplishments to the development of pride in the group. Such things as work tables, floors, blackboards, bulletin boards, the coat room, the toilet room, and lockers can become objects of group concern and of group action in keeping them clean and presentable.

Suggested Activities*

Primary Level

1. Show the 7-minute film, *Health: The Dirt-Witch Cleans Up* (Encyclopedia Britannica Educational Corp.), which encourages younger children to enjoy bathing and developing regular routines of washing hands, faces, bodies, and hair. Then discuss differences between a bath and a shower. Ask: How do you *feel* after a bath?

---

*For an extensive listing of teaching aids and sources to be used with these and the following major health topic activities, see Chapter 10.

2. Take turns dusting the room, books, bookcases, and arranging shelves and clothing racks.
3. Draw pictures that illustrate taking a bath, washing clothes, ironing shirts, and cleaning fingernails. A first grade child can draw a meaningful picture of washing the face in the bathroom at home without much difficulty. Have several children illustrate their own story of cleanliness by holding their pictures up for all to see.
4. Discuss the different ways people take baths (full tub, wash tub, shower, sponge, or steam baths). Read the poem "After a Bath" by Aileen Fisher.
5. Visit the school nurse for a personal inspection. This may be quite rewarding, especially if done with a little advance planning.
6. Have the students demonstrate to the class the proper method of:
   a. Washing and drying hands
   b. Combing the hair and cleaning the hairbrush
   c. Covering coughs and sneezes
   d. Blowing the nose properly
   e. Drinking from a drinking fountain
7. Have a child bring his or her pet cat or dog to school and show the class how he or she brushes it and keeps it neat.
8. Appoint all class members as "Health Detectives." Before the week-end begins, ask everyone to keep their eyes open on Saturday and Sunday and note what can be seen involving the cleanliness and appearance of people, animals, buildings, roads, walks, lawns, and gardens. On Monday permit everyone to tell what he or she saw. This may be made more interesting by having the group make little cardboard badges which may be worn right away on Friday afternoon.

9. Talk about personal experiences such as falling in the mud, walking through mud puddles, or getting covered with paint. When is getting dirty fun? When is it unpleasant? Have you ever felt embarrassed or out of place because you were dirty?
10. Give each child a coat hanger for his or her clothes and a large number cut from a calendar. Play a game with numbers until each child can tell his or her own. Then the child can paste it over the hook where his or her clothes are hung.

11. Appoint a committee to prepare an exhibit of different types of clothes for different occasions. Work clothes, rubbers, raincoats, riding clothes, snowsuits, and bathing suits are all designed for special purposes. Appoint another committee to collect various types of hats that express native customs, i.e., felt hat, cap, turban, straw hat, fez, fur hat, hood (applicable for third grade).

12. Create a classroom store and engage in buying and selling experiences which will help to provide a better understanding of the kinds of clothing best suited to health needs and appearance.

13. Talk about the protective covering of animals, fish, and birds: the fur of the bear, fox, squirrel, raccoon; the feathers of the wild duck; the shells of clams and oysters; the bark of the trees.

14. Invite the school custodian to class to talk about how the school is kept safe and clean.

15. Construct a Health Check Wheel. Use a wheel 20 inches in diameter. Use a brad to fasten an arrow to the middle of the wheel. Use pictures of health practices made by pupils or illustrations from magazines. Ask a pupil to spin the arrow to select a health practice to be checked for the day.

Intermediate Level

1. Raise questions about being careful in the use of certain cleaning solutions. Some products are harsh to the skin or highly flammable; some may damage the floor or furniture if spilled. List the cleaning solutions your parents keep at home. Are any dangerous if used in the wrong way?

2. Discuss ways of making the classroom more attractive.

3. Examine the skin on the back of the hand with a magnifying glass. See the creases and folds when the hand is relaxed. See also the dirt which will disappear after washing (good for a fifth or sixth grade class). Have the class note the pores and tiny hairs. Discuss perspiration and body odors. Note oil and hair glands and tell what they do for the skin and one's appearance.

4. Have the class bring in pictures from magazines depicting

how the skin senses changes in temperature. Pictures such as a man shivering from the cold or sweating from the noon-day sun or of a little boy burning his finger on a hot stove are good examples. Magazine advertisements for beauty aids may also be discussed. Do the aids do everything the ads claim they do?

5. Discuss injuries to the skin which may affect health and personal appearance. Talk about cuts, bruises, blisters, burns, and splinters. Show the class or have the nurse demonstrate how to treat a blister and remove a splinter of wood from a finger.

6. Prepare an article for the school paper on some topic of cleanliness.

7. Experiment with the wearing of wet clothes by taking a piece of dry cloth and a piece of wet cloth and placing both on the skin. Ask the class which feels cooler. Which takes more heat from the body? What conclusion should be drawn? Proceed from there to study types of seasonal clothing. Refer also to clothing used in tribal areas and other sections of the globe.

8. Discuss germs and how they cause disease when the hands, tableware, and family utensils are not clean. Use the microscope to see the germs. Point out that germs are both helpful and harmful and that washing with water may remove a few but only careful washing with soap and hot water will remove enough of the germs to protect our health.

9. Show how "hidden dirt" stays on the skin even when a pupil thinks he or she is clean by rubbing the back of the hand with a small piece of cloth dipped in alcohol. Let the class see the cloth before and after rubbing the skin.

10. Find out how Jenner, Pasteur, Koch, Reed, and others have benefited humanity.

11. Visit the school cafeteria to inspect and observe the methods used to maintain sanitary conditions. The same thing may be done at a park, picnic area, or public beach to note hygienic conditions.

12. Show the relationship of posture to personal appearance.

2. PHYSICAL ACTIVITY, SLEEP, REST, AND RELAXATION

Behavioral Objectives (Primary Level)

Explains how one balances exercise, play, work, sleep, and relaxation to provide for optimum achievement in physical and mental well-being,

Describes the need for play and large muscle activity, daily relaxation periods, and a wide variety of leisure time activities.

Identifies reasons why sound sleep in quiet surroundings is healthful and why quiet activities before bedtime or meal time are beneficial.

Behavioral Objectives (Intermediate Level)

Demonstrates how exercise builds and maintains health.

Explains the importance of outdoor play and recreational activities.

Analyzes the value of sleep and rest and how to rest and relax.

Personally observes regular hours of retiring and rising together with other requirements for sleep and rest.

Employs hygienic practices when engaging in physical activity at school and in the community.

Comments

Boys and girls at all age levels should reach the end of the day free from undue fatigue and irritability. They should rest a while before eating and engage in pleasant and quiet activities before going to bed. They should arise in the morning rested and ready for schoolwork or play. What could be more simple? Yet, getting this knowledge across to all elementary school pupils and having them modify their living practices accordingly is indeed a difficult task.

Health teaching on this topic includes a number of significant variables. Children vary in their sleep requirements. Those from four to eight years of age need a total of 12 or 13 hours of sleep. For 11 year olds, 10 hours is generally sufficient. By age 12 or 13, nine hours is usually enough. But the quantity of sleep is not nearly as important as the quality. The quality is affected by numerous home and community stimuli. In every neighborhood there are items such as street noises, factory noises, industrial odors, barking dogs, older children at play, and other factors which have a negative effect on the quality of the night's sleep.

Parents must have an understanding of sleep and rest needs, of wholesome physical activities, of signs of fatigue, and many more conditions conducive to adequate growth. When parents fail to guide their children properly at home, the efforts of the classroom teacher may seem quite meager. Late evening programs, movies, television shows, radio, and after-dinner visits tend to cut into the optimum sleep requirements for growing children. Over a period of time pupil behavior is affected. Children in such instances become more fatigued, lose their keen appetites, perform poorly in school, and frequently demonstrate a less social behavior. Fatigue in children is also sometimes a sign of anemia caused by insufficient iron in the blood. This can usually be corrected by better nutrition and prescribed medication.

Although children are more discriminating than they used to be in what they choose to watch on television, there are still many who spend hours per week sitting and watching. There are, of course, many excellent offerings on television but numerous children stay up too late watching.

There is an excellent opportunity for the teacher to work with the home and to see that all pupils receive their due share of vigorous growth-stimulating physical exercise, relaxation, and sleep each day. Probably more bacterial and viral diseases get a foothold in the human organism because of chronic fatigue than from any other hygienic shortcoming. Children need school activities which will point out the fact that satisfying school work, outdoor play, rest, sunshine, proper food, and happy associations at school and in the home neighborhood help them to secure a restful night's sleep.

Today more than ever, considerable attention must be given by the teacher to the role of physical exercise in the maintenance of organic health.

Physical fitness is the prerequisite to everything else pertaining to health. It is the wherewithal that permits movement; it is in a very real sense the capacity for any and all activity. Tyler says that the muscles are the "organs of the will." Since the muscular fitness variables of strength and endurance (which relate to organic health and mental-social health as well) cannot be stored, it is necessary that daily attention be directed to vigorous physical exercise. Although most students appear quite active, a knowledge of the benefits of exercise needs to be stressed in the classroom as well as directly on the playgrounds and gymnasiums. There are numerous boys and girls today who are well below a minimum level of strength and muscular fitness. Their physical efficiency is too low for them to live fully and function with a full display of energy. The quiet, chore-free activities of a somewhat sedentary adult population have affected the school-children. Even those pupils a few blocks from school ride the bus; other sit and watch much of the time instead of participating; still others are tense and emotionally on edge due in part to the rapid pace and stresses of modern civilization. With overeating and underactivity, it becomes clear that education for health is more important than ever. Suitable activities that are carried on in a pleasant atmosphere, free from the pressure and rapid pace of modern society, can be most profitable.

The role of the classroom teacher is to demonstrate clearly that exercise, nutrition, and rest build a quality of physical fitness that is a forerunner for all other activities. This means that the classroom teacher is a physical education teacher and as such is a teacher of health. The value of physical skills cannot be overemphasized, for fitness in later life is related to skills acquired during the early years. Emerson, in his *Essay on Education,* refers to "educated eyes in uneducated bodies." In so doing he makes a strong point in favor of physical efficiency and skills.[3] Thus each instructor of youth, particularly at the elementary level, teaches the mimetics and story plays, the games, the rhythms and dances, and the recreational skills that contribute to growth and understanding.

A large percentage of classroom teachers carry on their own programs of physical education. It is the minority that have the services of the trained specialist to teach activities. It is important, therefore, that each teacher be well acquainted not only with the behavior characteristics of the age group but also with the appropriate activities for each grade level, season, and facility. The program

[3]". . . let us have men whose manhood is only the continuation of their boyhood, natural characters still; such are able for fertile and heroic action; and not that sad spectacle with which we are too often familiar, educated eyes in uneducated bodies."

must be a broad and varied one so that all children have a number of experiences and find something that they are interested in. It is the learning associated with these games and dances that fosters social efficiency, cultural appreciations, and moral and ethical values. This becomes emphasized when one considers that activity—play, games, stunts, rhythms, and dance—is to the child as work is to the adult. It is serious, special, and full of meaning—the child's way of life. Through it the child learns about self and the people and things around him or her.

Student and teacher interactions are very much a part of the physical activity program. It has been determined that a teacher-directed approach appears to be best for the development of motor skills and a greater exposure to a range of activities. However, a student-sharing approach contributes measurably to the development of a self-concept.[4] When students share in decisions involving activity selection, time allotment, amount of student interaction, and student evaluation, there is a significant improvement in self-concept. Since the development of both motor skills and a self-concept are desirable, there should be a balance of teacher-directed and student-sharing activities.

In this connection, a word about movement exploration is appropriate. This is a relatively new direction in elementary physical education. It is taught by problem-solving methods, affording all children the opportunity to perform as individuals and to be creative as they discover new ways of handling their bodies and objectives. The teacher sets the problem. He or she may ask, "Can you jump *over* the beanbag?" "Now, can you jump over it again and *land* without making any noise?" Or he or she might say, "Show me how *high* you can bounce the ball. Can you make your body *low* and bounce the

[4]Martinek, Thomas J., Zaichkowsky, Leonard D., and Cheffers, John T. F. "Decision-Making in Elementary Age Children: Effects on Motor Skills and Self-Concept," *Research Quarterly*, 48:349–357, May 1977.

Figure 8–1. Children in physical education class prepare to jump to feet and raise parachute vigorously overhead. (Courtesy Baldwinsville, Baldwinsville, N.Y.)

ball?'' Original responses are encouraged throughout movement exploration activity. This builds concepts of level change, direction, force, speed, timing, and space relationships needed in mind-body understandings. Not only does it contribute to joy in activity, physical fitness, and motor development but it also measurably improves listening habits, creativity, and confidence in ability to adapt to the immediate environment.[5]

Suggested Activities

Primary Level
1. Talk about the relationship of physical activity to "feeling good." Show how overactivity relates to fatigue, sleep, and relaxation.
2. Have the class tell about the games and dances they enjoy playing most. Play one or two favorite games in the classroom as an illustration of something the children like to do or do the same thing on the school playground.
3. Put the following poem on the blackboard in big letters.[6]

> WE ARE PLANNING OUR DAY
>
> WE PLAN OUR WORK
> WE PLAN OUR PLAY
> TO MAKE A HAPPY
> BUSY DAY.

Have the class plan the work, play, and rest periods for the day. Point out the balance between these three items. Ask the class to tell why they think this kind of planning may make them happy.
4. Teach some exercise that will strengthen abdominal and back muscles and contribute to good posture and body

---

[5]See "Movement Education: Play With a Purpose" by Elsie Werra in *Instructor* 80:84–85, October 1970. See also "Creative Dancing" by Monica Pendergast in *Instructor, 81*:62–63, March 1971.

[6]Reprinted through the courtesy of the Metropolitan Life Insurance Company.

BALANCE BEAM

CAN YOU?

WALK FORWARD HOLD ARMS SIDEWARD

WALK FORWARD TO MIDDLE TURN AROUND WALK BACKWARD

WALK FORWARD HANDS ON HIPS

WALK FORWARD BEND PICK UP ERASER WALK TO END

WALK FORWARD STEP OVER ROPE WALK TO END

mechanics. Play games to release tensions built up in concentrated activities. Engage in fundamental rhythms such as walking, marching, skipping, hopping, sliding, twirling, and jumping to music (applicable to kindergarten and first grade). Use the balance beam. (Even a homemade 2″ × 4″ × 12′ piece of wood with side supports can be used.)

5. Try some exercises in class or on the playground. Demonstrate the three that follow from the American Medical Association booklet (see Figure 8–2).

6. Have a quiet period. Say to the class: "Stand up very slowly. Sit down very slowly. Go somewhere on your feet—now go a different way. Go somewhere on your hands and feet—

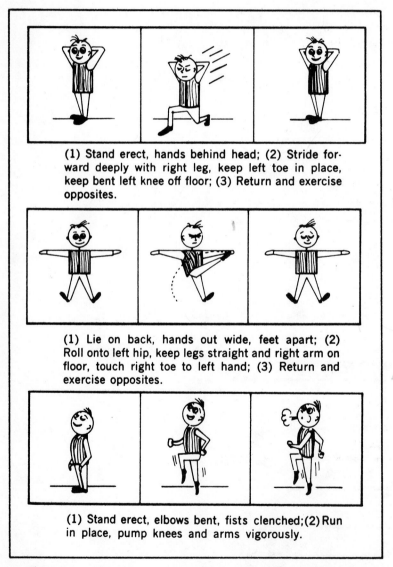

(1) Stand erect, hands behind head; (2) Stride forward deeply with right leg, keep left toe in place, keep bent left knee off floor; (3) Return and exercise opposites.

(1) Lie on back, hands out wide, feet apart; (2) Roll onto left hip, keep legs straight and right arm on floor, touch right toe to left hand; (3) Return and exercise opposites.

(1) Stand erect, elbows bent, fists clenched;(2) Run in place, pump knees and arms vigorously.

Figure 8–2. Adapted from the American Medical Association booklet, *Physical Fitness,* A.M.A., Chicago, Illinois.

now find a different way to go—go faster. Move somewhere on any part of your body. Find a space and make yourself small, very small, as tiny as you can. Now stretch every bit of your body way out. Squeeze up very tight. Stretch again and relax."

7. Bring a kitten to class. After the class has been underway awhile, tell everyone to look at the kitty. See how many children have pets. Have them tell how their animal friends rest or sleep. Ask where birds go to sleep.

8. Make a clock out of cardboard. Place the pointer at a reasonable bedtime. For first graders set it at 7 P.M. Inquire as to when the various children go to bed.

9. Bring a globe of the world to class. Explain daytime and nighttime by pulling the shades to darken the room and holding a flashlight over the globe to represent the sunshine. Notice in what countries people are sleeping when it is daytime in America.

10. Talk about the nice feeling of going to bed. Let the pupils suggest how nice the sheets feel and the softness of the bed (first grade).

11. Check on the number of children that have baby brothers or sisters. Have the children answer questions on how long the babies sleep, what awakens them, and why they need more sleep than older children (first grade).

12. Have someone demonstrate a cartwheel. Let everyone try a few. Then do cartwheels along a line, along a set of hoops on the floor, along a line and picking up an object in the process, over an object such as a rope, with a run, etc.

13. Take the opportunity to capitalize on the daily rest period in school. Listen to soft music before the rest period (kindergarten to second grade). Examples: *Lullabies for Sleepy Heads,* Dorothy Olsen (RCA Victor) or *The Swan* from *Carnival of the Animals* by Saint-Saens.

14. Construct a model bedroom on a large table. Use doll furniture and doll people. Show a comfortable room with clean bedclothing, an opened window, and other optimum physical factors. Put a clock on the wall set for bedtime. Vary the model according to the known socioeconomic level of the students.

15. Display activity posters during the teaching period such as the 22" × 28" colorful poster *Keep Physically Fit,* available free of charge from School Services Division, Florida Department of Citrus, Lakeland, Florida.

16. Make pictures or posters suggesting activities conducive to play, sleep, or relaxation.

17. Prepare a wall board with pictures brought to class depicting sleep, work, play, and relaxation (second and third grade).

Intermediate Level

1. Formulate a well-balanced daily schedule that makes ample provision for each of the functions of exercise, relax-

ation, and sleep which affect the growth and development of the human body.

2. Discuss the values of muscular work as a health measure. Point out that a muscle in good tone is firm and ready to act; muscle tone is the foundation for further development of strength and skill; sufficient strength and endurance reduce fatigue and permit a child or adult to keep going longer; agility, flexibility, speed, and precision are improved; increased heart action results in a more efficient heart with more blood being pumped together with fewer beats per minute; oxygen is better distributed to tissues; all organic functions in the body are improved; and general health is advanced (fifth or sixth grade). Discuss the difference between organic and dynamic fitness as set forth by the President's Council on Physical Fitness and Sports:

Organic Fitness. The foundation of fitness is good organic health—a body free of disease or infirmity and well nourished. This may mean an adjustment by the individual to certain physical conditions that cannot be reversed by medical or dental care—wearing properly fitted eyeglasses and dentures or using a hearing aid when prescribed.

Dynamic Fitness. A person may be free of disease but not fully fit. There is the additional dimension of dynamic fitness which involves the resources to move vigorously, to do, to live energetically. This dynamic quality has several components: efficiency of heart and lungs, muscular strength and endurance, balance, flexibility, coordination and agility.

3. Use a wall chart to show how the muscular system works and how its use puts demands on the other body systems;

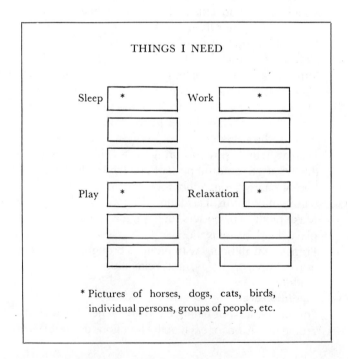

THINGS I NEED

Sleep [*]   Work [*]

Play [*]   Relaxation [*]

*Pictures of horses, dogs, cats, birds, individual persons, groups of people, etc.

Figure 8–3. Teacher-parent communication to promote proper sleep practices.

the demands in turn tend to keep the other systems organically and functionally healthy.

4. List on the board a number of physical activities that may be engaged in around the home. Number these activities according to the degree of vigor required. Do the same for occupations in the community and for sports and games in the school physical education program.

5. Display pictures of prominent athletes or pictures of athletes in action. Magazines such as *Sports Illustrated* abound in excellent picture of swimmers, golfers, tennis players, baseball batters, football carriers, and ice skating champions.

6. Plan a hiking, camping, or bicycling trip. Make the trip if possible.

7. Practice relaxing. Have the class stand by their desks with both arms extended above the head. On command, relax only the hand by allowing the wrist to "break." Then relax to the elbow joint, and then the rest of the arm. Repeat by relaxing the whole arm on command. Point out how difficult this seems at first (fifth and sixth grades).

8. Discuss the meaning of recreation. Ask the children what their parents do for recreation. Suggest and list on the board several reasons that play is not a waste of time.

9. Prepare a hobby exhibit. Show pictures of the hobbies of prominent people. Suggest to the class that they illustrate some of the hobbies of their older brothers and sisters and their parents.

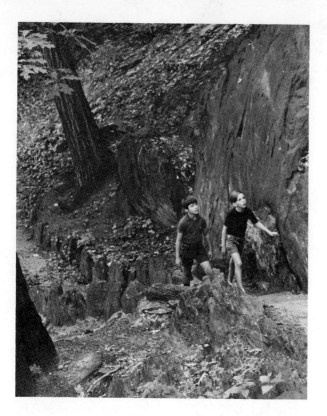

Figure 8–4. Exploration and relaxation: can they go together? (Courtesy U.S. Bureau of Outdoor Recreation.)

10. Encourage informal discussions of why we tire, how rest affects posture, work, and play, and why anxiety, fear, anger, and eating before bedtime may affect sleep.
11. Keep individual records for each child of the number of hours slept each night for one whole week with notations on "How I felt in the morning." Discuss the records at the end of the week. Bring into the discussion the advantages of sleeping alone, the kinds of mattresses slept on, restlessness in sleep, and sleep practices (sixth grade).

MY SLEEP RECORD		
Day	Hours Slept	How I felt in the morning
Monday		
Tuesday		
Wednesday		
Thursday		
Friday		
Saturday		
Sunday		

12. Count pulse rates before and after a period of exercise. Note also the respiratory rate, its increase, and return to normal. This may be made quite interesting. Have the children stand by their desks and count their own pulse beats for 30 seconds. Multiply by two and record on a piece of paper. Then run quietly in place for one minute and quickly take the pulse rate again for 30 seconds. Record in the proper place on the paper. Sit down and rest. Take the pulse two minutes later and record.

Find out who had the greatest rise in pulse rate. How many came close to returning to their original pulse rate? Discuss what has happened in the body, with particular reference to physical condition and fatigue. Plot individual line graphs.

13. Interview the school nurse regarding the relationship of excessive fatigue, inadequate sleep, and activity to the common cold.
14. Invite the physical eduation teacher into class to talk about athletes he or she has known. Encourage questions from the class relative to the eating, sleeping, and resting practices of athletes.
15. Appoint a committee of three to find out about the Harvard Step Test of Physical Fitness for elementary age pupils. Give the test and check individual student scores.[7]
16. Have an indoor track meet when the class needs a "rest-less" break.

The Hundred-Inch Dash: Draw a starting line and a finish line one hundred inches apart. Starting with their feet together, contestants move forward by touching the heel of one foot to the toe of the other foot.

The One-Minute Mile: Time each person for one minute as he or she runs in place, lifting feet at least twelve inches. Every time the contestant's right foot hits the floor, it counts as one. The child with the highest count within a minute is the winner.

---

[7]Adequate instructions may be found in Donald K. Matthews, *Measurement in Physical Education,* 5th ed., Philadelphia: W. B. Saunders Co., 1978.

The Paper-Bag Put: Grab a paper bag and crush it into a ball. You now have an indoor shot that can't damage anything. See who can throw it the farthest, using proper shot-putting form.

The Javelin Throw: Save a few straws from lunchtime—they make harmless javelins! Let kids experiment with different ways of throwing them.

17. Investigate insomnia and sleep and insomnia's relationship to chronic fatigue. Review the article by Carol Kahn, "Do You Dream (Perchance) of Sleeping?" *Family Health,* 9:36–43, September, 1977.

3. NUTRITION AND GROWTH

Behavioral Objectives (Primary Level)

✗ Explains that a variety of food is needed by the body for growth and energy.

✗ Investigates a variety of nutritious foods and demonstrates good eating habits and customary social behavior at mealtime.

Relates how energy is necessary for work and play and that some foods provide more energy than others. Outlines how appetite can be improved by careful planning of work, play, and rest.

Portrays how being tired, sick, and unhappy is often related to poor nutrition.

Describes a happy, pleasant mealtime.

Investigates how foods are used in other parts of the world and how food is handled, preserved, and stored.

Demonstrates ability to be able to personally choose suitable meals when child must select his or her own. Investigates common food fads, misconceptions, and superstitions.

Cooperates with others (including parents) in meal planning.

Behavioral Objectives (Intermediate Level)

Interprets the concept that well-balanced daily nutrition includes food from each of the four basic food groups.

Structures a well-balanced diet which helps to achieve success in work and play and shows how it relates to one's emotional outlook.

Selects foods that contain various nutrients, minerals, and vitamins necessary for prevention of disease, personal vigor, and enthusiasm.

Interprets the concept that the body is composed of cells which need wholesome food for proper growth and development.

Comments

Citizen surveys continually indicate a need for nutrition information. Only a few years ago, books and manuals on nutrition replaced those on sex as best sellers. But the increase in interest is deceiving. Many people are interested in food labeling, but in an Illinois study only 16 per cent could understand label information and only 2 per cent knew of the importance of protein in the diet.

Also, the McGovern Committee in the U.S. Senate analyzed eating practices and food content and discovered that people consume inadequate amounts of vitamins A and B—with as much as 34 per cent of schoolchildren receiving inadequate amounts of vitamin A and iron. The same Senate study called attention to sugar consumption. However, sugar in breakfast cereals is not the problem some consumer activists consider it to be. The consumption of sugar without considering nutritional value should be discouraged. However, the presence of sugar may motivate young children to drink milk and eat cereals. Since the 1880's, breakfast cereals have been useful, but they were never intended to be a full meal. In fact, Mr. Kellogg himself advocated his cereals for chewing exercise. Moreover, several studies have shown that there is no correlation between the consumption of presweetened cereals and increased tooth decay.[8]

The Society for Nutrition Education reports that the public's knowledge of nutrition is lower than ever, quackery is rampant, and the only solution is effective nutrition education starting in the elementary school.

Nutrition education is affected by changing lifestyles, government regulations, and a powerful consumer movement. One third of all meals are now eaten away from home. Over one half of all meals are prepared away from home. Convenience foods are popular and coffee and doughnuts are eaten too frequently. Motivation is necessary if improvements in eating habits are to occur. Knowledge alone is quite inadequate. There are probably just as many overweight people in the American Dietetic Association as there are in any other group.

One problem is that the public is willing to let government agencies and legislators decide how much money to spend on nutrition research. The government spends only $70 million per year on nutrition education while the food industry spends $400 million a year on television advertising alone, much of it directed at children. In a University of Minnesota study of the national television networks, 580 commercials were monitored during a 27-hour period. Some 78 per cent of the food commercials were aimed at children. Almost half of the commercials were for snacks, beverages, and quick foods, most of which were of low nutritional value. This research augments the findings of the Senate Select Committee on Nutrition and Human Needs. In this report, children were shown to be profoundly influenced in their eating practices by the approximately 13,000 food and drink commercials they are exposed to yearly. Testimony by experts indicated that the impact was largely detrimental to good nutrition. Coupled with this is the unfortunate fact that large numbers of people know little about nutrients even when well-educated. The poorest nutrition knowledge is in the lower socioeconomic, lower educational, and older age groups.[9]

---

[8]Glass, R. L. and Fleisch, S. "Diet and Dental Caries: Dental Caries Incidence and the Consumption of Ready-to-Eat Cereals," *Journal of the American Dental Association, 88*:807–813, 1974.

[9]Fusillo, Alice E., et al. "Consumer Nutrition Knowledge and Self Reported Food Shopping Behavior," *American Journal of Public Health, 67*:846–850, September 1977.

The White House Conference on Food, Nutrition, and Health called for ". . . a dynamic nutrition education program that begins in early childhood and continues through the early elementary and secondary schools." This was the cry as 1970 began. It hasn't changed; and the burden of nutrition education is on the teacher.

In a Los Angeles study to determine the effectiveness of a nutrition education program, 1,720 second grade pupils were divided into three groups for instruction: (1) those whose teachers were trained by nutrition educators and were given teaching materials; (2) those whose teachers were not trained, but were supplied with materials; and (3) a control group whose teachers were supplied with nutrition objectives only.[10] Pretesting was done for nutrition knowledge and its application in the selection of meals. Post-tests were given after the instruction was finished. The students in group one who had the trained teacher increased 360 per cent in knowledge and 150 per cent in ability to select balanced meals. No significant improvement was noted in the other two groups. It is clear from this study that elementary teachers can indeed help children if they broaden their general education with some work in nutrition. At present, little nutrition education will occur in the grades unless classroom teachers do it themselves.

These are major difficulties regarding nutrition to be overcome. One of these has to do with an adequate breakfast. For some time, research studies have indicated that about 25 per cent of the daily nutritional needs should be supplied at breakfast. An adequate break-

---

[10]Lovett, R., Barker, E., and Marcus, B. "The Effect of a Nutrition Education Program at the Second Grade Level," *Journal of Nutrition Education*, 2:80–88, Fall 1970.

Figure 8–5. Breakfast for the primary grade school pupil. (Courtesy Cereal Institute, Inc.)

fast permits one to do more work during the late morning hours, to be quicker in reactions, and not to tire as easily. How many children, even in affluent communities, meet this requirement? (See Figure 8–5.) A great number do not. In a recent study of 80,000 Massachusetts public school children, it was discovered that 24 per cent of all children came to school without an adequate breakfast. Even more startling was the finding that 13 per cent ate no breakfast; younger children did better than older children, and boys did better than girls. Moreover, food eaten for lunch was not all nutritious either.

Moderately severe and prolonged undernutrition in children can produce alterations in brain activity which may never be corrected. In addition, recent research indicates that malnutrition delays puberty and slows the development of mental ability. This ability, however, may be advanced in a stimulating environment. In fact, studies with primary grade children suggest that an adequate diet plus special physical and cognitive stimulation results in marked intellectual improvement but when an adequate diet is present with no special stimulation, there is little or no intellectual improvement.[11]

It is not easy to tell when a child is malnourished. It may help, however, to check the characteristic deviations in appearance and behavior listed in Chapter 5. A familiarity with these signs not only will be beneficial in terms of individual cases of malnutrition but also will suggest items for study in the food instruction program.

There are certain essentials one must bear in mind for effective nutrition teaching. The teacher may ask such questions as these.[12]

---

[11]Monckeberg, Fernando. "Malnutrition and Mental Capacity," *Nutrition, The Nervous System, and Behavior,* Pan American Health Organization, 251:48–54, 1972.

[12]Martin, Ethel A. *Roberts' Nutrition Work with Children.* Chicago: University of Chicago Press, 1972.

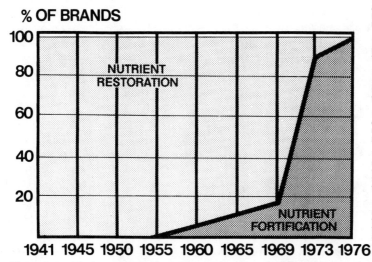

% OF BRANDS

NUTRIENT RESTORATION

NUTRIENT FORTIFICATION

1941 1945 1950 1955 1960 1965 1969 1973 1976

1941 Voluntary restoration of thiamine, niacin and iron to whole-grain levels.

1955 Introduction of the first protein- and vitamin-fortified cereal.

1961 The first cereal with 100% of the Minimum Daily Requirements for several vitamins.

1969-72 Accelerated development of nutritionally fortified products.

1973 More than 85% of all ready-to-eat cereals vitamin-fortified. Some are also protein-fortified.

1976 More than 92% of ready-to-eat cereals vitamin-fortified, excluding granola types. Some are also protein-fortified.

Figure 8–6. Ready-to-eat-cereal nutrition 1941–1976. (Courtesy *Cereal Foods World,* St. Paul, Minn.)

1. Do I relate classroom experiences and other activities to the daily food practices of children?
2. Do I make clear to the children the habits that are desirable for them to establish?
3. Do I provide parents with information and solicit their suggestions so that I may expect full cooperation from them in habit formation?
4. Am I guided by the needs of children and the community in selecting learning situations?

Most nutrition educators point out that to be most successful, nutrition teaching should begin early in the grades. This is the time when the school supplements the home, and here, perhaps more than ever again, there is mutual interest of parent and teacher. In this respect, a set of reasonably attainable primary and intermediate level behavioral objectives have been arranged by the National Dairy Council.

In the primary grades, there is a wealth of teaching possibilities built around growing big and strong, such as farm and market visits, growing vegetables in the classroom or school garden, preparing, tasting, and enjoying foods, and emphasizing the sociability of the occasion. The list of possible teaching units in nutrition is lengthy indeed. One can fire the imagination of the enthusiastic child with such headings as, "Getting Ready for Our Picnic," "The Animal Way," "Off to the Farm," "To Market with Mother," or "Making Butter the Hard Way." Moreover, the list of available top-rate films on nutrition is extensive; many are excellent. (See Chapter 10).

The nutrition area is rich in teaching materials available from commercial organizations. The Cereal Institute, for example, has several kits which include colorful cartoon filmstrips, records, and duplicating masters for activity sheets. In *Alexander's Breakfast Secret* (Alexander is a talking dog) there are music and sounds of the morning to go along with a number of activities. The same organization makes the booklet *Breakfast Cereals–Part of Modern Life,* available for intermediate grade level children. Here again a transparency master is free of charge along with duplicating masters for student worksheets. The Florida Citrus Commission also makes duplicating masters available to teachers at no charge. These help call attention to vitamin products. (See current addresses of companies referred to in Chapter 10.) The posters and charts of the National Livestock and Meat Board are the most realistic made. Meats and other foods as depicted look real enough to eat right off the paper.

A list of other organizations that supply teachers with nutrition education materials follows. The National Dairy Council is the organization most prolific in dispensing teaching aids, with everything from posters and leaflets to white rats for animal feeding experiments (a *Nutrition Learning System* is now available from this organization to make foods exciting. It comes with an excellent scope and sequence chart that sets forth nutrition education in a step-by-step approach that is geared to learner outcomes.) H. J. Heinz Company with *Facts About Foods;* American Institute of Baking with many colorful pamphlets and *The Wonder of You*—an informative 12-page manual for the teacher and intermediate pupils; General

Figure 8–7. More children make their own breakfast and often eat it alone. (Courtesy Cereal Institute, Inc., Chicago, Illinois.)

Mills, Inc. with *Nutrition Guide* developed to help the new teacher; Pet, Inc. with the carefully detailed *Meal Planning Guide;* and Sunkist Growers and their filmstrips, posters, and big orange booklet for the teacher, *Build a Better You With Fresh Citrus.* A noncommercial manual designed for the elementary teacher, grades kindergarten through six, is *Focus on Nutrition.* It may be obtained from the Massachusetts Dept. of Education, 182 Tremont St., Boston, at a small cost. It is a complete curriculum guide loaded with fine ideas on how to make the subject of human nutrition alive and vital to younger children.

Suggested Activities

Primary Level

1. Show the *Guide to Good Eating* and stress the need for food each day from the four basic groups (third grade). The *Guide to Good Eating* (in color) is made available by the National Dairy Council (see Figure 8–8). It also is available in Spanish.

2. Keep a record of height and weight. Interest in growth, especially through the individual pupil's readily visible characteristics, is generally high. Particularly useful charts which may be hung on the school wall for groups of children to use may be obtained from Travelers Insurance Company, Hartford, Connecticut (second grade activity).

3. Establish the EE and FF club. Copy the daily lunch menu on the board. Children read this and compare the food items with a food chart also on the board. Everyone goes to the cafeteria knowing what they are eating and *why.* On their return, the pupils report themselves as EE (eat everything) or FF (fussy feeder). Then they discuss why they think they acted the way they did (first and second grades).

4. Prepare a flannelboard presentation about foods (first

A Guide To Good Eating
USE DAILY. . .

Most people are motivated to follow a food guide more closely when they understand why certain foods are em-phasized. On the next pages you will find ideas that may help you explain the importance of each food group.

DAIRY FOODS

3 TO 4 GLASSES—CHILDREN
4 OR MORE GLASSES—TEEN-AGERS
2 OR MORE GLASSES—ADULTS

CHEESE, ICE CREAM AND OTHER MILK-MADE FOODS CAN SUPPLY PART OF THE MILK

2 OR MORE SERVINGS
MEATS, FISH, POULTRY, EGGS, OR CHEESE—WITH DRY BEANS, PEAS, NUTS AS ALTERNATES

MEAT GROUP

VEGETABLES AND FRUITS

4 OR MORE SERVINGS
INCLUDE DARK GREEN OR YELLOW VEGETABLES; CITRUS FRUIT OR TOMATOES

4 OR MORE SERVINGS
ENRICHED OR WHOLE GRAIN ADDED MILK IMPROVES NUTRITIONAL VALUES

BREADS AND CEREALS

This is the foundation for a good diet. Use more of these and other foods as needed for growth, for activity, and for desirable weight.

The nutritional statements made in this guide have been reviewed by the Council on Foods and Nutrition of the American Medical Association and found consistent with current authoritative medical opinion.

Figure 8–8. A daily reminder. (Courtesy National Dairy Council.)

grade). *Ollie and the Orange* and *Smile, Ralph, Smile* are excellent stories with complete teacher instructions which may be obtained free from Sunkist Growers, Inc. in Los Angeles, California.* The same company puts out the filmstrip, *Vitamin C Makes the Difference*—an interesting narrative on vitamins and disease.

5. Visit the local milk bottling plant or bakery to see how foods are preserved through sanitary and other processes. Arrange for samples of the product ahead of time. Be certain, also, that the class knows what to look for.

6. Study color in foods. Begin by asking the class to bring in colored pictures of foods. In the fall, a blue hubbard squash cut down the middle is brilliant. So is a pumpkin, a sweet potato, a box of freshly picked cranberries, or a handful of sweet apples.

7. Ask the class where their food comes from. Some foods come from seeds, others from fruits, leaves, stems, roots, and animals. The class may bring in special foods to illustrate this point.

8. Display several animal bones and human teeth. The children may have samples of first teeth at home and are usually happy to bring them to school. Then discuss the makeup of bones. Calcium and phosphorus are obtained from a number of items which the teacher may take, one at a time, from a large basket on a table at the front of the class: milk, celery, hard cheese, eggs, almonds, dried beans, turnip tops, broccoli, peanut butter, and a piece of lean meat (liver, kidney, or heart). See also the excellent wall chart, "For the Calcium You Need," Evaporated Milk Corporation (free) and the *Nutrition Guide,* available free from General Mills, Inc., Minneapolis, Minnesota.

9. Make clay and cardboard food models which can be used in building combinations for meals. Models already made in appetizing colors may be obtained from the National Dairy Council. Make place mats and place cards for the table. Discuss and arrange flowers for the table (first grade).

10. Make paper cups by folding clean sheets of paper. Enjoy drinking water from them.

11. Visit a farmer in the chicken yard or in the fields raising grain. See turkeys at Thanksgiving time. Have one brought to class in a cage if the class cannot visit a farm. Notice how foods like milk, butter, cheese, and bread are kept safe from dirt and flies.

12. Play grocery store; pool the knowledge of the class for an efficient operation. Use real canned goods and solid vegetables such as potatoes, onions, and carrots.

13. Subscribe to *Food News,* available from the National Dairy Council. Copies are fifteen cents apiece, or $7.50 per hundred; it is for students and teachers to use together.

---

*All addresses of companies referred to may be found in Chapter 10.

14. Prepare and taste fruit and milk drinks. Milk may be flavored with honey, chocolate syrup, peanut butter, or bananas.

OUR CHILDREN suggest

15. Look over various food advertisements brought to class. Post the better ones so that they may be seen. Discuss accuracy. Talk about food values, truths, and half truths (third grade).
16. Prepare a cookbook made chiefly of pictures instead of words. Each pupil will collect all kinds of colored pictures of foods. Past issues of popular magazines may be cut up at home or in class. These pictures are then pasted on sheets of paper in groups and the sheets may be combined into one small booklet.
17. Conduct an experiment in which two tomato plants are used—both plants to be given sunlight, air, and water, but one to be planted in poor soil and the other in good soil.
18. Use the clock when talking about regular meal habits, sleeping, work, and play.
19. Make large posters showing the body engine in action, such as hopping, running, dancing, skating, swimming, or playing games. Other posters depicting active children and relating to food and rest are available from General Mills, Inc., Minneapolis, Minnesota.
20. Ask about appetite. What makes a person eat well? Draw rough sketches of two kinds of eaters and display in the classroom.
21. Make butter in class; then spread it on crackers to eat as a midmorning snack. (Obtain instruction leaflets for all class members from the National Dairy Council.)
22. On different days, prepare and serve raw vegetables: cauliflower, carrots, turnips, lettuce, celery, spinach, broccoli, cabbage, and tomatoes. Serve a small bit of the vegetable which is broken and washed by the children.

Eats a good, big breakfast

Leaves much of his breakfast

23. In discussing breakfast foods, make a display or "store front" of empty cereal boxes brought from homes of the children.

24. Using a large map of the United States, find and mark the places from which meat comes. Locate the sources of the different kinds of fish.

25. Keep a weekly record of the basic four groups eaten every day. (Use chart distributed by Maltex Company, Burlington, Vt.)

26. Hold a parent-child breakfast at school.

27. Use a committee of interested parents and children to do planning. Follow up with a breakfast discussion. How about breakfast appetite and the rule that 25 per cent of the daily calorie requirement should be eaten at breakfast?

28. Have a "Crazy Milk Day" in the classroom. Help the children make butter to eat on crackers, buttermilk, cottage cheese, yogurt, and cream cheese. Call attention to cheese with some "Did You Know?" posters:

DID YOU KNOW?

. . . that in Switzerland, when a baby is born, a wheel of Saanen cheese is marked with his or her name? On all the holiest occasions of his or her mortality this private cheese is served. When he or she dies the mourners consume the last of this ceremonial Wheel of Life.

. . . that the holes in Swiss cheese form themselves naturally through the chemical changes that take place during aging?

---

29. Coloring books, *Jane and Jimmy Learn About Fresh Fruits and Vegetables,* are available with *Tips for Teaching* from United Fresh Fruit and Vegetables Association. Coloring familiar foods is still a first grade activity that holds interest.

Intermediate Level

1. Discuss the statement, "It's smart to eat a good breakfast." How much breakfast should one eat, and what kind? The

Iowa breakfast studies and a number of others show that 25 to 30 per cent of the day's nourishment should be provided by breakfast. The bacon and eggs type of breakfast can be equaled by one consisting of milk, cereal, toast, and butter. Present-day cereals have a far greater food value than most people realize. A single serving of Cream of Wheat, for example, contains as much iron as a serving of liver. And many cereals are rich in high-vitamin wheat germ.

2. Prepare several breakfast menus. Divide the class into "Try Out" committees. Each committee will try out two or three menus, considering such things as ease of preparation, taste, cost, food values, and personal preferences (sixth grade). Further discussion might center around the factors involved in establishing personal preferences.

3. Study food dishes from other lands. Consider the nationalities represented by pupils in the classroom. Possibly an Italian dinner, Greek lunch, or Brazilian breakfast could actually be served in the school with or without parental assistance. In the dairy areas of Brazil, for instance, a breakfast would consist of a hard roll *(pãozinho)*, butter *(manteiga)*, mineiro cheese *(queijo mineiro)*, and warm milk flavored with coffee. A Chinese meal complete with chopsticks, plate, and spoon affords quite an experience. See *It's Always Breakfast Time Somewhere* (National Dairy Council) for suggestions and facts of particular interest to middle grade children.

4. Hang the *Orange Is Beautiful* mobile in the classroom or cafeteria and then discuss empty-calorie snacks versus nutritious ones. Mobile available free from Sunkist Growers, Inc. in Van Nuys, California.

5. Have the local or county agent visit the class to explain some of the problems of local agriculture and animal husbandry. Before he or she arrives, have the class prepare a list

---

Can't Danish pastry or doughnuts be considered an adequate breakfast for some people?

It may be "breakfast," but it probably won't get you through the morning. If you eat two Danish pastries, with two pats of butter, you've consumed some 400 calories, but only five grams of protein. This negligible amount of protein in a high-calorie breakfast may provide a quick pickup but can result in symptoms of hypoglycemia (low blood sugar) in two or three hours. As a result, you'll feel tired, despite the fact that you've eaten "breakfast." Ounce for ounce, doughnuts have even less protein than Danish pastries. Two plain doughnuts (250 calories) provide three grams of protein; two raised doughnuts (also 250 calories), four grams. Nutritionally speaking, neither Danish nor doughnuts adds up to a good breakfast.

of questions that they would like to have him or her answer (fifth and sixth grades).

6. Request the state agricultural college or county agent to send some samples of various types of soil for use in the classroom. Fertilizing additives may be used to stimulate plant growth and to demonstrate why the farmer must employ crop rotation to insure the return of certain elements to the soil after a crop has been harvested. One New England school has for years demonstrated the necessity for proper fertilizers by having an experimental garden in the classroom. Seed quality may also be demonstrated this way.

7. Correlate such factors as rainfall, temperature, altitude, and frost dates with the food belts for corn, wheat, cotton, or dairy products.

8. Look over a simple diagram of the digestive and elimination tract. Answer questions on digestion, appetite, hunger, assimilation, and the elimination of waste. Most children enjoy talking about appetite—good and bad.

9. Post the following poem for all to see. What do you suppose it means?

There was a fat lady from Eye...

who felt she
was likely to die;

But for fear
that once dead
She would not
be well-fed,

She gulped down
a pig,
a cow,
a sheep,
twelve buns,
a seven-layer cake,
four cups of coffee,
and a green apple pie.

10. Secure several recordings of music and experiment with each while the class eats. How do marches compare with soft string music as a background for eating?

11. What is meant by a pleasant, cheerful atmosphere at meal time? Post the following poem just before lunch period.

When supper's almost ready

We rest a little while

And think of something funny

That will make the family smile.

12. Grind some dried corn kernels in class. This may relate well to a study of Indian life (see Figure 8–9).

13. Conduct an animal feeding experiment with white rats, hamsters, or baby chicks.[13] This is especially good for a fourth grade class. Two 65-gram rats, weighed each Monday over an eight-week period, may yield startling results. In an Indiana classroom, one rat was fed the regular school luncheon diet and grew to 180 grams. The other rat was fed only hard candy, vanilla wafers, unenriched bread, jelly, and soft drinks; he wasted away to 55 grams. (For more on this see Chapter 9.)

14. Investigate food fads, dieting, and calories. Build calorie charts for typical quantities of common foods. List foods

---

[13]Local National Dairy Council offices are generally able to meet requests for these experimental animals (free). See also *White Rat of Hawkins Halls,* a story of a white rat experiment, Evaporated Milk Association.

Figure 8–9. Discovering foods by grinding corn the Indian way. (Courtesy *Instructor* magazine.)

consumed during previous three days and calculate calorie intake. Excellent calorie lists which may be obtained in quantity free of charge are contained in the following booklets.

Day	Breakfast	No. of Cal.	Lunch	No. of Cal.	Dinner	No. of Cal.	Snacks	No. of Cal.	Total Calories For Day
1									
2									
3									
								_____Total Calories	

Breakfast Source Book. Cereal Institute, Inc.
Your Guideline to Nutrients and *The Wonder of You.* American Institute of Baking
Choose Your Calories Wisely. Kellogg Co.
Compare differences within the class. Compare daily activities of the various pupils at home and at school and relate to food intake.

15. Become calorie conscious for a time. Post a chart for all to see (see Figure 8–10). Relate calories to daily activities (6th grade). Estimate the number of calories used to perform an activity: (1) Multiply body weight by number of calories used per pound per hour. (2) Multiply this figure by the fraction of an hour actually spent on the activity.

Activity	Calories Per Pound Per Hour
Dressing and undressing	0.7
Eating meals and snacks	0.2
Sitting in classes	0.4
Dancing	2.0
Laboratory work	0.5
Walking	1.1
Walking rapidly	1.8
Running	3.7
Piano playing	0.9
Typewriting	1.0
Housework	1.2
Carpentry	2.0
Swimming	4.1
Writing	0.4
Ping-pong	2.5
Sleep	0.1

EXAMPLE
If you weigh 80 lbs. and play ping-pong for 15 minutes, you will be working at the rate of 200 calories per hour. Thus, in 15 minutes you will use about 50 calories. (Would a tablespoon of peanut butter provide enough energy?)

16. Collect food superstitions and discuss these in terms of scientific knowledge.
17. Discuss the terms "enriched," "restored," and "fortified." Flour and bread were first enriched in 1941. The law re-

IMPLEMENTING THE HEALTH CURRICULUM

Figure 8–10. Figuring nutrients on the spot. (Courtesy National Dairy Council.)

HOW WE IN THE UNITED STATES GET OUR CALORIES

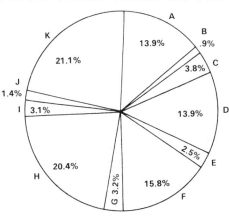

A. Meat, poultry, and fish

B. Leafy, green, and yellow vegetables

C. Other vegetables and fruit

D. Dairy products, excluding butter

E. Eggs

F. Sugar and syrups

G. Dry beans and peas, nuts, soya flour, and cocoa

H. Fats and oils, including pork, fat cuts, and butter

I. Potatoes and sweet potatoes

J. Citrus fruit and tomatoes

K. Flour and cereal products

about 200 CALORIES

Cake, plain . . . . . 3x2x1 ½ inches
Doughnut, cake type . . . . 1 ½
Ice cream . . . . ⅔ cup
Meat, except pork . . . . 2 oz.
Peanut butter . . . . 2 tablespoons
Potato chips . . . . 20 medium
Sherbet . . . . ¾ cup

about 300 CALORIES

Cake, frosted
   layer . . . . 2-inch wedge
Chocolate
   candy bar . . One 2-2 ½ oz. bar
Cookies, plain and assorted . . . 3
Frankfurter and bun 1
French fried potatoes . . 16 pieces
Ham . . . . 3 oz.

Hamburger and bun 1
Milk shake with
   ice cream . . . . ½ serving
Peanuts, roasted . . . . ⅓ cup
Pie, 9-inch diameter . . . . . ⅐ pie
Spaghetti, with
   meat sauce . . . . ¾ cup

Figure 8–11. Calories do count. They come from many sources.

quires the enrichment of flour and bread in most states. The American Bakers Association reports that 80 to 90 per cent of all commercial bread is currently enriched. Bring food packages to class.

18. Ask pupils to help you prepare *behavioral objectives* that can be measured at a later date. A sixth grader might suggest the following:
    a. Identify the information required on a food package label in front of the class.
    b. Give an example of the difference between a factual and a misleading sales presentation for a given food item.
19. Show intermediate level filmstrips, *Project A.M.,* which shows how food scientists relate to one's daily nutrition. Available from Cereal Institute, Inc.; a Spanish version is also available.
20. Place a number of up-to-date colorful booklets on a side table for independent study use. Most can be obtained free from companies. Five examples:

Food for Growing Boys and Girls—Kellogg Company
Vitamin Supplements and Their Correct Use—American Medical Association
Citrus Fruit and Nutrition—Florida Citrus Commission
Build a Better You—Sunkist Growers
Meal Planning Guide—Pet, Inc.

21. Cook dried fruit. Make a fruit salad. Make chopped vegetable sandwiches using dark bread. Serve in class following a discussion of the food values involved. Arrange a centerpiece of vegetables for a classroom table.
22. Appraise the school lunch program. Read and talk about the article, "Would You Eat Your Child's School Lunch?" by Nat Benezra in *Family Health/Today's Health,* September 1977, p. 40.
23. Conduct an experiment using chickens to show the need for green, leafy, or yellow vegetables. Give one chicken feed without vitamin A. Give the other the same diet, but add one of the many sources of vitamin A.
24. Discuss "organic" foods. Do they have special values? To promote a good discussion, obtain a copy of "It's 'Organic'!—So What?" from the United Fresh Fruit and Vegetable Association in Washington, D.C. (free).
25. Review the film *Let's Eat Food* (McGraw-Hill Films). It talks about salt, sugar, and coconut oil being added to processed foods and points out why coconut oil is unsaturated and is completely solid at room temperature.
26. Interview officials of the local health department regarding food protection practices.
27. Read and report about some of the harmful effects of overweight and underweight (sixth grade, independent study).
28. Under committee leadership, conduct an "experimental

kitchen"; prepare and try out nutritious snacks, sandwich spreads, and drinks. Example:

Hot Spiced Cider
Heat apple cider with lemon slices and lemon peel. Spice with cinnamon sticks, cloves, and allspice.

29. Ask the school nurse to explain red cell blood count. Have pupils study foods which provide iron and protein needed to maintain a normal red cell blood count (fifth grade). Note that certain cereals now contain 100 per cent of daily iron requirement.
30. Try some food experiments. For ideas see Ethel Austin Martin, *Nutrition Education in Action*. New York: Holt, Rinehart, and Winston, 1972.

---

4. DENTAL HEALTH

Behavioral Objectives (Primary Level)

Demonstrates how to brush the teeth using the toothbrush.

Explains without apprehension what the dentist does, some information about the equipment, and where he or she is located.

Rinses the mouth with water after eating when at all possible. Investigates how raw foods help clean the teeth.

Distinguishes clean teeth from dirty teeth.

Behavioral Objectives (Intermediate Level)

Explains clearly that dental health is a significant part of one's total health.

Compares crooked teeth with straightened teeth in terms of appearance and efficiency.

Describes the causes of toothache and the need for immediate treatment. Explains how diseases in the body may be related to diseased teeth.

Evaulates dentifrices through reading and discussions with dentists.

Illustrates how water fluoridation functions to reduce tooth decay.

Depicts practices that may injure the teeth.

Comments

About 97 per cent of all children in the United States are affected with dental caries and half of them under 15 never have been to a dentist. By age 16, the average youth has 7 decayed, missing, or filled teeth involving 14 tooth surfaces. Moreover, a large number have broken front teeth. This accident most frequently occurs in the 8 to 11 year age group and is particularly serious because the treatment is very difficult.

The makeup of a thorough dental program consists of dental information for the general public, including educational material for civic groups, a patient education program in the dentists' offices, and a dental health program for schools. These three means of improving dental health have a strong bearing on classroom activity.

As a result of a two-year pilot program in the San Antonio schools sponsored by the U.S. Public Health Service, it is now considered feasible to train children in effective personal dental care practices in the elementary classrooms. Through a series of workshops, 36 teachers were trained in small groups and then they taught 1100 elementary grade children the proper practices. In ten weeks, 88 per cent of the students showed improvement in gum tissue health and reduction in plaque scores. Brief classroom exercises took place to integrate dental health concepts with pupil training in tooth cleaning techniques. This study developed a package curriculum which could be transported to any elementary school in the state. Films, models, and guides for teachers and parents were developed and used. Prepackaged toothbrushing kits containing brushes, dental floss, disclosing wafers, mirrors, and models for a 16-week program were assembled.

Cusato and Kaplan showed that when a dental consultant team works with the elementary school teachers and reinforces proper toothbrushing skills, there is a significant reduction in plaque on the teeth, thereby reducing the incidence of gum disorders and dental caries.[14] According to Green's Index for plaque scoring, 81 per cent of the students had a reduction in plaque following the program and the average decrease in the amount of plaque per child was 36 per cent. It is the concept of brushing *properly* every day that is significant. Greenberg stresses this point as a result of his studies with students having high plaque readings and gingivitis.[15] He found that oral health could be improved by having the parents reward their children weekly for brushing and flossing every day. Getting parents to teach their own children properly results in better oral health, less expense to the school, and the development of a parent-school partnership in the process of health education. Calling for parental help is not new but it has been slow to take hold. In studying five modes of dental health instruction (parent-applied, student-centered, teacher-dominated, dental hygienist-dominated, and a combination mode), Greenberg found the parent-applied behavior modification program to be the most promising.[16]

A number of programs of fluoride mouthrinsing in schools have recently been sponsored by the National Institute of Dental Research of the U.S. Public Health Service. Benefits from mouthrinsing with dilute solutions of neutral sodium fluoride have been repeatedly demonstrated during the past 12 years. Children who rinse weekly

---

[14]Cusato, James L. and Kaplan, David E. "An Elementary School Program in Preventive Dental Health," *Journal of the Massachusetts Dental Society, 23*:256–259, Fall 1974.

[15]Greenberg, Jerrold S. "A Study of Behavior Modification Applied to Dental Health," *Journal of School Health, 47*:594–596, December 1977.

[16]Greenberg, Jerrold S. "An Analysis Of Various Teaching Modes in Dental Health Education," *Journal of School Health, 48*:26–32, January 1977.

may expect to have 20 to 50 per cent fewer cavities than without the mouthrinsing program. The procedure costs about 50 cents per child per year and requires only 5 minutes a week and few materials. The advantage of having this self-applied fluoride program in schools is that schools operate on a more rigid schedule than most families do. Moreover, it works, and more than four million elementary school children are mouthrinsing once a week or taking a fluoride tablet once a day in school.[17] In an Arizona study, 90 per cent of the grade school children participating in the mouthrinsing program experienced fewer dental caries than the nonparticipants and had an attack rate 50 per cent less than that of the nonparticipants.[18] (The attack rate represents the percentage of permanent teeth that are attacked by the carious process in relation to the total number of susceptible teeth.)

The American Dental Association's oral health program, *Learning About Oral Health,* appears to be effective in improving oral health behavior. So does the learning modules program set forth in *Yes, You Can Teach Dental Health* distributed by the American Alliance for Health, Physical Education, and Recreation. Much depends, of course, on the nature of the teacher.

Several commercial organizations make teaching kits available that are used in numerous school health programs. Colgate-Palmolive Company has a program for students in grades K-4 which includes a filmstrip and record, "The Mouth I Live In," a disclosing tablet for checking teeth cleanliness (excellent for home use), and a teacher's guide. This kit is made to serve 35 students. A similar kit, together with step-by-step instructions to the third grade teacher, is available from the Procter and Gamble Company. A class toothbrushing chart for posting is used along with a dental health quiz. First-rate, large, colorful posters can be obtained from the company at no cost. Dental health posters for classroom display are also available from the Florida Citrus Commission (free). Available from Floxite Company, Inc. are lighted mirror sets that permit children to look far into their mouths to see how they look before and after cleaning (see Figure 8–12). The individual student sets certain flash lights, reflectors, and mirrors. This permits regular attention to be paid to the teeth with only a few minutes of teacher time. Toothbrushing record charts are available for each student to take home.

Most state health departments, as well as the American Dental Association and the numerous companies that make dentifrices, are very willing to make available for the teacher's use a variety of teaching aids, brochures, and suggested learning experiences. The majority of these are good when used in the right way. It must be remembered that some elementary schoolchildren have heard about tooth decay and have drawn pictures about teeth for several years. Yet tooth decay is present today as much as it ever was. One might ask what is wrong with the effort. For one thing, the effort has been a

---

[17]For program details, secure a copy of *A Guide for Implementing Self-Applied Fluoride in Schools,* DHEW Publication No. (NIH) 77–1196, National Institute of Dental Health, Bethesda, Md. 20014.

[18]Petchel, Karen A. and Mello, Arthur F. "A School Fluoride Mouthrinse Program," *Journal of School Health,* 47:557–559, November 1977.

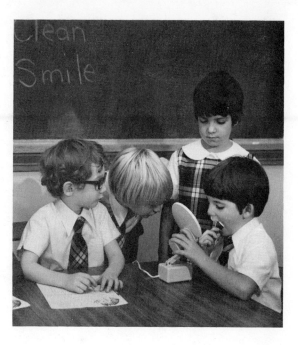

Figure 8–12. Special mouth mirror and reflector shows hidden details of the mouth. (Courtesy Floxite Co., Inc., Niagara Falls, N.Y. 14303.)

weak one. For another, when it has been made, its importance has not been made *vital*. There has been too much talk and not enough action. Experiences have not been lifelike. There has been little imagination employed.

Suggested Activities

Primary Level

1. Ask the class to tell what they know about teeth—How the teeth chew food, how they help in talking, and how they look.
2. Show the primary grade film *Health: Toothache of the Clown* (Encyclopedia Britannica Educational Corporation)—the story about a circus clown who is not happy because he is suffering from a toothache. An excellent teaching script is available for the teacher using the film. The same organization puts out a 9 full-color 8mm loop film dealing with oral health, grades K-6.
3. Talk about toothbrushes. Are some better than others? Have a few samples of new and well worn brushes on hand to look over. Discuss proper care of the brush.
4. Teach about teeth in an incidental way, especially when a child loses a baby tooth or has just returned from a trip to the dentist.
5. Bring animal and human teeth to class. The local meat market may have teeth and the local dentist will be happy to lend teeth. Bring a live cat and dog to class so that the teeth of pets may be seen. Or show pictures of the teeth of different animals.

Figure 8–13. The toothbrushing drill—a pleasant experience.

6. Demonstrate and practice proper toothbrushing. Recent studies reported by the American Dental Association show that a total of one hour of instruction (in four sessions) usually is adequate. Drills may be executed by the whole group right in the classroom. This is easy when below-cost toothbrushing kits are available. A free publication with full instructions for a toothbrushing drill is available from the American Dental Association entitled, *You Can Teach Toothbrushing.* Post brushing diagrams shown in Figure 8–14.

7. Discuss reasons for considering the dentist as a friend. Write the statements formulated by the class on the board. These may be copied later on a ditto sheet for each pupil to carry home. This may alert the parents to take their child to the dentist right away instead of waiting until there is toothache or other complaint.

8. Have each child look into a well-lighted mirror to see if the mouth is clean and to see what the dentist did or can do.

9. Demonstrate decay in an apple. Start with two sound apples. Break the skin of one and place both on the window ledge for daily observation. After a few days, observe what has occurred. Compare this to tooth decay when a "break" in the tooth occurs.

10. Illustrate ways to protect teeth, such as using the drinking fountain correctly and being careful when playing ball. Ask if anyone knows someone who has broken a tooth.

11. Demonstrate how acid can dissolve calcium in tooth enamel. Place a whole hard-cooked egg in a bowl of vinegar (acetic acid) for about 24 hours. As vinegar decalcifies the shell, it becomes soft. Before the experiment, try

DOWN FROM THE TOP inside and out . . . starting on the gums

UP FROM THE BOTTOM inside and out . . . starting on the gums

ACROSS THE TOPS (chewing surfaces)

Toothbrushing using the Bass technic. Use the soft-textured multi-tufted brush. Place all of the bristles where the teeth and gums meet. Rotate the brush until the bristles are gently spread between the teeth. Then while maintaining pressure against the teeth and gums, vibrate the bristles using back and forth strokes.

With the Bass method, the biting surfaces of the teeth must be cleaned separately. Use short back and forth strokes. Be certain to clean all of the teeth.

Figure 8–14. Diagram to post. Regular method continued with Bass method.

pushing the egg through the top of a milk bottle; after decalcification the egg can be pushed into the bottle easily.

12. Mimeograph a chart such as the accompanying one on 8 inch × 11 inch paper. Post the charts in class. Every time pupils brush their teeth—breakfast (B), lunch (L), or dinner (D)—they may color the proper square. They may use different colors (first grade).

Sunday	Monday	Tuesday	Wednesday
B			
L			
D			

13. Practice (play telephone) making appointments to see a dentist. The student playing the dentist should ask proper questions about whether there is an emergency toothache, accident, or need for a regular checkup.

14. Have all class members take the "Tablet-test." Procter and Gamble distributes free two little tablets containing a harmless coloring agent. Colgate also supplies these disclosing tablets. The pupils first brush their teeth the way they always do. They then chew one tablet, letting it dissolve in the mouth. They swish the solution around in the mouth, then rinse the mouth. When they look in a mirror the children will see red areas here and there indicating harmful, decay-producing deposits that were missed in brushing. Rebrushing, of course, will remove the stains.

15. Post a list telling how much sugar there is in some common foods. Then discuss factors influencing wide use of sugar (third grade).

BRUSH UP ON YOUR BRUSHING

TAKE THIS ● TABLET-TEST ●

16. Give children a daily record of toothbrushing to keep in the home.

17. Encourage parents to supervise the brushing of teeth at home. Consider sending an information letter to the parents.

Intermediate Level

1. Examine the wall chart showing a sound tooth. Refer early to three factors associated with tooth decay: nutrition,

brushing, and individual differences (hardness of teeth and hereditary strengths or weaknesses). This last factor is important. There will always be people, exceptional cases, who eat poorly and appear to have good teeth. Children see them and often draw erroneous conclusions. Thus these exceptions, together with other examples of variation, need discussion in the classroom.

2. Have a student committee visit a local dentist and report back to the class with their findings regarding tooth decay, extractions, dental tools, filling materials, and anesthetics.

3. Make tooth powder. Have the class members mix one part of salt to three parts of baking soda. Put a few drops of wintergreen extract into this to give it a pleasant smell. Let it dry, then try it out. Everyone may comment. Perhaps the group will want more wintergreen added to a new batch of powder, or another flavor may be desired.

4. Show pictures of crooked teeth, diseased teeth, and bright, clean, sound teeth. Learn the parts of the teeth. Investigate the functions of the joints and heart for the purpose of associating disease in these areas with infected teeth. Show how decayed teeth are bathed by the blood stream so that one's total efficiency may be reduced through poor teeth.

5. Teach dental health in connection with a study of foods and nutrition. Emphasize the necessity of eating bone-building foods.

6. Formulate and record by way of tape recorder a list of reasons why teeth are important and how teeth should be cared for. Play back the tape and appraise it in terms of its effectiveness in changing behavior. Encourage suggestions for shortening the recording and making it appealing. Compare it to radio and television advertisements for dentifrices and foods.

7. Collect toothbrush and dentifrice advertisements; study the claims made. Gather information to determine whether the claims are reasonable and accurate.

8. Prepare, as a group, such snacks as apple slices, dried fruit, celery, carrot sticks, and nuts that can be eaten between meals. Talk about how satisfying they are to the appetite and the values of each kind of snack. Note how celery and carrot sticks help keep the teeth clean (fourth grade).

9. Have a dentist or dental hygienist come to class. Have a panel of students on hand to ask questions. From such an interview, the class should find that the dentist does at least the following important things: makes a complete health inventory and dental history; cleans and scales the teeth; x-rays every tooth, locating the cavities no matter how small; detects abnormal conditions of the gums or mouth; and gives a full explanation of his or her treatment plan, number of visits, and proposed fees.

10. Stress the relationship of good grooming, appearance, and pleasant breath to success both in school and in the com-

munity. For upper grade pupils this approach may hold more interest and shape more attitudes than the approach through foods, disease, and body physiology.

11. Show the Johnson and Johnson film, *Take Time for Your Teeth*. Have each pupil list the essential points when the showing is over.

12. Using small pocket mirrors, or Fluxite mirrors (see Figure 8–12) one for each row of pupils, have each child look at his or her own teeth and try to answer the questions, "How do our teeth work?" "What work do the different-shaped teeth do?" "Do my teeth meet evenly when I close my mouth?"

13. Make wax impressions of the teeth. Use household preserving wax, 2 inches × 2 inches and ¼ inch thick (molds may be made in class to this size from heavy aluminum foil). For further hints on this project, secure a copy of the free booklet, *The Way to Smile,* from Procter and Gamble Co.

14. Find out how much sugar is in many of the popular foods. There is more than a casual relationship between excessive sugar consumption and dental decay. Most children hear about this at an early age but they do little about it because of other more impressive factors. Discuss these other factors; the pupils will know what they are.

There is a substantial amount of sugar in most popular foods. For example:

		Sugar
Coca-Cola	6 oz. bottle	4⅓ tsp.
root beer	10 oz bottle	4½ tsp.
candy bar	1–5 oz.	5–10 tsp.
angel food cake	4 oz. piece	7 tsp.
ice cream sundae	1	7 tsp.
cherry pie	1 slice	10 tsp.

15. Post this sign at the front of the classroom:

> PAUL REVERE MADE FALSE TEETH FOR GEORGE WASHINGTON AND ADVERTISED HIS PRACTICE IN THE *BOSTON GAZETTE* IN 1786! WHAT ELSE CAN YOU FIND ABOUT THE EARLY PRACTICE OF DENTISTRY?

(See the book by Esther Forbes, *Paul Revere and the World He Lived In*. Boston: Houghton-Mifflin Co.)

16. Include dental words in spelling lessons. Fourth and fifth grade pupils should be able to spell words such as:

erupt	enamel	fluoride
cuspid	pulp	abscess
bicuspid	decay	malocclusion
calcium	tartar	orthodontist
molar	bacteria	
permanent	Novocain	

17. Do not overlook the opportunity to point out that water fluoridation is a classic example of the public health ap-

proach to dental disease control (sixth grade). Over three decades of brilliant research have shown that the community may reduce the dental caries attack by over 60 per cent by fluoridating the water supply.

18. Distribute a 10-inch piece of dental floss to each pupil. Have the class practice using the floss to clean the area between the teeth. A leaflet suitable for grade four or above may be obtained (free) from Johnson & Johnson. It is entitled *How to Use Dental Floss.*

19. Examine "before" and "after" plaster of Paris molds of sets of teeth showing malocclusion and the results of orthodontia. Local dentists are usually helpful with the loan of materials. Have the class relate malocclusion to a number of mouth problems. How may halitosis occur here? Will mouthwashes overcome effects of crooked teeth and an unclean mouth?

---

5. BODY STRUCTURE AND OPERATION

Behavioral Objectives (Primary Level)

Describes the basic bone and muscle structure of the body and compares it with the framework of other structures such as automobiles and buildings.

Shows where vital organs of the body are located and what they do.

Identifies elements in health examination and tests of seeing and hearing.

Demonstrates proper posture in sitting, standing, and walking.

Relates key ways to protect the eyes and ears from injury.

Behavioral Objectives (Intermediate Level)

Explains how sound body structure is a prerequisite to proper functioning.

Investigates and describes how exercise and recreation tend to relax tensions caused by strong emotions and overambitious living.

Identifies the structure of cells, tissues, organs, and systems.

Portrays what is meant by normal growth.

Chooses scientific terms to describe the body and its functions.

Interprets the close relationship existing between systems of circulation, respiration, digestion, and elimination.

Applies an understanding of the special senses to the care of eyes, ears, and mouth.

Comments

According to Abraham Maslow, one of the characteristics of a healthy, self-actualizing person (his term for maturity reaching toward the fulfillment of the individual) is that he or she has an understanding and appreciation of his or her body which lead to less actual body consciousness and greater use of the body *as an extension of the whole personality.*[19] If this is true, then educators for years have been missing an oportunity to influence human effectiveness through a study of the physical self.

A study of the body structure and its function is a fundamental one. It is a biological topic that should be carried on as soon as the class is ready for it.

Primary graders require very little reference to body function. Short general answers to questions of "why" usually suffice, but the upper grade pupils very often want a detailed reason. This is the time to bring in elementary anatomy and physiology—not in a cut and dried approach but with familiar examples and choice references to personal well-being and appearance. In fact, in many cases boys and girls are impressed more with how they look to others and feel on special occasions than they are with the circulation of blood or the physiology behind good sight and hearing.

Children of all ages tend to be interested in their posture and their general body mechanics if the topics are presented in terms of personal growth, appearance, and well-being. Measuring growth in the classroom by checking height against the wall and weight on the scales seldom fails to ferret out a number of excellent questions, especially in grades one to three. Here the teacher has an opportunity to demonstrate good standing posture, to discuss ligaments, tendons, and muscles that maintain this posture, and to relate this function to sound nutrition, adequate sleep, and freedom from disease-causing organisms. It may readily be shown that poor eating and fatigue cause many problems and that postural attitudes tell much about a person's mental health.

Upper grade children will be especially fascinated by a study of how the foot works, the nature of the longitudinal and metatarsal arches, why the policeman is called a "flatfoot," why sneakers are not advisable for use on hard pavements, the benefits of good shoes and foot exercises, why top-rate athletes practice proper foot hygiene, and how overweight can cause pain in the feet. Of course, merely lecturing to a class about the position of the feet in walking or how they should stand or sit will not in itself change the body mechanics of many children. In fact, talking is not enough. In every class, one finds a child whose poor posture represents a kind of rebellion against nagging parents and teachers who have overpreached on this topic. Postural changes are brought about when children hear, see, and *feel* what optimum posture is. Bring a mirror to class. Have boys and girls take a side view look at themselves. Have them back up against a flat wall and with their hand feel how much space there is between the hollow of the back and the wall. Let them "stand tall" and walk away from the wall to the mirror so that they can reinforce the way they feel with what they *see.*

---

[19]Maslow, Abraham. *Motivation and Personality.* New York: Harper and Row, 1960, p. 196.

In the case of the tall girl who is seen stooping a bit while talking with a number of friends, it may be that her defect is due strictly to an intense desire to "keep up with the Joneses" by lowering the body to the level of her shorter friends. Such an illustration is rich in instructional ideas. Tall children should know that many a tall person has a kind of upright bearing and grace in movement that is the envy of others.

Included in this particular topic of structure and function is the care of the special senses. Primary grade children need to discuss in detail how to protect their eyes and ears. They should understand the relationship of light and glare to seeing and eye comfort, and they should know how eyeglasses work and how to watch television. Intermediate classes should have a simple understanding of how the eyes and ears work as well as how to take proper care of them. Fifth and sixth graders almost always show interest in a large model of the eyeball or ear, especially if the parts as shown are immediately related to abnormalities shared by members of the class. For example, nearsightedness (myopia) or farsightedness (hyperopia) are readily explained. A simple eyeball sketch on the blackboard showing a convex or concave lens which is used to correct the particular difficulty will be effective. This is especially true if it is used with actual eyeglasses which the children are permitted to examine. The flexibility of an eyeball can be demonstrated by noting the properties of a hard boiled egg. A Snellen Test chart, employed to measure simple visual acuity or accommodation, can be used in the classroom as both a screening instrument and a teaching device. Some reference should be made, when the special senses are being investigated, to the relationship between safe driving and optimum seeing and hearing. Good eyesight has much to do with personal safety—riding bicycles, crossing streets, and reading roadside signs and markers. The question of how blind and deaf boys and girls behave and how they feel is one that provokes discussion.

Help is available for the teacher who is concerned with the care of the special senses. The primary grade film, *Health: Eye Care Fantasy* (Encyclopedia Britannica Educational Corp.), runs eight minutes and usually provokes a number of good questions and student observations. Perhaps the finest teaching manual, *Teaching About Vision,* was developed by the American School Health Association and the National Society for the Prevention of Blindness, Inc. especially for classroom teachers. Lessons are suggested and all scientific words are explained in simple terms. Also, when discussing the skin as a sense organ, the American Alliance for Health, Physical Education, and Recreation has a very popular intermediate grade level filmstrip, *Every Body's Skin Makes Everybody Kin;* it deals very well with appearance, sensation, and feeling.

The body structure and its operation simply cannot be taught in terms of systems, processes, and mechanics to elementary school children. It has to be taught quite personally with pertinent questions being answered as they are raised by the class. Good teaching motivates the questions the teacher knows to be important. Most children want to know sooner or later what they look like with the

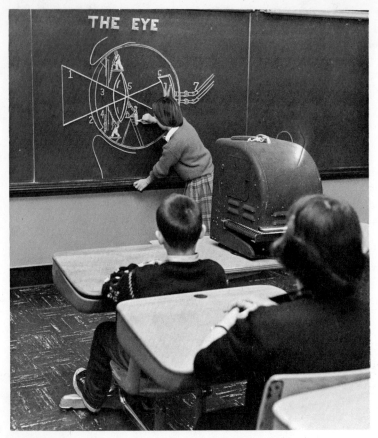

Figure 8–15. Intermediate students are ready for detailed work. (Courtesy Cincinnati Public Schools.)

skin off and why their bodies function as they do. They want to know how the heart beats and what it sounds like, why they perspire in summer, how the arms move, and a hundred other such practical questions. Without the teacher's moralizing, the class can be shown that the body, in the words of the poet, is the "temple of the soul" and the "organ of the will." It is, by simple statement, an amazing machine with intricacies so numerous that man has not yet figured out all of its actions. Finally, and this is significant, children will not treat the body as a fine instrument until they learn to appreciate it for what it is.

A number of teachers like to discuss essential organs such as the heart under the body structure-function topic. This provides an opportunity to discuss pain and other heart attack symptoms as well the relationship of high blood pressure to the stresses of our society. Children can be taught that when a family member or friend experiences difficulty breathing, nausea, vomiting, cold sweat, paleness, weakness, and anxiety, he or she may be undergoing a heart attack.

School Days, Inc., 2361 Jefferson Davis Highway, Arlington, Virginia 22202, distributes a fine kit that promotes a positive awareness of the body. It was designed following a pilot testing program involving 150,000 youngsters in 13 states. The introductory kit deals with muscles and bones.

Suggested Activities

Primary Level

1. Post baby photographs around the classroom. A set that shows development through the years is most valuable. Pictures of babies, children, and young people may be cut from magazines and brought to class by the pupils. These can be graduated in such a way as to depict the story of a steady growth.

2. Bring pictures of machines to class and discuss similarity to body functions. Feel arm and finger bones and shoulder and hip joints and see how they move. Choose a pupil to bend, twist, and straighten his or her backbone to show that the spine is made up of many little bones (second grade).

3. Measure each child for height and weight at intervals. Tie this activity in with body growth. Refer to the growth of the hair, fingernails, and toenails. An excellent "How Tall" wall chart for measuring height is put out by the Travelers Insurance Co., Hartford, Connecticut (free). It is hung on a wall or door, 2½ feet above the floor. The names of the children may be written in at the head of the height column. Each time a meausrement is made, add the date near the height mark. Seven charts will service a class of 28 pupils.

4. Using this growth measuring activity, show the relationship of height to standing posture; stress standing tall without affecting a braced type of posture. Illustrate this by dropping a string plumb line from the ceiling of the classroom. The line should run approximately through the tip of the ear, the center of the shoulder, the hip joint, the knees, and the

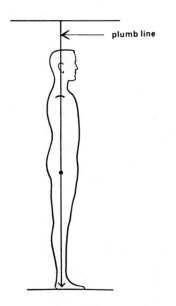

plumb line

outside ankle bone. Let each class member try this. (A window pole held vertically may be substituted for the plumb line.)

5. Play a game where everyone chooses an animal and mimics its movements by carefully moving about the classroom or recreational area. Then stop and discuss what animals and humans have in common relative to movement.

6. Listen to the beat of a heart. A stethoscope may be borrowed from the health service department so that each child can hear a heart beat. This is a good project to engage in just before visiting the school physician for a medical examination.

7. Compare the function of the ears with an ordinary telephone receiver. A simple demonstration can be made with an upright telephone. This may be borrowed from a secondary school science department or the local telephone company office. First graders will be amused; third graders will want to see the telephone taken apart.

8. Identify objects by taste, odor, or sound while blindfolded. This can be carried out after the initial demonstration by making a game out of it. In a class of 28 children, four teams of seven children each may, for example, listen to a particular sound. The first child in each group guesses first. The first to give the correct answer scores a point for his or her team. He or she then moves to the end of the line. The game continues with different sensory items being introduced. This game motivates the class to want to talk about their senses of smell, taste, and hearing and how these work with the important sense of sight. Material to have on hand for this game might include a piece of chocolate, a spoiled orange, sour milk, or a musical record.

9. Use bellows to demonstrate breathing. Compare a sponge to the lung structure. Look at an x-ray picture of a pair of

normal lungs (third grade). A school physician or local health department will usually be able to supply a no longer needed negative for classroom use and storage. Have pupils breathe in deeply, holding their hands on their sides to feel the ribs.

10. Talk about reading books which are printed in a type which is easy to read and sitting in a comfortable position while reading in order not to get tired. Examine some fine print with a reading glass or ordinary magnifying glass.

11. Check sight in class by using the Snellen chart. Use it more as an object lesson than a screening device. Have children talk about their own seeing problems and what they should consider doing to correct the difficulty. (See reference to Snellen chart in Chapter 3.)

12. Let the class hear high and low vibrations to show that certain sounds are more readily heard and recognized. Use whistles, pipes, or a flute to compare with the sound of a tuba, cello string, or low note on a saxophone. One of the many records on the individual instruments of the orchestra may prove helpful here.

13. Teach special senses safety. Point out that only a clean handkerchief should be used near the eyes, that one should refrain from pointing objects such as scissors, pencils, or sticks at anyone, and that nothing should be put in the ear.

14. Show why it is necessary to play carefully so that the ears and eyes will not be injured. Point out that running while carrying sharp objects or glass is not a good practice. Warn pupils about shouting into ears. Make pictures of objects that may injure the eyes and ears, such as pencils, scissors, paper clips, snowballs, BB guns, slingshots, or rubber bands. Have children talk about their pictures to the class.

15. Distribute bookmarks so that each class member has one. These are available free from the American Optometric Association. (See opposite illustration.)

16. Find out what to do in case of earaches. Bring the school nurse into the classroom to help.

17. Collect pictures of different kinds of eyes from magazines and newspapers. Put together a large mural-sized montage of the pictures. Be sure to get pictures of fish, birds, animals, and insects, as well as humans.

Intermediate Level

1. Discuss growth. Of what does it consist? Look over body diagrams or wall charts (Dennoyer-Gebhart wall charts of body systems are available in many schools). Refer briefly to the relationship of the various areas of body, i.e., circulation to respiration, digestion to elimination. This should be brief and merely introductory in nature.

2. Point out that 23 million Americans, including many young children, have high blood pressure. Take the children's blood pressure and discuss how it is affected by stress, tobacco smoking, obesity, heredity, and excess sodium

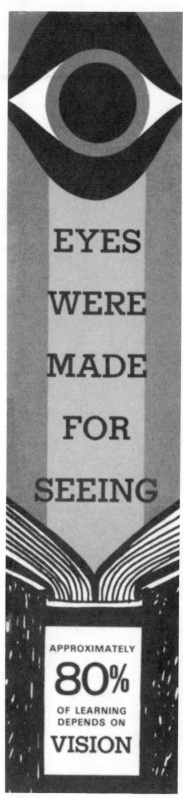

EYES WERE MADE FOR SEEING

APPROXIMATELY

80%

OF LEARNING DEPENDS ON

VISION

from too much salt in the diet. Explain systolic and diastolic pressure.

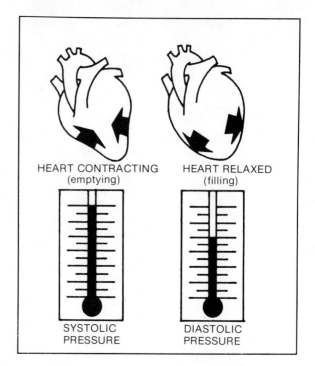

HEART CONTRACTING
(emptying)

HEART RELAXED
(filling)

SYSTOLIC
PRESSURE

DIASTOLIC
PRESSURE

3. Listen to the heartbeat with a stethoscope. Study a simple diagram of the heart. Have one pupil jump up and down for 30 seconds. Then notice the increased heart action by listening again with the stethoscope. Notice also the increase in breathing. Show how the lungs perform the function of securing oxygen for the blood.

4. Locate and feel the pulse beat; relate this to the heart beat. Point out which arteries near the surface of the body may serve to measure pulse. Note the notch along the side of the chin, the artery under the upper arm, in the groin, and near the ear on the side of the head. Check these pressure points and indicate briefly how severe bleeding may be controlled by causing pressure over these points.

5. Post an open map on the wall alongside a diagram of the body showing the road or path followed by the blood stream. Point out such items as:

   a. Blood, bathing an infected tooth area, can carry germs to the lining of the heart, to another organ, or to a joint.

   b. The force and rate of the heart beat has a bearing on the efficiency of the system.

   c. Vigorous physical exercise calls for more oxygenated blood to be supplied to the muscles.

   d. An effective brain depends as much on the blood and oxygen supply as on the muscles.

6. Show the effect of fatigue, food, rest, disease, emotions, and exercise on the pulse beat. Let the class add to this by telling

their experiences. Answer the "why" questions in terms of elementary physiology.

7. Illustrate, through experiment, the relationship of physical fitness (strength and endurance) to heart efficiency. Set up a simple exercise test which is related to the rise and fall of the pulse rate.

8. Discuss the relationship of body posture to body function. Let the class point out that poor nutrition, inadequate sight or hearing, and personal feelings have a bearing on posture.

9. Illustrate the connection between poor standing and sitting posture and general fatigue. Have two pupils stand at the front of the classroom with their left arms extended horizontally to the side. Continue with the lesson and about five minutes later ask the two pupils where they are tired. They will mention the extended arm together with the opposite side of the body. Point out that they have expended considerable energy while in "poor posture" by trying to keep from falling away from the line of gravity. Illustrate this further by using kindergarten building blocks. (See illustration.)

Show that there is less strain in the building block molecules when they come close to approximating the line of gravity *B* than there is in figure *C,* and that there is more stress and strain in the materials of the blocks in C. This is similar to the stress and strain in boy *A* who is attempting to stay on the gravitational or "fall" line. Then have several pupils walk across the classroom, illustrating a number of pronounced postural defects such as a head forward position, rounded shoulders, a high shoulder, and a hollow back curve. Relate these conditions to *A* and *C* and fatigue.

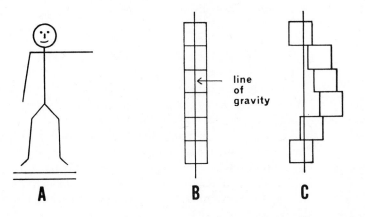

10. Discuss the mechanics of walking, sitting, and sleeping. Show the relationship of poor sleeping posture, mattresses, and beds to chronic fatigue and irritability. Further discuss the social benefits of correct posture. Practice sitting down and getting up from a chair.

11. Display some animal bones, which may be obtained from a meat market. Show longitudinal and cross sections.

12. Choose a girl to respond to the role of *Jane,* and another for the role of *Sue.*

13. Organize a posture contest. This might develop into a full elementary school assembly program. Some preparation should precede this event. Fourth, fifth, and sixth grade posture contest entrants may be checked at each of seven stations:
    a. Sitting (at a desk)
    b. Walking (across the platform)
    c. Exercises (for coordination and flexibility)
    d. Posture screen (by school nurse)
    e. Plumb line test
    f. Foot and leg alignment (by the nurse)
    g. Roaming judgment (by a judge who judges posture at all times in between the stations)

Score on the basis of 70 points for a perfect score. Many good activities and experiences may be derived from such a contest.

14. Talk about good foot health. Secure an animal's foot or the bones of a leg and foot from the local meat market. Show a cow's knee joint. Have a leg and foot of chicken on hand to show how muscles and ligaments are associated in the human foot. Explain the longitudinal and metatarsal arches and the relationship of their functional efficiency to gait, shoes, and posture.

15. Measure a footprint angle with the protractor (fifth grade activity). Supply each child with a piece of brown paper, a ruler, pencil, and protractor. Have each child step on a damp towel and then stand on the brown paper. Do the same for each foot. Before the paper dries, draw lines A-B and C-D. Measure the angle formed by these lines.

This is a project that will promote all kinds of foot questions.

What is a good arch? What is a flat foot? Why should police officers sometimes do foot exercises while standing on the corner? Are sneakers and moccasins harmful to the feet? How should the heels wear down on the shoes? How should we walk? Is pigeon-toed walking harmful or helpful?

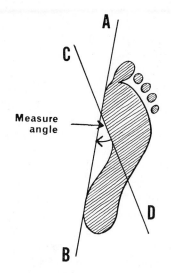

16. Make a large, simple diagram or picture that shows the parts of the human eye. Assign parts of the eye for several pupils to define. An encyclopedia, health texts, and eye booklets may be laid out on a side table for independent use. Compare the eye to a camera. Discuss the rods and cones of the retina and their relationship to good nutrition, disease, and body poisons. The eye of a sheep is especially useful for classroom use.

17. Smear a drop of blood on a glass slide and examine it through a microscope to observe the structure and arrangement of blood cells.

18. Collect and display pictures that depict people from all walks of life taking part in various work and play activities in which good eyesight, good hearing, and a fine sense of balance are necessary. Supplement the display with pictures that show how certain handicaps and inadequacies can be compensated for by the use of such devices as braces, hearing aids, artificial limbs, and eyeglasses.

19. Tell stories to illustrate how the emotions affect the body. Show how stress items such as fear, anger, jealousy, hate, and worry increase the pulse rate and make people tense. Read a particularly exciting and suspense-filled story or show such a movie. Stop the class at the critical moment to have them notice their heart and respiration rates.

20. Match up everyone with a partner. Blindfold one partner and have the other serve as the guide. One by one each blindfolded pupil should try to explore the classroom, locate his or her desk, identify other persons and objects in the room, etc. Then have the partners switch places so that everyone will have a turn to be blindfolded.

21. Dramatize the story of Thomas Edison and his hearing problem.

22. Demonstrate the use of an audiometer by the school nurse.

23. Draw and label parts of the respiratory system. Follow this with a demonstration of how mouth-to-mouth breathing is administered to a person in need of artificial respiration. Leaflets for class distribution are available from Johnson & Johnson (free).

24. Play a game linking language and thought through sensory awareness activity. Prepare a paper bag, putting in such objects as a smooth stone, a rough stone, a small piece of metal, hard bread, a piece of wax, soap, and modeling clay. Blindfold a pupil and let him or her take an object out of the bag and discuss its texture. To further illustrate sensory awareness, create other bags with different materials such as burlap, cotton, silk, velvet—or honey, butter, relish, and detergent powder. A fun activity.

---

6. PREVENTION AND CONTROL OF DISEASE
Behavioral Objectives (Primary Level)

Describes how children go freely to visit the nurse and other medical personnel.

Explains a few activities carried on by some health workers in the community who protect the health of others.

Relates elementary disease conditions to personal unhappiness.

Drinks properly from a water fountain and does not share glasses and straws.

Describes germs and relates them to sneezes, sore throats, and similar occurrences.

Identifies hospitals as important factors in the process of recovery from disease.

Explains the necessity for proper healthful practices concerning oneself and others and shows favorable attitudes toward the school physician and nurse and their equipment, thereby overcoming any fear of medical personnel.

Demonstrates several practices which will protect the individual and others from common diseases and illnesses.

Behavioral Objectives (Intermediate Level)

Differentiates between germs that are harmful, others that are harmless, and some that are helpful.

Describes how germs may be spread and their relationship to common communicable diseases.

Explains how the body defenses react to disease and that scientists are laboring to obtain more information about disease.

Demonstrates understandings by staying home when ill, keeping immunizations up to date, covering coughs and sneezes, keeping appointments with physicians and dentists, and practicing cleanliness in the preparation, serving, and storage of food.

Identifies the disease prevention value of professional health workers in the community.

Analyzes sources of infection: bacteria, viruses, and fungi from people, animals, climate, insects, water, and food.

Distinguishes people in science for what they have done to conquer disease.

Comments

Disease prevention and control have more than a slight bearing on the lives of schoolchildren of all ages. Illustrations of this are everywhere and disease experiences come to every pupil. This fact should do at least one thing for the teacher; it should contribute significantly to the pupil interest level.

Teaching the concept that germs cause disease and that disease can be prevented through the control of germs may seem like uphill work in the elementary grades. Yet children have been successfully taught that microorganisms are everywhere and can be controlled. But because they are not completely controlled, they cause such things as upper respiratory infections, sometimes leading to hearing impairment, pneumonia, colds, and stomach and intestinal upsets. "Strep" germs alone can cause sore throats, tooth decay, and heart damage. Today, some of these germs can "come alive" in the classroom through the use of special slides, films, filmstrips, overhead transparencies, and powerful microscopes.

An especially effective film, entitled *Spot Prevention* (color, sound, 13½ minutes), designed to show the chase and capture of the measles "germ," is available for showing to children in kindergarten through second grade. It is distributed by the U.S. Public Health Service, Audiovisual Facility, Atlanta, Georgia 30333. The films *Germs and the Space Visitor* and *Your Protection Against Disease* (Encyclopedia Britannica) are also good.

As far as the primary grade children are concerned, the prevention and control of disease might well come under the area of personal cleanliness and appearance. Certainly disease control is related to one's personal practices of cleanliness. Children in the first three grades are quite capable of understanding this, especially if the subject is treated lightly and tied in directly with such routine health practices as covering the mouth when coughing, washing the hands before eating and after going to the bathroom, drinking properly from the drinking fountain, keeping away from others when ill, and staying at home when ill.

During the primary grades, the teacher is especially concerned with day-to-day signs and symptoms of infectious diseases and defects. He or she is alert to note deviations from normal health and performance. There is an excellent opportunity to make clear to pupils that they should remain at home when ill and not place too great a premium on perfect attendance. Third grade pupils, for example, may be interested in preparing a note to their parents encouraging them to make careful observation of their children before sending them to school. Third graders are also interested in the first stages of the common communicable diseases such as measles and chickenpox as well as immunization and simple first aid procedures. Upper graders, of course, may want to talk about specific immunization for whooping cough, tetanus, typhoid, diphtheria, and smallpox (see Chapter 5). Since several million children are inadequately protected against common childhood diseases, the film *Immunization Now* may be helpful in provoking class discussion. It is available from American Educational Films, Beverly Hills, California 90212.

As one grows older and must accept additional responsibility, the topic of disease control and its prevention takes on greater meaning. At the intermediate level it offers discussion possibilities greater than the topic of cleanliness and personal appearance. An effort is now made to use scientific knowledge and give decisive answers to "why" certain practices are helpful or harmful. Children show interest in scientific materials. The mystery surrounding bacteria, why some kinds are difficult to see even with powerful microscopes, and such questions as whether or not bacteria are useful arouse much comment.

It would be a mistake to miss an opportunity to present real case studies to a fifth or sixth grade class. Two case studies, such as the following, could be used to initiate a unit and provide immediate kindling of interest and discussion.[20]

CASE 1—Seventeen persons aboard a ship became ill within 8 hours after eating a noon meal. Nausea, vomiting, cramps, and diarrhea were the symptoms. Macaroni had been cooked prior to the meal, and chopped

---

[20]From *You Can Prevent Foodborne Illness.* U.S. Public Health Service, Publication No. 1105, Washington, D.C. 20201.

pimentos, lettuce, boiled eggs, mayonnaise, and mustard were hand-mixed by two mess cooks. One of those cooks had several minor cuts on two fingers. These finger cuts yielded *Staphylococcus aureus,* the same kind of bacteria found in the salad.
PREVENTION.—*Never use your hands to mix foods when clean sanitized utensils can be used! Never work with food when you have infected cuts because the germs causing the infection may be a source of foodborne illness!*

CASE 2—One hundred and fifty-five persons became ill with severe diarrhea and stomach pains. The suspect meal, roast beef and gravy, had been eaten by 170 persons. This beef and gravy had been prepared the day before and allowed to cool in open trays without refrigeration for 22 hours. *Clostridium perfringens* organisms were found in the beef and gravy.
PREVENTION.—*Potentially hazardous (readily perishable) foods should be thoroughly cooked and then either kept hot (140°F. or above), or cold (refrigerated to 45°F. or below) until serving.*

When upper elementary grade school children review the long and stimulating record of medicine and hygiene practices, there is a good opportunity to impress them with the historical emphasis on disease prevention and control. The control efforts came first, for people were plagued with sicknesses. Even today, in countries like Egypt, some 80 per cent of the population is disease-ridden. Problems of control are of first importance, followed quickly by prevention techniques. The first project is to save the life of the afflicted, then set out to prevent the disease in others. It is suggested, therefore, that intermediate graders take a look back through the pages of history and see what has gone on in the past. Superstitions, magic, and witchcraft in primitive society, the worship of special gods during the early days of Egypt, Greece, and Rome, and the slow transition from alchemy and astrology to the science of chemistry and astronomy are items that challenge the imagination of eager fourth, fifth, and sixth grade pupils.

Studying sickle cell anemia can be very practical in inner city areas where there are predominantly black schoolchildren. Such a discussion is appropriate from the fourth grade up. Information relative to this genetic disease needs to get around. Moreover, anemic children suffer shortness of breath and tire easily. Unfortunately, too few parents and their children know if they have sickle cells in their bloodstream.

There is an opportunity in the disease prevention area to relate disease to occupational activities and to environmental pollutants. The teacher has to decide whether to attack disease problems and methods of control (including government regulations) here or in the environmental health section. In either case, the discovery of disease agents and what is being done about them can be interesting. Relating disease to the workplace by looking at medical, personal, family, and occupational histories can set the stage for a further look at factors determining frequency and distribution (epidemiology) of illnesses and deaths in certain population groups. Studying the prolonged exposure to a substance such as coal dust can be enlightening as one learns its connection with crippling lung disease—black lung or pneumoconiosis.

Primary Level

1. Consider germs from a general point of view. Ask if all germs are harmful. Talk about helpful microorganisms that give cheese its wonderful flavor. If possible, emphasize this point by giving each child a little cube of milk cheese to eat on a small cracker. Talk about the yeast that makes bread rise and the microorganisms helpful in turning apple juice into vinegar. Ask how many children have tasted apple cider. Follow this discussion with some information on harmful germs that make canned fruit spoil and milk and cream turn sour. Continue by relating germs to disease—the common cold and sore throat.

2. Ask someone to tell the class what measles, chickenpox, or some other common communicable disease is like. Why do people feel sick when they have a disease? What are some of the ways to keep germs away from the body? Emphasize cleanliness, injections by the doctor, vaccinations, good food, rest, and sleep.

3. Post on the board an enlarged picture of the common housefly. Or employ an opaque projector to enlarge a real fly a dozen times on the screen. Discuss other disease-carrying insects and rodents. West of Colorado, rats, squirrels, and rabbits spread more disease-causing organisms than in the East. Examine a fly under a magnifying glass. Note the hairs. Discuss how flies spread disease.

4. Build a simple exhibit of items about the house that help people control germs. A number of items, including a garbage can, a trash basket, a refrigerator, a clean toilet bowl, a bath tub, or a garden hose may be made from cardboard (third grade).

5. For one week keep a record of the people who have been

absent, taking notice of the reasons people are not in school. Emphasize improved health, not improved attendance.

6. Call attention occasionally to an opened box of clean paper tissues on the corner of a classroom table.

7. Have class members describe personal cleanliness and its relationship to the transmission of diseases. Call attention as often as needed to the manner in which germs travel among boys and girls:

   a. By coughing and sneezing.
   b. By dirty hands and fingers of one person touching those of another
   c. By picking up and eating food that has fallen on the floor or sidewalk.
   d. By failing to refuse food that has been bitten into by another person
   e. By sharing individual cups, glasses, and straws
   f. By coming to school with a bad cold

8. Call on a scout to describe his or her part in a cleanliness campaign. Perhaps the class could talk over how to organize a small one.

9. Have the class find how the early American settlers kept clean in such settlements as Jamestown or Plymouth.

10. Make a list of all the housekeeping chores engaged in by the parents to help keep the home clean. Then have each pupil choose a chore and illustrate it in mimetic form, or the chores may be selected by the class members as a topic for a drawing.

11. Engage in pupil-teacher planning of ways to keep the school washroom clean.

12. Demonstrate how to use the soap dispenser and towels.

13. Build a model hospital on a small classroom table. Dress several dolls as the doctor, nurse, and patient. Have a garage where a toy ambulance is ready and waiting. A total class project can be planned by having the children, voluntarily or by assignment, secure the necessary items.

14. View the color film *How to Catch a Cold*. It may be obtained on a free loan basis from Kimberly-Clark Corporation (Kleenex) or Associated Films, Inc. Following the movie discuss the 2000 year old problem, the common cold.

15. Hang an attractive sign from the ceiling which may readily be seen by all pupils (see illustration).

    Point out colds are related not only to cleanliness but also to getting overtired, wet, or chilled, and that balanced diets, sleep and rest, and fresh air and exercise help prevent colds.

16. An independent research project for some children is to find out how nursing started. A student may want to talk to some nurses. The teacher may read the booklet, *Florence Nightingale* (Metropolitan Life Insurance Co., free). Or,

ceiling

string

Common Cold

**Treat It Like A Secret
Keep It To Yourself**

sign (blue
or yellow)

the 35 mm filmstrip of the same title available from the same source may be shown.

17. Hold a clinical thermometer up for all pupils to see. Ask questions. Do you have a thermometer at home? Is it an oral or rectal thermometer? What does it tell? Should we encourage our parents to get a thermometer if they do not already have one?

18. Discover how dishwashing affects the family health. The commonplace food utensil is a potential carrier of many infectious diseases. Discuss hand washing, proper rinsing of dishes, hot water, soap, detergents, drying, and machine washed dishes (third grade). The machine washed dishes are the cleanest, according to the research results available from the American Public Health Association.

19. Create drawings to illustrate ways in which children can avoid infection, supplying appropriate captions for each poster, for example:
    a. "Catch That Sneeze" (a child may be shown coughing or sneezing into a disposable tissue).
    b. "Cut the Apple to Share It" (indicate the danger that can result from several persons taking bites from a single article of food).
    c. "Use Your Own" (show a child drying his face with his own towel or combing his hair with his own comb).

20. Look into the ways in which people live around the globe. They have special ways for living in hot, dry deserts; in hot, wet jungles; and in snow-covered lands. Are diseases different there than in the USA?

Intermediate Level

1. Prepare immunization record forms for parents to complete and keep at home. An excellent sample form may be obtained from the U.S. Public Health Service, Washington, D.C. 20402. Have pupils enlarge these forms and discuss their meaning.

2. Collect newspaper clippings concerning communicable diseases and community sanitation and cleanliness and magazine advertisements having to do with health protection, cleanliness, and disease. Post these accounts and compare the number of magazine advertisements with the

GUIDE FOR FUTURE IMMUNIZATION

THIS IS A GENERAL GUIDE ONLY. See your doctor or health department for your own schedule of immunizations.

SHOTS FOR ▼	CHILD'S NAME ▶	
• **DIPHTHERIA**	AT AGE 2 MOS.*	
• **TETANUS**	2 MOS. LATER	
• **WHOOPING COUGH** One immunization (one shot each date) can immunize for all three if doctor recommends.	2 MOS. LATER	
	12 MOS. LATER	
	BOOSTER 4-6 YRS. OLD	
• **POLIO** One oral immunization each date.	AT AGE 2 MOS.*	
	2 MOS. LATER	
	2 MOS. LATER	
	12 MOS. LATER	
	BOOSTER 4-6 YRS. OLD	
•**MEASLES** •**MUMPS** •**RUBELLA** (German measles) {Triple immunization (one shot for all three). Measles booster at 15 mos. if first immunized before 1 year.	AFTER 1 YEAR OLD	
	AFTER 1 YEAR OLD	
	AFTER 1 YEAR OLD	
	*For children already beyond infancy, don't delay. See your physician and start series now.	

number of advertisements used for other topics. The soap and beauty ads alone will be quite plentiful.

3. Experiment with bacteria. Show that the germs "like" a warm, moist, and dark atmosphere in order to thrive and multiply.
    a. Crush several dried beans. Place half of the beans in each of two containers. Cover with water. Store one of the containers in a warm, dark place and the other one on the classroom sill. After several days note the results.
    b. Secure two apples. Peel one and place it in a dark, moist, and warm place; leave the other exposed to the air and sunlight on the teacher's desk. Note the results in a few days.
    c. Indicate how the human skin acts as an envelope somewhat like the apple skin to protect the body.

4. Using a magnifying glass, study the molds that have grown on stale bread, fruit, or other material. Point out that there are other bacteria so small that only a microscope can magnify them enough for the human eye to see. Bring a microscope to class. Let each child use it. Talk about Leeuwenhoek's discovery of the microscope.

5. Identify and be able to use correctly such words as:

contagious	bacteria	scientists
disease	dangerous	laboratory
harmless	superstition	infection
sterilize	microscope	immune
pasteurize	health	ferment
quarantine	science	illness

6. Analyze the poem, *Stictly Germ-proof,* by Arthur Guiterman.

7. Demonstrate the ways in which drinking water differs. Illustrate the passage of water through stones and sand. Have a committee of several persons build a stone and sand model for class use: pour muddy water in at the top of the box; see how much cleaner it is when it comes out at the bottom.

8. Post and encourage comments regarding local rules about dogs and rabies immunization.

9. Inquire about raw milk. What are the dangers in drinking it? What is meant by tuberculin-tested cattle? How does this compare with pasteurization in terms of health protection?

10. Read excerpts from the stimulating book by Hans Zinsser, *Rats, Lice, and History.* Here is a man who did a great deal of research and writing on typhus fever and wrote a best-seller. Follow this reading by discussing head lice. What are nits? What are graybacks? How may lice be controlled? Name other small insects and animals responsible for carrying disease.

Pediculus humanus or head and body louse

Ye Ugly creepin' blastit wonner,
Detested, shunn'd by saunt and
sinner!
How dare ye set your fit upon her,
Sae fine a lady?
Gae somewhere else, and seek your
dinner
On some poor body.

from To a Louse
by Robert Burns

11. Search out illnesses attributed to meats. Point out such things as the following:
    a. Meat killed in the woods is not always properly refrigerated in time.
    b. To prevent spoilage of meats a farmer sometimes coats it liberally with salt. Notice how salty country hams taste.
    c. Look for the federal or state inspection stamp on meat that has been processed under favorable conditions.
    d. Many animals are capable of carrying undulant fever and diarrhea to people. Swine spread hookworm, tapeworm, and muscle worms (trichinosis). All animals may spread tuberculosis.
    e. The first meat inspections were made by early Egyptians and Israelites. Mohammedan food regulations today are similar to those of years ago. Meat inspections by the Federal Government began in 1890.

12. If at all possible, visit a meatpacking plant and see what takes place in the way of inspections, cleaning, and refrigeration. Post two large stamps of approval.
13. Assign library research reports on the stories of the lives of such scientists as Koch, Jenner, Pasteur, Reed, and Salk.
14. Ask a restaurant owner or any food handler to come and speak to the class on the rules and regulations for protecting the public from spoiled foods and inadequate sanitary practices.

15. Set up the huge wall chart on cancer cells. This superb chart is available (free) from Eli Lilly and Company. Investigate the 7 warning signs of cancer shown. Develop the concept that the risk of abnormal cell growth can increase because of personal health practices.

16. Investigate several dimensions of cancer. Show the American Cancer Society film *From One Cell*. Discuss how cancer spreads. Illustrate uncontrolled growth in plants (galls). Plants can be induced to develop cancer-like growths by applying chemicals. Encourage school laboratory or home experimentation: Paint the stems of growing tomato, castor bean, or sunflower plants with diluted tar or with a solution of ammonia in water. Irregular masses will form on the stems.

17. Post the words

MENS SANA

IN CORPORE

SANO

and ask the questions:
What does this mean?*
What are the implications for our lives?

18. Using the common cold as an example, describe and illustrate the stages of infection (see next page):

19. Demonstrate how skin surface wounds should be disinfected to kill bacteria. Discuss the function of antiseptics. Then touch the skin on the back of the hand, where an imaginary cut might be, to a Petri dish containing nutritive

---

(*A sound mind in a sound body)

Figure 8–16. Sickle cell anemia needs attention. (From *Where's Herbie?*, Children's Bureau, U.S. Department of Health, Education, and Welfare.)

material and cover the dish. Next to it place a sterile second Petri dish and cover it. Store the dishes in a warm dark place for four days. There should be some bacterial growth on one dish and none on the other.

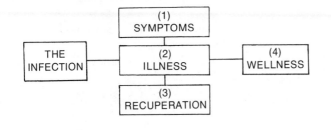

---

7. SAFETY AND FIRST AID

Behavioral Objectives (Primary Level)

To understand and be able to practice such items as the following:

Crosses the street safely.

Travels the safest route from home to school.

Demonstrates ability to give name, address, name of school, and name of parents.

Demonstrates ability to get on and off the bus safely and behave safely when riding on buses, cars, and trains.

Walks and runs in the right places.

Shows what to do in cases of illness or injury to self or a companion. Describes how to report accidents and emergencies to an adult.

Uses swings, slides, and other playground equipment properly.

Recognizes the need for keeping buildings, walks, gymnasiums, and playgrounds safe.

Demonstrates ability to use and properly store items such as saws, scissors, hoes, rakes, pins, needles, and other school-home equipment.

Does not accept rides with strangers.

Accepts responsibility for helping protect younger children.

Acts properly in case of fire and practices simple rules of fire prevention.

Chooses safe bicycle practices.

Explains why one should refrain from teasing pets and playing with strange animals.

Chooses to practice safety at home as well as at school.

Behavioral Objectives (Intermediate Level)

Crosses streets at intersections, obeying traffic signals, lights, and traffic rules.

Practices safety in free play situations.

Demonstrates safety in using a bicycle, the school bus, and all forms of public transportation, tools, electricity, and playground game equipment; and in flying kites where there are no power lines and no danger from automobile traffic.

Shows skills required to administer first aid for slight injuries, such as sprains, fainting, insect, dog, or snake bites, burns, blisters, or nosebleed.

Describes safety precautions needed while swimming, fishing, boating, canoeing, and water skiing.

Explains fire prevention in the home and in the community.

Comments

According to The National Safety Council, accidents to children outrank all other causes of death, killing more children between the ages of 5 and 14 years than cancer, congenital malformations, pneumonia, and poliomyelitis combined.

Recognizing the enormity of the problem, the U.S. Public Health Service expanded its accident prevention program, making it officially equal with the study of mental illness, cancer, and heart disease. This is understandable in view of the fact that there was a 12 per cent increase in drownings in the last decade; 500 children die each year from poisoning; and out of 800,000 dog bites a year there are thousands of children who haven't learned not to pet strange animals and not to tease a dog or take away its bone. Also, there are over 50,000 children injured a year in pedestrian accidents. Those children in the first three grades fare poorly as compared with older groups (see Figure 8–17). These figures are not surprising since

Figure 8–17. Percentage of school children killed or injured in pedestrian accidents. (Courtesy American Automobile Association.)

primary graders are prone to cross streets at the wrong time, pass between parked cars, and dart into the street during their informal play activities.

Certainly the school, where half the accidents to children occur, has a definite responsibility in the area of safety instruction. Teachers must be cognizant that young people usually seek adventure and excitement. This is as it should be, for it is through adventure, challenging experiences, and bold activities that young people grow and develop their personalities. Frequently, however, children become absorbed in their classwork or in their play and forget to exercise precautions essential for their personal protection and the protection of other children around them. It is the little things sometimes that cause the greatest trouble and alert the teacher to a health teaching need. For example, among the non-hospitalized accidents to youngsters, injuries caused by cutting and piercing instruments and those involving bicycles exceed even the accidents due to motor vehicles. Falls in and about the school occur continually. Firearms explode at the wrong time. Drownings occur in every community where there is a body of water. Primary grade children become victims of their curiosity when it comes to poisons. The newly-formed poison centers in one state alone handled 470 cases of poisoning in a recent year. There were 48 cases of children drinking kerosene, 40 eating roach tablets, and 92 eating too many aspirins. These are incidents the school can do something about. In this respect, an excellent teaching guide is available from the Division of Accident Prevention, U.S. Public Health Service. It is entitled *Teaching Poison Prevention in Kindergartens and Primary Grades.*

About a quarter of a million products designed for use in the home contain toxins and many of these seem to be attractive to youngsters for chewing, drinking, and eating. Products such as cleaning and polishing agents, detergents, shoe polish, cosmetics, paint, plant and food sprays, and a variety of medicines have all been involved in accidental poisonings. Efforts to decrease the number of home poisonings led to the passage in 1960 of the Hazardous Substance Labeling Act. It requires the labels of household aids and medicines to include poisons, antidotes, and recommendations for use. An important innovation in poisoning treatment procedures is the poison control center, organized by physicians and coordinated by the Department of Health, Education, and Welfare. There are almost 500 such centers in hospitals throughout the nation. Here the poisonous contents of thousands of trade-name products are cross-indexed. These are primary information centers.

Teachers have an important role to play. Once a year they should be instrumental in getting the message to all parents of primary grade children that poison hazards can be reduced by:
1. Placing drug cabinets high on the wall and locked or securely fastened.
2. Keeping carbon tetrachloride, contained in dry-cleaning fluids and polishes, out of the way of children.
3. Keeping aspirin out of the reach of the young.
4. Checking the labels on children's toys to be sure that the

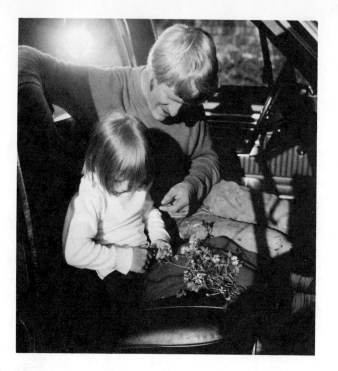

Figure 8–18. Buckling up for safety: can parents help teachers?

paint used for the often bright and cheery colors is not deadly.

5. Determining whether or not unused medicine should be saved. To avoid hazards, unused medicine should be thrown away.

Accidents occur because of the human factor. Related to this at the elementary school age are essentially four elements:

1. Lack of knowledge and experience regarding the laws of cause and effect—the underlying reasons behind accidents and accident topics, i.e., fire, electricity, and water safety
2. Lack of skill in such activities as swimming, using playground apparatus, shop equipment, and crossing busy highways
3. Improper attitudes and personal traits—a "daredevil" or foolhardy manner that makes it easy to "take a chance"
4. Inadequate emotional health, coupled with unrestrained emotions and yielding an "accident-prone" state.

The last factor is especially interesting. A close study of accident causes shows too often that injuries are not as accidental as they first appear. A small number of people have a higher percentage of accidents. Even when they move to new locations they keep on getting hurt. These individuals are termed "accident-prone." They have an accident habit or pattern which usually develops early in childhood. Accidents have become their way of solving problems and frustrations. Thus the careless child who has frequent injuries and many minor accidents becomes the concern of medicine, psychology, and safety education. More specifically, this child has more emotional outbursts, lacks self-control to a greater degree, is apt to be more impulsive, and acts more hastily than other children. With such children, close school-home cooperation is needed.

What is suggested here should be quite clear; that is, avoiding accidents is not a simple matter. Overcautious teachers, for example, may fill a child's world with "don't"—"don't swim alone," "don't run down the stairs," implying that if children sit in the corner they will be safe. In reality safety requires skill, judgment, and common sense to meet daily problems with successes. The relationship between feelings, emotions, and actions is fundamental. Thus accident prevention involves the promotion of good mental health, as well as day-by-day opportunities for children to practice safe behavior.

The school safety effort also calls for the provision of a safe school environment, one that is supervised and surveyed periodically. Across the land there are 800,000 accidental injuries to school pupils while under school jurisdiction. There should also be an accurate accident reporting system. First aid, medical procedures, and fire drills must be set up on "standing orders." Community personnel must cooperate with the schools. And finally, the classroom instruction program must be carefully structured so that pupils completing a unit of work on safety will be quite aware of hazardous situations in the school and community and how to adjust to them satisfactorily. Edith Vincent points out that the ability to identify and evaluate safety hazards must begin early in the grades with opportunities to actually practice accident prevention.[21]

At the primary and intermediate levels, the accentuation is as follows:

Primary Level

1. Safety in the home
2. Safety to and from school
3. Classroom safety
4. Playground safety
5. School building safety

Intermediate Level

1. Safety patrols
2. Bicycle safety
3. Traffic safety
4. Fire prevention and drills
5. Home and farm safety
6. First aid procedures
7. Harmful substances

By the sixth grade more attention is directed toward firearms safety and other significant aspects of safety within the community. Certain, in a town or city where there are a number of lakes and streams, some specific instruction is called for in the area of water safety. A growing number of the newer elementary schools have

---

[21]Vincent, Edith P. "Early Safety Education," *Health Education,* 7:30–34, July/August 1976.

excellent swimming pools. In such cases instruction pertaining to personal safety is taught directly to pupils of all ages. This is done through the development of skills in swimming and the handling of boats and canoes. These experiences in physical skills are followed by classroom discussions. This kind of "skill-knowledge" experience is extremely effective. Carryover value, in terms of practices and attitudes, is long lasting. Excitement-loving fifth and sixth grade boys and girls are sometimes repelled by the idea that being safe means avoiding all risks but they may be intrigued with the idea that it takes smartness to recognize and appraise risks and good judgment and skill to overcome them. Almost anything may be accomplished either in a hazardous or a comparatively safe manner. In class discussions teachers can help their pupils to realize that what counts in accident prevention is the ability to anticipate risks and the willingness to prepare to meet them with clear thinking and personal skill.

Teaching first aid to boys and girls permits the teacher to strengthen attitudes concerning how a person should react to emergency situations. Injury and sickness should be dealt with calmly and with an air of confidence. Fortunately, pupil interest is high. They give instant attention to accidents by asking, "Did he have to go to the hospital?" "Did he go in an ambulance?" "Will he be O.K.?" The teacher should have some training in first aid and be familiar with first aid supplies and the emergency practices in the school. The teacher should also be able to capitalize on the curiosity aroused by individual first aid occurrences in the classroom. Taking advantage of interest by holding a group discussion on a topic

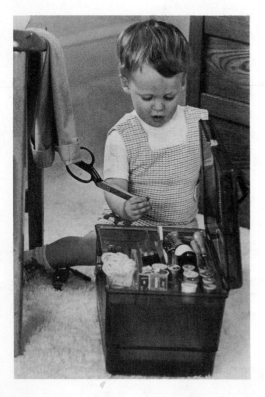

Figure 8–19. Children will talk about very curious toddlers.

growing out of an emergency situation is good teaching. As an example, an appropriate time to consider the control of bleeding and the precautions which should be taken to prevent it is when a pupil cuts his or her finger and requires immediate first aid. Likewise, when a child gets a blister or burns himself or herself, there is an opportunity to make safety education a vital subject in the health curriculum. Moreover, the teacher should be able to capitalize on a local community occurrence involving emergencies such as choking and cardiopulmonary resuscitation (CPR). Many American Red Cross headquarters offer a short citizens' course in emergency practices covering these items. A helpful booklet, *Teaching Safety in the Elementary School,* by Peter Yost, is available for the classroom teacher. It may be obtained from the Department of Classroom Teachers, N.E.A., Washington, D.C. 20036. Another excellent classroom teaching aid is the programmed instruction manual, *First Aid,* developed for sixth grade use by Behavioral Research Laboratories and distributed as a public service by Johnson & Johnson. This company also makes available (free) copies of *First Aid for Little People.*

Sixth grades boys and girls should be given instruction in artificial respiration. Many of these students will also be able to learn cardiopulmonary resuscitation well enough to be helpful in an emergency situation. There is support for this from the American Heart Association and the National Academy of Sciences. In teaching these procedures, the newer model of *Resusci Anne* or a similar mannequin should be used. (*Anne* may be obtained from Laerdal Medical Corporation, 1 Labriola Court, Armonk, N.Y. 10504.)

Considerable instructional assistance is available to any teacher who requests it from the National Safety Council. The materials are informative and are carefully designed to create and maintain student interest in personal health and safety. The 60-page booklet, *Improving Elementary School Safety—Here's How They Did It,* is a compilation of safety success stories, poems, songs, etc. from elementary teachers throughout the country. The Council periodically distributes leaflets illustrating unique experiences in elementary safety education. Teachers who want to meet safety needs should:

1. Make an analysis of the temporary and permanent hazards in the student's environment.
2. Make an analysis of the hazards connected with the pupil's activities.
3. Study the records collected through the usual student accident reporting system.
4. Study the hazards associated with the various seasons and with such special days as Fourth of July, Halloween, and Christmas.
5. Carefully consider individual student abilities, limitations, and difficulties.

Thus, proper safety programs provide for many experiences in the classroom involving textbooks, audio-visual aids, and pupil-made materials. They also involve experience with school equipment, school buses, emergency drill, physical education activities, and such other major motivation items as junior safety councils, safety patrols, safety committees, monitors, and bicycle clubs.

It should also be pointed out that *Safety Magazine* is a periodical of high caliber which is worth reading each month for new ways of making instruction on this topic more effective with children.

No study of safety would be complete without referring to bicycle safety. The need for bicycle safety education is emphasized by the fact that three out of four youngsters between the ages of 6 and 15 ride a bicycle. There are more than 75 million bicycles on American streets and highways. Every 19 minutes, day and night, a cyclist is injured; every 21 hours a cyclist is killed by an automobile . It is recommended that all communities establish a sound procedure for testing, registering, and licensing bicycles.

Numerous communities, working through the schools, have developed quite satisfactory bicycle safety programs. In Hamden, Connecticut, for example, a standard bicycle safety test record is kept on boys and girls. Once the examination is passed, a wallet-size card is issued. Teachers interested in working out similar programs will discover the materials from the Bicycle Institute of America, Inc., quite exciting to use. The game book, *Bike Fun,* the *Bike Quiz Guide,* and the several colorful posters should be seen to be appreciated.

The suggested activities which follow on safety and first aid, instead of being grouped together, have been set up in categories. This is because safety embraces so many phases of the school and community environment. The categories are home and community safety, bicycle safety, school safety, playground and gymnasium safety, and first aid. Of course, some items overlap and tend to apply to more than one category. Bicycle safety, for instance, could easily have been incorporated under the home and community area or under school safety. However, because bicycle safety is such a major problem, the activities and experiences are treated separately.

Fire safety might well be treated as a separate topic. It is included here as an item under home and community and school safety. With over a million fires a year and 11,000 fatalities (one third of them children), it becomes necessary to prepare lessons in fire prevention, many of which can be integrated with classes in history, science, and social studies. Fire safety materials for classroom use may be obtained for a small cost from the American Insurance Association in New York and the National Fire Protection Association in Boston. The latter organization has a great variety of materials prepared for school use; the *Sparky* fire prevention program is complete with a coloring book, posters, quizzes, and booklets. Helpful materials are also available from the American National Red Cross.

Suggested Activities

Home and Community Safety—Primary Level

1. In the winter, appoint several pupils to put sand or ashes on icy steps or pavement. Show young pupils how this reduces the danger of slipping. Show also how calcium chloride melts and helps break up ice.

```
BICYCLE SAFETY TEST RECORD


_____
         Name of Pupil                    Initial
                                            of
                                         Inspector
```

	Initial of Inspector
Written Test	
Mechanical Condition	
Test #1-Balance	
Test #2-Obstacle Course	
Test #3-Precision	
Test #4-Braking	
Test #5-Maneuvering	
Test #6-Hand Signals	
Certificate	

HAMDEN PUBLIC SCHOOLS
BICYCLE OPERATOR'S CERTIFICATE

———

This is to certify that

_____   _____
PUPIL'S NAME   SCHOOL

has passed an examination on Rules of the Road
for bicycle riders and has passed the Bicycle Riding
Test.

Matthew Barberi
_____   _____
SUPERVISOR OF PHYSICAL AND HEALTH   PRINCIPAL
           EDUCATION

Figure 8–20. Promoting bicycle safety through testing and certificate.

2. Make an exhibit of familiar items which have rough surfaces to reduce the danger of slipping. This exhibit might include sport shoes, automobile tires, tires with snow treads, bicycle tires, rubber gloves, and rubber-backed throw rugs or mats.

3. Have pupils make suggestions relative to the causes of street accidents; not looking in either direction, running after a ball, dashing from behind parked cars, or crossing the street diagonally or in the middle of the block (third grade).

4. Draw an imaginary street with intersections on the classroom floor. Use the children as buses and automobiles, a traffic officer, and people. Teach how to cross the street safely and obey signals (kindergarten or first grade).

5. Use the sand table to build a community complete with streets, playgrounds, and houses. Put in traffic lights and stop signs. Use small toys for community equipment such as bulldozers, derricks, trucks, police cars, and fire engines. Build an airport on the outskirts of the town. Use twigs and sticks as trees and telephone poles.

6. Make a stop and go sign for class use. Place a small inexpensive flashlight behind each piece of colored paper. Have the class practice operating and responding to the light changes.

Red paper

Yellow paper

Green paper
Cardboard

7. Play a game such as "grab bag game." Produce a big bag filled with various items. Have students draw from the bag pictures of pins, scissors, matches, nails, and sharp instruments, and tell how each should be taken care of.

8. Practice calling the fire department by telephone.

9. Build a model of a house that is open on one side, or borrow a large doll house for class demonstration of the relationship of space to accidents (third grade). Falls and poisonings may be traced to the unwise use of space. With the model show:
Small objects left on stairs
An open window on second floor
An open basement door
Medicines left where toddlers can "try" them

Say—

"I want to report
a fire."

"My name and
address are _____
_____"

Electric toaster partly plugged into outlet
Ladder against the house
Milk bottles sitting on window sill
Bubbling coffee pot on edge of stove (with model of small baby standing under it)

10. Discuss "Our Friend the Fireman." Read or tell stories about brave firemen. Have children check off a list of fire hazards in their homes.

11. Demonstrate that a candle will not burn after it has used all the air under the glass jar which is put over it. Point out that if clothes catch fire, the fire can be smothered by wrapping the person in a rug (third grade).

12. Prepare an enlarged chart for a fire drill, marking exits in red. Talk over the importance of the fire drill and then conduct one.

13. Organize a fire brigade with the following duties:
    a. Inspect the school premises. Gather up papers and other waste materials and put them into metal containers. Watch for anything that might cause fire and report the condition to the teacher.
    b. Confiscate matches brought to school by boys and girls. Emphasize the need for thinking of others.
14. Have the class list ways in which falls may be prevented. Here are some examples:
    Keep toys where they belong
    Keep rugs straight
    Ask grownups to reach things on high shelves
    Keep shoelaces tied
    Do not play on window sills and porch railings
15. Visit a drug store. Have the pharmacist point out poison labels and caution children regarding tasting substances they know nothing about (third grade). Return to the classroom and talk about how children have put the following into their mouths:
    Aspirin
    Tranquilizers
    Sleeping pills
    Iron pills
    Furniture polish
    Cleaners and lye
    Insect or rat poisons
    Weed killers
    Kerosene

Home and Community Safety—Intermediate Level

1. Make a class survey of the community agencies for recreation. Discuss the facilities available and some of the hazards involved in their use.
2. Study the beaches and swimming pool, noting sanitation, supervision, safety devices, and the presence of lifeguards, and inform children about these conditions. The suggestions prepared by the American Red Cross may be quite helpful.
3. Build a model of a safe well, showing that it should be dug properly, lined, and covered to protect the water from pollution; a model of the local inspection and purification plant might also be made by a committee of about three who would arrange to visit the plant manager and make sketches.
4. Encourage extensive discussion on safety in the use of fire. Point out that over 2000 children die each year in home fires. Discuss lighted cigarettes, bonfires, electrical appliances, candles, gasoline and kerosene, rubbish, defective chimneys, stoves, fireplaces, and furnaces. Display the poster, *Don't Give Fire a Place to Start*. It may be obtained from National Fire Prevention Association.
5. Have a student demonstrate how to roll over and over on

the floor in case the clothing is on fire. Have another pupil demonstrate how to wrap someone in a rug, blanket, or coat. "Never run. Inform an older person at once or turn in the alarm and wait for the firemen at the alarm box."

6. Demonstrate through group action fire fighting methods such as the bucket brigade and the volunteer system. Follow this with a description of the way the big city system is operated.

7. Invite the local fire chief or director of public safety to visit the class.

8. Have a pupil roller-skate into the class, preferably at a most inopportune time. Discuss roller-skating safety.

9. Have a pupil bring his or her pet dog or cat to a class. Talk about safe practices in handling animals and about avoiding strange dogs. Discuss rabies and, if appropriate (in the southern states), talk over animal hookworm.

10. Plan a clean-up campaign in each home. Let the class hear some of the plans.

11. Check the daily paper for one week for accidents of all kinds. Note types of accidents and age classification.

12. Either organize a school safety council or consider ways of improving the one in existence (sixth grade).

13. Secure a list of city ordinances which pertain to public safety. Study these to find what they are all about.

An interesting activity, particularly for fourth graders, is to list and talk about dangerous products in our everyday life, which bring

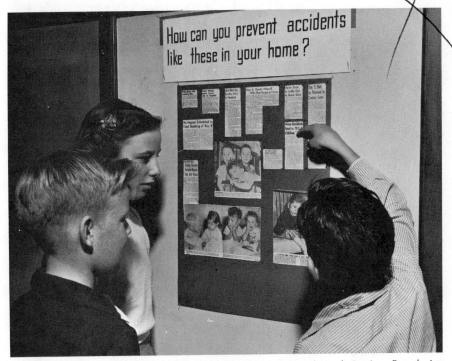

Figure 8–21. Hazards are everywhere. (Courtesy Safety and Youth Services Branch, Los Angeles Schools, California.)

about 30,000 deaths and 20 million injuries every year. As studied by the National Commission on Product Safety in 1969 and more recently by the Senate Commerce Committee, among "unreasonably hazardous" products were: glass doors, color television sets, fireworks, gas-fired floor furnaces, glass bottles, high-rise bicycle handlebars, hot-water vaporizers, household chemicals, stepladders, power tools, football headgear, rotary lawn mowers, toys, wringer washing machines, electric blankets, electric driers, hot plates, bathtubs, extension cords, lead paints, propane gas, eyeglasses, swimming pools, boats, and aerosol containers. Look at each.

14. Discuss "the grownups." Do they always set a good example?

Display in front of the class the following poster:

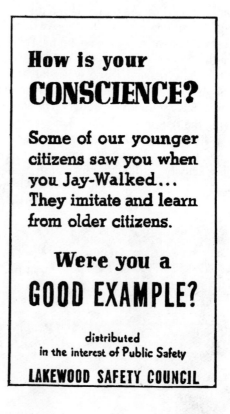

Tell the class that this is a reproduction of a jay-walking ticket actually distributed in Lakewood, Ohio. Discuss its implications (fifth or sixth grades).

15. Discover the hazards of pesticides. They are potentially dangerous both in diluted and concentrated form. Accidental swallowing by children has been responsible for most deaths from pesticides. Read the labels carefully (see Figure 8–22).

16. Investigate smoke and fire detectors. They may be a life-saving item for the family. There are many models to be looked at in a variety of stores and discussed later in class.

Figure 8–22. Pesticide label study.

The label diagram shows numbered sections:

3 PRECAUTIONARY STATEMENTS
HAZARDS TO HUMANS
(& DOMESTIC ANIMALS)
CAUTION

ENVIRONMENTAL HAZARDS

PHYSICAL OR CHEMICAL HAZARDS

2 DIRECTIONS FOR USE

GENERAL CLASSIFICATION

It is a violation of Federal law to use this product in a manner inconsistent with its labeling.

RE-ENTRY STATEMENT
(IF APPLICABLE)

STORAGE AND DISPOSAL

STORAGE

DISPOSAL

5

6

PRODUCT NAME

ACTIVE INGREDIENT: _____ %
INERT INGREDIENTS: _____ %
TOTAL: 100.00%

THIS PRODUCT CONTAINS   LBS OF   PER GALLON

KEEP OUT OF REACH OF CHILDREN

CAUTION

STATEMENT OF PRACTICAL TREATMENT

IF SWALLOWED
IF INHALED
IF ON SKIN
IF IN EYES

SEE SIDE PANEL FOR ADDITIONAL PRECAUTIONARY STATEMENTS **4**

MFG BY
TOWN, STATE
EPA ESTABLISHMENT NO.
EPA REGISTRATION NO.
1
NET CONTENTS

CROP:
CROP:
CROP:
CROP:
CROP:

WARRANTY STATEMENT

---

1 **EPA Registration Number:** Look for this number on every product you buy. The number is your assurance that the product has been reviewed by the EPA and should be safe and effective when used as directed on the label.

2 **Directions for use:** Before you buy any pesticide, make sure the product is labeled for use against the pest(s) you are trying to control. Read all label directions thoroughly before you open the container. Use only the amounts recommended, at the time and under the conditions specified, and for the purpose listed. (Don't think that twice the dosage will do twice the job; it won't. You may harm yourself or whatever you are trying to protect. It is also a violation of Federal law.)

3 **Precautions:** Read the precautions carefully. The most toxic products will be labeled DANGER-POISON. The word WARNING on the label means the product is less toxic, but extreme care must be exercised in its use. The word CAUTION will appear on those products which are least harmful when used as directed. Pay particular attention to warnings about keeping children and pets out of treated areas and about special clothing that should be worn when using certain chemicals.

4 **First Aid Instructions:** Know what to do if someone is accidentally poisoned by a pesticide. Check the label for Statement of Practical Treatment. This information will give instructions for immediate action. Then, ALWAYS call or get to a doctor or hospital right away. Be sure to take the pesticide label with you. The label will help your doctor prescribe treatment.

5 **Storage and Disposal:** Read and follow all directions for storage and disposal of pesticide products carefully. Keep all pesticides out of the reach of children, preferably under lock and key.

6 **Classification Statement:** After October 21, 1977, all pesticide products will be classified for either "general" or "restricted" use. Restricted use pesticides are highly toxic or require special knowledge or equipment for application and, therefore, will generally not be available for sale to the homeowner. Look for the statement "General Classification" on the label at the beginning of the directions for use to ensure that the pesticide is classified for use by the general public.

Bicycle Safety—Primary Level

1. Display a large poster of a bicycle with lines going to all significant parts. Excellent posters may be obtained free from the Bicycle Institute of America, Inc.

2. Talk about bicycle safety aids. Discuss the *bell or horn* as an important signaling device which should be used to warn of approach. Discuss the *headlight,* so essential for safe bicycling at night. Stress, however, that night riding should be held to a minimum. Illustrate how the *reflector* brightens when a headlight beam hits it and how it serves as a warning signal to protect riders from unforeseen dangers. Show how the *basket* or *carrier* keeps the hands free for the proper control of the wheel. The Bicycle Institute of America will furnish an excellent four-color poster which wisely illustrates these bicycle aids.

3. Practice giving hand signals. Have several class members illustrate these by riding a bicycle on the playground for all to observe:

   a. Left arm *pointed up* for turning to the right.

   b. Left arm *straight out* for turning to the left.

   c. Left arm *pointed down* for slowing or stopping.

   Posters in green and orange about bicycle hand signals may be obtained free from Bicycle Institute of America.

4. Bring a bicycle into class. Stand it on a table where all pupils can see it clearly. Discuss "How to care for your bicycle." Include the saddle, wheels, brake, handle grips, reflector, chain, pedals, warning devices, level of handle bars, fork bearings, light, spokes, tire pressure, and tire valves (third grade).

BELL OR HORN
Be sure it works properly, loud and clear.

HANDLE BARS & GRIPS
Adjust for your comfort, stem well down in fork. Tighten securely. Replace worn handlegrips. They should fit snugly.

SADDLE
Adjust height so leg bends slightly with ball of foot on pedal at bottom of stroke. Tighten saddle and seat post nuts securely, leaving at least three inches of seat post in the frame.

LIGHT & REFLECTOR
Must be state-approved for night riding. Though requirements vary, most states require headlight to be visible 500 feet, rear reflector for 300 feet.

FENDERS
Be sure they are undamaged and securely fastened.

COASTER BRAKES/ HAND BRAKES
Must brake evenly every time, no slippage. Have brakes adjusted by a trained serviceman.

TIRES
Inflate to correct pressure. Check frequently, removing imbedded glass, cinders, nails, etc. Don't ride on "bald" or soft tires; inspect valves often for leaks.

WHEELS
Adjust cones and tighten wheel nuts for a straight, steady ride.

CHAIN
Check for damaged links and a snug, but not too tight, fit. Clean and lubricate frequently with light oil.

PEDALS
Be sure they are securely fastened to cranks. Replace worn or bent pedals.

SPOKES
Replace broken ones promptly. Keep them tight.

5. Have class members demonstrate the method of getting on a bicycle, the means of guiding it, applying the brake and coming to a stop, and parking the bicycle (first or second

grade). Discuss using the horn or bell. Do not use the horn or bell as a brake.

6. Encourage pupils to send for safety materials from state motor vehicle departments and other sources. Materials designed to assist those working with bicycle safety are available from:
   a. American Automobile Association
      Traffic Engineering and Safety Department
      1712 G Street, N.W.
      Washington, D.C. 20006
   b. Bicycle Institute of America
      122 E. 42nd Street
      New York, New York 10017
   c. Insurance Institute for Highway Safety
      1725 DeSales Street, N.W.
      Washington, DC. 20036
   d. National Safety Council
      425 N. Michigan Avenue
      Chicago, Illinois 60611

7. Talk over how to ride sidewalk vehicles:
   a. Ride alone on a tricycle, not double.
   b. Be especially careful when there are pedestrians on the sidewalk.
   c. Watch cars backing out of garage or driveway.
   d. Stay on sidewalks or in own yard—streets are made for fast-moving vehicles (kindergarten or first grade).

8. Play an obstacle game such as Bicycle Slalom. Set six poles in the ground about 10 feet apart. The participant races from the starting line about 20 yards to the first pole. He goes to the right or left of the poles to the finish line. Try a Potato Race or Tug-Of-War on bicycles. See *Bike Fun,* distributed free by Bicycle Institute of America.

Bicycle Safety—Intermediate Level

1. Administer a bicycle test at the start of this topic to see how much the class actually knows about their bicycles and how to use them. The *Bicycle Safety Quiz,* distributed (free) by Aetna Life Affiliated Companies, is a good one.

2. Post a readily visible list of bicycle safety rules on the bulletin board. Typewritten rules on white paper pasted to a black background are easily noticed. Call attention to these rules and have the class check themselves to see how many they sometimes violate. Here is a sample list of rules:
   a. Observe all traffic regulations—red and green lights, one-way streets, stop signs.
   b. Never hitch on other vehicles, "stunt," or race in traffic.
   c. Have satisfactory signaling device to warn of approach.
   d. Ride at a safe speed.
   e. For night riding have a white light on front and a danger signal reflector on rear.
   f. Wear white or light-colored clothes at night.
   g. Give pedestrians the right of way.
   h. Avoid sidewalks; otherwise use extra care.

i. Watch for car pulling out into traffic.
j. Look out for sudden opening of automobile doors.
k. Keep to the right and ride in a single file.
l. Keep a safe distance behind all vehicles.
m. Do not carry other rides.
n. Do not carry packages that obstruct vision or prevent proper control of the cycle.
o. Slow down at street intersections; look to the right and left before crossing.
p. Check the brakes for good working condition. Keep the bicycle in perfect running order.
q. Ride in a straight line. Do not weave in or out of traffic or swerve from side to side.
r. Always use proper hand signals for turning and stopping.
s. Park the bicycle in a safe place.
3. Invite a safety specialist or member of the police department to talk on bicycle safety, including mechanical condition of the bicycle.
4. Prepare a bicycle skill test to be given on the school playground or play yard. Several of the pupils in the class will be especially eager to help in such a project. The following test, for example, is not hard to set up.
a. Begin at point A.
b. Ride slowly, being careful not to touch border lines.

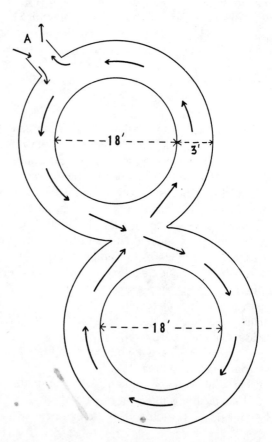

School Safety—Primary Level

1. Help the class analyze the essentials of good fire drill. Teach the importance of a cool and immediate response, how to send in the alarm in the community (in the absence of an adult), and where to find the fire hose and extinguisher in the school. Tour the school, corridor by corridor, to see these locations.

2. Talk about the safest route home from school. Early in the school term, practice crossing the street.

3. Play the little game, "Who Are You?" Line the class up in the front of the room. Appoint one pupil to ask the question of anyone he or she chooses, "Who are you?" The pupil selected gives name, address, name of school, and parents. If this is done satisfactorily, the person becomes "it" next.

4. Use the school bus to practice safe behavior on a bus. Have the school bus driver speak to the pupils, especially in connection with a field trip.

5. Discuss what to do if a stranger offers a ride. Know that one should not accept rides from strangers.

6. Organize the class on a daily basis to put away their toys and other materials when they have finished using them.

7. Make an attractive cut-out to use with a school safety jingle. The one below, for example, could be used with third graders:

   a. Have the pupils step on a piece of colored paper. With a pencil trace the outline of the shoes.

   b. Cut out the footprints and in the space available write a safety jingle.

School Safety—Intermediate Level

1. Discuss school fire hazards. Make a survey of the school building.

2. Prior to an extended vacation period (Thanksgiving, Christmas), make charts of safe practices to be followed during vacation activities. For example, what are the hazards to be

aware of while on Christmas vacation, both indoor and outdoor?

3. Engage in safety poster construction. Each row or small group of pupils should be made responsible for a particular phase of safety; completed posters could be exhibited in the school corridor or multi-purpose room.

4. Participate in a school safety patrol. Train leaders so that everyone will eventually have a chance to be a patrol-person; local traffic officials are usually available to assist the school safety patrol in setting up acceptable standards. This may well be a total elementary school project with classroom representation. Patrol standards and particulars are available from National Safety Council.

5. Describe an accident that may have happened in the school. Write down all the facts and decide what might have been done to prevent it. Compare pupil findings.

6. Safety is not an isolated topic. The help of a parent or a group of parents may be enlisted in a discussion of school, home, and community safety. The children may enjoy preparing a play or reading a report on their safety activities before a group of interested adults.

7. Try "on the spot" safety messages over the school intercom system. A special event of the school day is connected to the safety message and relayed to the students.

Playground-Gymnasium Safety—Primary Level

1. Talk over the many sources of danger from playground accidents. Call attention briefly to items such as the following:
   a. *General:* Broken glass, protruding nails, tin cans left on ground. Unnecessarily rough play, tripping, pushing, climbing fences, shelters, trees. Congestion of activities. Bicycle riding across the playground, especially during games. Children with contagious skin diseases mingling with others. Activities not adapted to grounds. Dogs on grounds. Pools of water remaining after rain. Need for first aid kit.
   b. *Swings:* Jumping from moving swings, running or playing between or around swings. Climbing on frame while swings are in use. Holding baby brother or sister while swinging. Improper use of swings. Other activities too near swings. Swinging too high causing chains to slap and yank. Climbing across top of frame.
   c. *Sandboxes:* Glass, cans, and broken or unbroken bottles in boxes. Throwing sand or blocks; concealing hard or sharp objects in the sand. The importance of using of a sandbox lid or cover when box is not in use. Looking for nails working loose and splinters.
   d. *Drinking fountain:* Pushing or crowding. Molesting the drinker. Unsanitary conditions of the bubbler.

2. Set up a number of situations to study. Refer to them as cases. Example:

3. Appoint a weekly clean-up squad for the play area.
4. In winter, when there are snow and ice, stress safe places to skate and slide. Point out the dangers of interfering with others. Encourage the use of targets in snowballing. Purposely set up targets and let everyone throw all the snowballs they want.
5. Plan an outing and, after the fun and food details have been considered, talk over the safety precautions:
   Provide safe transportation
   Use school bus if possible
   Have the school nurse go on the trip
   Check the availability of a telephone
   Take a first aid kit along
   Consider safe cooking, water supply, provisions for shade and rest
   Shelter from rain
6. Study the natural surroundings at a picnic or outing area. Give information on such matters as poison ivy, poison oak, snakes, insects, and overexposure to the sun. Caution against eating unknown plants. Each year 12,000 children swallow parts of potentially poisonous plants.
7. Select from several volunteers a group of children to help mark off the danger area around swings and to warn other children about entering it while swings are being used. Consider, also, other safe practices and equipment safety rules.
8. Demonstrate the importance of proper footwear on a gymnasium floor. Stress that sneakers are cleaner than shoes, they give better traction while shoes slide, it is difficult to be agile and quick when wearing shoes, and our athletic skill is improved when we wear good sneakers.

Playground-Gymnasium Safety—Intermediate Level
1. Appoint a small committee to inspect the playground or gymnasium area, its equipment, and game boundary lines. Have these people report back to the class. Point out that faulty and hazardous conditions should be remedied immediately or the play area should be closed from further use.
2. Have boys and girls discover how clear rules and definite boundary lines help make a game safe.
3. Have a painting project. Gaily colored swings and slides help reduce playground injuries. In addition, the attractive colors

Figure 8–23. Posters promote both laughs and questions. (Courtesy Employers Mutuals of Wausau.)

help entice youngsters to the playground and away from the street.

a. Slides—paint them green to counteract excessive sunlight. Paint the steps to the top of the slide yellow to draw the children's attention.

b. See-saws—paint green, with edges painted yellow to give greater visibility and reduce chances of children running into them.

c. Swings and swing rings—paint seats and swings yellow. Green is best for upright and overhead bars.

d. Sandboxes—paint green.

e. Jungle gyms—paint a cool restful blue.

f. Trash cans—paint gray with a white star. This emphasizes neatness and encourages youngsters to help keep the playground or gymnasium area tidy.

4. Have pupils make a list of the many sources of danger on playgrounds and in gymnasiums, such as:

   a. *Baseball:* Playing too near the street and chasing balls into the street. Spectators too near baseline during a game. Batting fly balls in too small an area. Throwing the bat after hitting the ball. Playing catch too near swings, sandboxes, and other activities. Older children playing on an area adapted only for younger children.

   b. *Horseshoes:* Running in front of the pitcher. Careless pitching and throwing too near other activities. Pitching distance too great for control. Locating stakes where children are likely to pass between.

   c. *Gym Floor:* Unnecessary running and pushing. Interfering with others who are on equipment. Playing unsafe games. Wearing shoes without rubber soles in gym. Wearing poor quality sneakers, especially for heavy children. Safe playing facilities: Do doors open outward? Are end walls padded? Is the heat of the water in the shower room automatically controlled? Are the radiators screened or set back into the wall? Does the gym floor have a smooth, non-slip surface?

5. Show the relationship between good sportmanship and safe play activities.

6. Demonstrate with pupils the safety rules for the most popular games. Example: Soft-ball: (a) The batter who throws the bat is automatically out, (b) catching behind the bat without a mask is prohibited, (c) sliding into a base is not permitted, (c) always signal that you are about to catch a fly ball so that someone else will know that you are after it and avoid a collision.

First Aid—Primary Level

1. Discuss the ways in which small children may get burned. Example:

   a. Surface burns may be caused by falling on hot radiators or by touching hot stoves, electric irons, or toasters.

   b. Burns may be caused by hot liquids falling off the stove, by bumping into a person with a hot substance, and by careless playing with matches.

Point out what to do when a burn occurs.

2. Show pictures or exhibit real cans of varnish, paint, kerosene, and gasoline. Have pupils give reasons for not touching or tasting these liquids.

First Aid—Intermediate Level

1. Plan and equip a first aid cabinet for the school. Consider also the items one might need on a day-long hike or trip into the country. Local needs should be considered.

2. Discuss the ways of acquiring a sun tan. Refer to the dangers.

3. Demonstrate care of ordinary cuts and bruises.

4. Practice the control of bleeding (fifth or sixth grade).

5. Practice giving artificial respiration. Blankets or heavy paper may be placed on the floor and children divided into pairs to work on each other. See the American Red Cross Water Safety or First Aid Manual for the approved manner of giving mouth-to-mouth breathing. Complimentary copies of *The Breath of Life,* with clear drawings of how to give mouth-to-mouth breathing, may be obtained from Aetna Life Insurance Co., Johnson and Johnson, Metropolitan Life Insurance Company, and American Insurance Association, all make first aid guides available at no cost. The Johnson and Johnson film, *First Aid Now,* is also appropriate (no charge). Both the American Heart Association and the National Academy of Sciences have recommended that children learn artificial respiration techniques in the fifth grade.

6. Make a list of first aid practices that might be employed in the winter sports scene. Consider accidents while coasting, skiing, and skating. Do the same thing for summer safety. Discussing diving into unknown waters, picking strange fruit, treating sunburn, and dangers involved in using an axe or knife.

7. Practice giving the *Heimlich Hug* for a choking victim. This may save one of the 2500 people a year who choke to death.
   1. Ask the victim if he or she is choking. They may nod, for they cannot speak.
   2. Stand behind your victim and wrap your arms around him just above his waist.
   3. Make a fist with one hand and place it against his abdomen just below his breast bone.
   4. With your other hand grab your own fist.
   5. Bend the victim forward.
   6. Press your fist into his abdomen with a quick squeezing, upward thrust.
   7. This should pop the piece of food out forcefully, but if it does not—
   8. Try the squeeze again or reposition your hands.

If the victim has already passed out or fallen to the floor you still can give the "hug."
   1. Place the victim on a hard surface on his back.
   2. Kneeling, straddle the victim facing his head.
   3. Place one fist on the victim's abdomen and the other hand over it.
   4. Thrust your hands into the victim's abdomen, and the food should come up. It may then be removed with your fingers.
   5. Usually, after the food is dislodged your victim will breathe on his own. If not, you may need to give mouth-to-mouth resuscitation until help arrives.[22]

---

[22]Adapted from "What is Your First Aid I.Q. on Choking?" *Current Health,* September 1976, p. 25.

MENTAL HEALTH

Behavioral Objectives (Primary Level)

Explains what it means to be accepted by classmates and school.

Demonstrates some ability to adjust in part to the demands of daily living and establish satisfactory relationships with others.

Identifies new interests and new friends.

Shares work and play materials with others and accepts some responsibility for actions.

Overcomes difficulties and adjusts to minor disappointments.

Chooses to help others and gains personal satisfaction from this action.

Behavioral Objectives (Intermediate Level)

Distinguishes between responsible and irresponsible actions as a member of the school and member of a family.

Employs ways of showing specific regard and respect for the welfare of others and for oneself. Serves sometimes as a leader and sometimes as a follower in school situations.

Enjoys working with others in play and work activities and realizes that routine changes and unexpected failures and successes are to be taken in stride.

Explains how mental health and personal feelings have a bearing on the way the whole body works.

Describes the close relationship between mental health, recreation, and rest.

Sets personal goals and shows how to attain them while maintaining proper mental health.

Comments

It has been said that the mentally healthy person possesses the three grand essentials in life—something to do, someone to love, and something to hope for. Despite the long-time existence of the National Institute of Mental Health and its hundreds of local centers serving 40 per cent of the population, there are still 21 million mentally disturbed individuals across the country who enter every day into the lonely, private world of their despair. And many of them are children.

Learning to live together harmoniously is still the number one problem for the people of the world to solve. Moreover, the hospitals and physicians' offices of the country are crowded with thousands of people who are ill enough to seek the assistance of a physician but whose illnesses are emotionally conditioned and frequently do not involve organic disease. This area of medicine is concerned with somatic symptoms (pain, rapid heart-beat, loss of appetite, undue fatigue) and psychologically or emotionally induced reactions. One out of two persons today who seeks the help of a physician has emotionally induced illness. Such individuals may be classed in one way or another as emotionally immature; they are not able to face life as it really is and their illness serves as a measure of their vulnerability to these stresses. Unfortunately, the steadily rising tempo of American life brings on growing tensions, frustrations, and complexities. And these in turn create the physical masks of stress (see Figure 8–24) leading to ulcers, high blood pressure, coronary attacks, allergies, and other disorders.

Mental health is more than the absence of mental illness. It is a style of life characterized by a capacity to adapt—a growth of the ability to cope with a wider range of changes in a complicated culture. Moreover, individual evidences of failure to adapt can not only be interrupted and reversed but they also can be *prevented*. This is why human dignity must be nurtured right in the local community, especially if children are to be guided toward sound mental health. In the more populated areas, teachers can get help from the Community Mental Health Centers established by Congress to intercept emerging crises in the home community.

There are few endeavors in the school curriculum of more im-

ANGER

FEAR

JEALOUSY

ANXIETY

WORRY

Figure 8–24. The masks of stress. (Courtesy American Alliance for Health, Physical Education, and Recreation, and Parke, Davis & Company, Detroit, Michigan.)

portance than the one concerned with the development of mental health. This is admirably set forth in *Mental Health in the Schools.*[23]

When a realistic perception of self is added to a realistic perception of the world, the possibility of effective and productive interaction is reasonably assured. The mentally healthy person's relationships with people and the world produce certain constructive consequences. Two consequences are especially significant to the school. First, the mentally healthy person perceives reality with minimal distortion and is able to communicate these perceptions effectively. Second, the possession of self-esteem contributes to intellectual functioning.

Back of the teenage difficulties and the compulsive search for happiness are unresolved problems that have to do with living with oneself and others during the formative elementary school years—when the classroom teacher's influence in the child's community is most effective. In the early grades, there are opportunities to encourage children to come out of isolation so that they can find themselves. When Ivan Illich talks about "de-schooling," he is stressing the need to get away from institutions and toward individuals. Each in his own way, Piaget, Erickson, Silberman, Bruner, and John Dewey have made the same point.[24]

Although sound mental health is related to the family background, the elementary school is in an excellent position to influence boys and girls. The chief reason for this is that personalities are defined early and children frequent the elementary grades during the most formative years. Early habits of response to teachers and classmates, to simple requests, to ideas, and the like are established during these elementary school years. The needs of children and the interrelationship of these needs are impressive at this time. Maslow suggests six groups of needs to keep in mind when teaching. These are: (a) physical needs, (b) safety needs, (c) love needs, including the need for affection, belonging, and mutuality, (d) esteem needs, including the needs for mastery, achievement, recognition, approval, and self-respect, (e) the need to solve problems and have sources of information, and (f) the need for self-realization, including the need to develop a sense of personal identity, to accomplish the tasks for which one is best fitted, and to function at a level in keeping with one's capacities.[25]

In recent years, *death education* has become associated with mental health programs for children. Certainly this is a humbling lesson to be learned—a lesson that John Donne preached in 1622 when he said, "Death comes equal to us all and makes us all equal when it comes." It is the final stage of growth, but paradoxically, "by learning about death many people become more aware of the values of life."[26] Therefore, learning activities permit students to deal more

---

[23]Joint Committee Report. *Mental Health in the Schools,* 32 pages, 1966.

[24]For greater detail see "Mental Health at an Early Age" by Carl E. Willgoose, *Instructor, 81*:58–59, October 1971.

[25]Maslow, A. H. "Theory of Human Motivation," *Psychological Review, 50*:370–376, 1953.

[26]Russell, Robert D. "Educating About Death," *Health Education, 8*:8–10, November/December 1977.

openly with the death of people whom they love. This is not easy to accomplish because we live in a death-defying and death-denying culture. But children can understand death and know that it is inevitable. They can read about John Brooke's funeral in Louisa M. Alcott's *Little Men* and express emotion. As Rabbi Grollman points out, death education begins when life begins.[27] It need not be an anxiety-ridden area if it is discussed during the child's formative years. It is a good mental health activity for 10 year olds to enter the woods in the springtime to understand the seasonal and life cycle of small plants, trees, and animals and to begin to accept death as an inevitable and universal part of life.[28]

Setting up a health curriculum that includes instruction in mental health is both challenging and formidable. One can begin to teach personality adjustment and wholesome participation in the classroom, for this is where the child spends most of his or her time outside of the home. Instruction in mental health, therefore, must permeate the *total* program. In a sense, it is not a subject at all, but a way of teaching. Curriculum cannot be divorced from method.

Since personality cannot be compartmentalized, every subject matter area has experiences and activities, often too subtle to measure, which consciously and unconsciously promote mental health. Every essential skill and learning, when coupled with worthwhile feelings and attitudes, tends to build a wholesome personality. Practically all classroom and school environment activities serve as social science experiences. In the laboratory of the classroom, gymnasium, lunchroom, workshop, and playground are to be found opportunities for attaining emotional maturity. Mental health is fos-

[27]Grollman, Earl A. "Explaining Death to Children," *Journal of School Health*, 47:336–339, June 1977.
[28]Everett, Marianne G. "Helping Parents Teach About Death," *Health Education*, 7:27–30, July/August 1976.

Figure 8–25. Togetherness can foster self-esteem—and be fun.

tered through learning the rules of sportsmanship and learning to play together in physical education. It is enhanced when pressures to succeed are relaxed a bit in arithmetic and reading. It is encouraged when scientific appreciations are deeply felt, for personal adjustment in the modern world is more than slightly related to our understanding of scientific advances. Music and art, when taught as recreational or diverting activities to be enjoyed, are rich items in the promotion of mental health. In addition, it seems true that the *way* we teach has much to do with relieving "pressures" and permitting the pupil to work up to his or her potential.

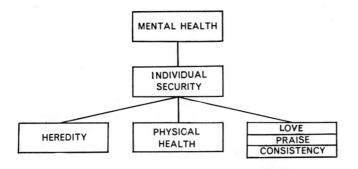

Instruction in mental health requires that the teacher know the pupils not as entities in the classroom but as living personalities. The instruction, to be effective, must involve each pupil in a number of activities designed to bring out personality. This is an ongoing process which is further enhanced by the teacher's own mental health. By example and precept, children are helped to make optimum adjustments in school and most of all to *feel wanted*. Youth is a time for reaching for human contact points; a time for searching. It is not always a joyous time, for sometimes one reaches and there is no one to touch. As one older pupil said, when looking back on his elementary school years: "I felt alone . . . I felt different . . . I was popular on the outside but shy and insecure on the inside . . . I needed friends . . . I needed to be accepted . . . I needed to feel valuable and important somewhere . . . I needed to be close to someone. . . ." At any age life is bound to be full of disappointments. Even so, wrote the Irish playright Sean O'Casey, ". . . each of us one time or another, can ride a white horse, can have rings on his fingers and bells on his toes, and if we keep our senses open to the scents, sounds, and sights all around us, we shall have music wherever we go." How to help young people discover the "scents, sounds and sights" is the inspiring task here.

Primary grade children love movement. They love to play. In fact, they play because they must. Their running, jumping, and dodging have potential values beyond the purely physical ones. Play contributes immeasurably to personality growth. Play and game situations in the classroom, therefore, have a vital part in building mental-emotional health.

Primary grade instruction and learning activities foster and deal primarily with:

A feeling of belonging	Affection
Inspiring self-confidence	Respecting the rights of others
Assuming responsibility	Etiquette
A feeling of importance	Facing up to fears
Making decisions	Keeping healthy
Realizing limitations	Pride in family
Learning to profit by mistakes	Getting along with others
Consideration for others	New experiences
Making others happy	Sharing with others

Exploring these kinds of mental health activities should provide a degree of built-in motivating power that will foster some creative ways of learning. Research has indicated for years that almost any kind of human functioning can be improved by increasing motivation. In this instance creative growth is the issue. Torrance and Myers make it clear that one of the most important conditions for creative growth is that pupils feel that *their* teacher is on *their* side.[29] Following along from this point, Sylwester and Matthews would have the children ask many questions—especially these four:[30]

1. What am I like?
2. How am I changing?
3. What will I be like?
4. How will I affect others and how will they affect me?

Peeking at one's feelings at the primary level may even be more important than waiting until later on. In the Brookline, Massachusetts schools, for example, the emphasis on mental health and personality development has been shifted from the junior high level to the elementary. Here, the Dimensions of Personality series is used.[31]

Additional intermediate grade instruction and learning activities which promote mental health deal primarily with:

Leadership and ability to follow	Accepting oneself
Assuming responsibility	Emotional controls
Knowledge of how to act	Making friends
Desirable pesonality traits	Working together
Worthwhile interests	Coping with living problems
Extending areas of interest	Reducing stress
A chance to create something	Identifying abilities and skills

A number of sources of substantive information and teaching ideas are available relative to the topic of mental health which are readily available to teachers. The Child Study Association of Ameri-

---

[29]Torrance, E. Paul and Myers, R. E. *Creative Learning and Teaching.* New York: Dodd, Mead & Company, 1971, p. 110.

[30]Sylvester, Robert and Matthews, Esther. "Four Big Questions Children Need to Ask," *Instructor, 81*:46–50, February 1972.

[31]Published by Pflaum/Standard, 38 West Fifth Steet, Dayton, Ohio 45402.

ca, the American Medical Association, and the American School Health Association have printed materials. There are many excellent films such as "Mr. Finley's Feelings" (Metropolitan Life Insurance Co.) and filmstrips for elementary school use. The colorful filmstrips on mental health topics of prejudice, envy, and criticism are part of a seven-part series designed by Image Publishing Corporation (Box 14, North Station, White Plains, N.Y. 10603) to develop deeper insights regarding mental attitudes.

In order to pinpoint more specifically what has already been stated rather generally, the following *teacher activities* are set forth as follows:

1. Create a desirable classroom atmosphere by making the room as cheerful, attractive, and healthful as possible.
2. Observe the relationship between each child and his or her companions. Where a pupil avoids another or fails to make friends, attempt to discover the cause.
3. Arrange group activities so that children showing the greatest difficulty in making friends may have a chance to participate.
4. Encourage the confident child to make friends of the timid.
5. Promote good fellowship through the art of listening and of cooperating in carrying out group ideas.
6. Develop opportunities for leadership. Group children so that all have a fair opportunity for recognition. Change groups so that leadership is not restricted to just one or two children whose leadership qualities are already developed.
7. Plan for children to share to a maximum degree in planning classroom activities. Try to give each child the feeling that he or she has something to contribute.
8. Provide opportunities for original effort. Avoid doing things for children which they can do themselves.
9. Give credit to pupil ideas and suggestions.
10. Challenge the pupil's creative imagination by having available a number of simple craft materials such as wood, fiber, plaster, and metal. Provide a time and place to work with these materials in an atmosphere conducive to creative work.
11. Encourage wholesome curiosity. Aid children who wish to explore and ask questions.
12. Use tests to help judge each pupil's intellectual capacity so that neither too much nor too little is expected of him or her.
13. Create a classroom atmosphere of fairness. The teacher should see that rules and regulations are reasonable. Have only a few rules but see that all observe them. This is also true in games played in the gymnasium or on the playground.
14. Keep the classroom atmosphere calm and serene, businesslike but unhurried.

Primary Level

1. Hang a printed sign or large poster in front of the class for a few hours prior to discussing its meaning:

> A GOOD LAUGH
> IS SUNSHINE
> IN THE HOUSE
> —William Makepeace Thackeray

2. Explain something that is painful to the teacher. Have the class suggest means of solving it.
3. In order to help children understand how people express what they are thinking and feeling, have individuals and groups demonstrate how a person moves when angry, excited, afraid, sad, happy, and so on.
4. Make a list of the qualities admired in other people.
5. Use every opportunity to practice using terms such as "please," and "thank you" (kindergarten or first grade).
6. Share toys and materials.
7. Send cards, pictures, or class letters to classmates who are ill.
8. Read and discuss stories which show thoughtfulness of others.
9. When a new pupil joins the class, plan several ways to make him or her feel at home.
10. Bring pets to class and talk about how one treats pets.
11. Work as a group on several projects. Point out to the class what each individual has done so that everyone will appreciate the contributions of others.
12. Encourage serving on committees and taking turns as leader.
13. Encourage children, especially at the start of the school year, to talk about themselves, what they like most at home, and what they think they will like around school.
14. Cooperate in keeping the room attractive.
15. Plan picnics and school parties. Talk about and demonstrate good manners and decide how everyone should act on the bus, on the street, in the stores, and on visits.
16. Do something about others less fortunate. Secure large scrapbooks and let the class cut colorful pictures from magazines and paste them in the books for sick children in the hospital.
17. Talk over taking turns on playground equipment.
18. Permit pupils to talk about their families. Encourage them to tell what they do to keep their home a happy place.
19. Talk over diseases that cause death and discuss the death of a pet or person one loves. Concentrate on ways of dealing

with feelings. Raise questions about men and boys crying, how one feels when someone in or near the family dies, how dead persons can live in one's memory, and how people help each other deal with feelings.

20. Keep a collection at school of something that each child cherishes.
21. Collect and post pictures of people showing kindness and of happy children and families.
22. Draw cartoons of various facial expressions in order to show feelings. (See Masks in Figure 8–24.)

Intermediate Level

1. Write, tell, read, and discuss stories about emotions. Particular instances of interest may be dramatized.
2. Discuss spontaneous situations that arise to develop understanding of emotions of other children. Use interesting stories involving emotional problems to stimulate discussions on the importance of controlling our emotions.

3. Participate in creative activities, such as finger painting, drawing, painting, clay modeling, and rhythmics, as acceptable means of expressing emotions. Encourage children to "talk it out" with sympathetic listeners.

4. Arrange for parent and child to each explain his or her feelings toward the other on a tape recorder and listen to each other's tapes (5th-6th grades).

5. Send a sunshine package to someone who is ill. This may contain cards, pictures, and various objects presented by the class.

6. Share hobbies. Have pupils tell about and demonstrate their special hobby before the class (sixth grade).

7. Make up some everyday problems and give correct and incorrect ways of solving them. Also use "open-end stories" regarding a problem, using class members' names.

8. Choose a class hospitality committee and set up a procedure for operation.

9. Have each class member pick out his or her worst habit or worst fault and tell how he or she hopes to overcome it.

10. Set up a question box and encourage questions concerning worries and fears of class members. A "What's on Your Mind?" box precipitates some excellent discussion.

11. Hear reports on famous handicapped persons such as Keller, Edison, and Baruch who have succeeded in spite of their handicaps.

12. Study moving in relation to feelings of loss and separation. Since 45 per cent of the nation's population moved last year, this is a timely topic. Distribute cards or sheets of paper on which each student fills in the blank spaces:

I think I would feel _____ if I had to move away

from where I live because _____.

The thing that would bother me the most is

_____. I think (or do not think) I

should feel this way because _____.

13. Collect newspaper clippings depicting cases of mental problems. Note, also, the numerous articles which appear

in the paper that have to do with personal unhappiness. In the course of a week, check to see if news items of an unhappy nature are more or less prevalent than those of a happy nature (sixth grade).

14. Employing role-playing, set up situations in which to study death and how it affects people. Look at:
    a. death and anger
    b. death and its denial
    c. death and bargaining to live
    d. death and depression
    e. death and its acceptance

15. Distribute cards and have pupils write down several ways they think they are different from others. Divide into small groups of four to six persons. Swap cards and discuss the accuracy of individual perceptions (sixth grade).

16. Emphasize good sportmanship and fair play. This may be done through a project dealing with a group game situation.

17. Find out why fatigue or illness can make us "fussy" or irritable.

18. In a fifth grade Cincinnati school classroom, the topic of mental maturation was discussed, with students in the leadership role. The leader has a 3' × 4' chart entitled "How Mature Am I?" It carried the following list:
    1. When someone pokes fun at me.
    2. When someone disagrees with me.
    3. When I want attention.
    4. When I am confused.
    5. When I don't get what I want.

At the right was a column for each day of the week, in which ratings could be entered.

19. Have everyone in class write some personal items on a card. Then place all student cards in an envelope. Two or three months later, return the cards and complete a second column. Note the interesting changes:

	Now	Later in Time
My name	_____	_____
My weight	_____	_____
Best Friend	_____	_____
Newest friend	_____	_____
Favorite song	_____	_____
Favorite food	_____	_____
Favorite game	_____	_____
What I worry about most	_____	_____
Other items	_____	_____

20. Risk-taking and trust-building can bring a class closer together and help develop mental health. Try the following activities with partners:
    a. Trust a partner by permitting him/her to lead you about over a variety of terrain while blindfolded. Then reverse

roles and repeat as before. Describe feelings after both
partners have had the experience.

b. With arms extended sideways and eyes closed, fall
backwards into arms of partner. Change so that partner
has a chance.

9. SEX AND FAMILY LIVING EDUCATION

Behavioral Objectives (Primary Level)

Describes a happy home and explains how one acts in it.

Shares work as well as recreation in the home.

Explains how animals protect and feed their babies.

Identifies with other living things—life with life, both plant and
animal.

Investigates how living things come from other living things—
plant life, baby animals, and mothers and babies.

Chooses a variety of activities that bring about good times in the
home and happy family living.

Behavioral Objectives (Intermediate Level)

Evaluates the specific role of each family member in maintaining
a happy home.

Interprets the cooperative and unique contributions of both
sexes to society.

Relates how life begins and how physical growth advances.

Describes the relationship of children's behavior to social living
and to family-community life in general.

Analyzes the different interests and activity choices of boys and
girls.

Describes the function of menstruation and conception and how
life begins from a single cell.

Employs several means to demonstrate that social and emotional growth are an essential part of the process of maturation.

Comments

It has been wisely stated that sex is not something we do—it is
something we are. Therefore, sex will never be thoroughly understood until it is related to the total adjustment of the individual in the
family and society. Ultimately, everyone must define his or her
sexual role and establish a value system. The combined efforts of the
home, church, and school are required in order to bring about a full
understanding and acceptance of human sexuality at all age levels. In
fact, the concept of sharing this responsibility is significant. Continuing to "dump" the problem of enlightenment on the schools and
expect miracles is unrealistic. Educating parents about sexuality and

encouraging church and social groups to make a contribution is a worthwhile endeavor that improves children's sex education and makes the role of the teacher more effective.

Sexuality and the feelings involved cannot be eliminated at any age. They can only be accepted and cultivated. It is the cultivation that is difficult in a society with pluralistic moral codes regulating childhood sexuality and in which attitudes toward both sex and aggression frequently reflect psychological conflicts. Sex is both loved and hated in our culture, so that a variety of people are constantly influenced in opposite directions. Parents frequently reject the concept of sexuality when raising their children, presumably to create a "sex-free" environment for children to grow up in.

Throughout the country, sex education has often been initiated because of the astounding prevalence of venereal disease. It is true that venereal disease is a major health problem. Gonorrhea is pandemic with several million cases a year, two thirds of which involve young people in the 15 to 24 year age group. One fact stands out: each year the number of cases increases, but the average age of those infected declines. Information about the sexually transmitted diseases should be given in the early years. Syphilis, gonorrhea, non-gonococcal urethritis, *Trichomonas* infection, monilial vaginitis, and herpes progenitalis (herpes II) are not disappearing. However, teaching about venereal disease is only part of the total sex education responsibility.

Interest in sex occurs at all ages. Whether sex education is formal or informal, a part of the home life or a part of the "gang talk" on the street corner, it is of vital concern to all growing boys and girls. Knowledge and appreciations in this area are every bit as important in terms of future behavior as they are in other health areas. More and more research indicates that the school is in an excellent position to carry out a sound sex education program. Here children gain values from peer-group discussions under competent leadership which is difficult for parents to duplicate.

Since attitudes are formed at an early age, it is important to start sex education at a time prior to the building up of personal inhibitions—inhibitions which tend to limit frank discussion. Foster has shown in a study of age and grade level inhibitions that children at the fifth grade level or below normally do not possess reticence toward matters of sex. He states that, "only if sex education is delayed . . . will the feeling of improperness influence his thinking since the child will have incorporated all of the fears and incorrect thoughts of his peers and perhaps his family. . . . It is better to be a year early in our provision of sex education during pre-adolescence than to be a day too late in adolescence.[32]

There is an immediate need for an educational program to offset the half-truths and general misinformation that children are constantly exposed to through the commercial exploitation of sex and erotica by modern mass media. Children have grown up to become

---

[32]Foster, Greg R. "Sex Information vs. Sex Education: Implications for School Health," *Journal of School Health, 37*:248–250, May 1967.

adults who believe that sex is simply a plaything or at best a biological phenomenon—a reproductive item. They have not understood it as an integral part of total personality. Quite the contrary, they see it as genital-centered—the exact opposite of what should be the goal.

It is difficult to develop responsible sexual morality in personal and family situations when the "anything goes" philosophy of life permeates the minds of primary graders and adults alike. As the old taboos die and the permissive society takes shape, only a calculated sex and family living education can hope to be an effective counteracting agent. This is not easy. It is a difficult undertaking in an era of obscene language, increasing nudity, suggestive posters and films, and an almost constant celebration of the erotic life.

Confusing genital-centered sex with true sexuality is recognized by the major faiths and parent groups as an unfortunate contemporary fact. Its relationship to sexual experimentation, venereal disease, promiscuity, pregnant teenagers, and unwed mothers is clear. The statistics are frequently overwhelming. (Review the evidence in Chapter 1.) Moreover, the numerous expressions of sex are as important to the health of the marital relationship and to the solid foundation of the family in twentieth century society as are its procreative aspects.

The Role of the School

It is the function of the school to cooperate with community leaders in the early exploration and planning of a curriculum in sex and family living education, from the kindergarten through high school. Failure to do so has almost always resulted in misunderstandings and less than adequate programs. Local groups of citizens should realize that they do indeed have a say in what the school does. Also, they have a responsibility to back the school in its efforts.

From the start it should be made clear that the objective is to eliminate anxieties and misunderstandings pertaining to sex through the development of an adequate knowledge of the physical, mental, social, emotional, and spiritual processes involved.

Sex education is to be distinguished from sex information. It implies that one's sexuality is integrated into total life development as a health entity and a source of creative energy.

Historically, the learned organizations and their prophets have been urging the schools to get started. In 1941 the American Association of School Administrators recommended that sex education be included in the school curriculum. It was recommended again in 1960 at the White House Conference on Children and by the middle 1960's a number of state and national groups called for action. Although less than a dozen states mandate the teaching of sex education in the public schools, there are many that permit it to be taught on an optional basis. Several have developed excellent policy statements regarding sex and family living education. One of the finest, put forth in a 24-page booklet and complete with 26 admirable objectives, is the one from Illinois.[33] Pennsylvania and Iowa also have especially noteworthy policy statements. Another policy statement, short and clear, was prepared by the New Jersey State Board of Education and given wide distribution throughout the state and beyond. The full statement follows:

A POLICY STATEMENT ON SEX EDUCATION

(Adopted by the State Board of Education on January 4, 1967)

Sex education is a responsibility which should be shared by the home, church, and school. The State Board of Education and the State Department of Education support the philosophy that each community and educational institute must determine its role in this area. Therefore, the State Board of Education recommends that each Local Board of Education make provisions in its curriculum for sex education programs.

Sex is a major aspect of personality. It is intimately related to emotional and social development and adjustment. Being boy or girl, man, or woman, conditions one's sense of identity, ways of thinking and behaving, social and occupational activities, choice of associates, and mode of dress. Sex cannot be understood simply by focusing on physiological processes or classifying modes of sexual behavior. Human sexuality—the assumption of the individual's sex role—can best be understood by relating it to the total adjustment of the individual in his family and society.

The primary purpose of sex education is to promote more wholesome family and interpersonal relationships and, therefore, more complete lives. It is not a subject that lends itself readily to "lecturing" or "telling." An approach which encourages open discussion and solicits the concerns of the individual is needed to help young people develop appropriate attitudes and understandings regarding their sex roles. This approach is possible if parents, clergy, teachers, health personnel, and others responsible for the education of children are informed and secure in their own feelings about sex.

Sex education is a continuing process throughout life and therefore must be planned for during the entire school experience of the child. Schools are important agencies in the development of health habits of living and moral values. Therefore, the Department of Education recommends that appropriate programs in sex education be developed by educational institutions cognizant of what is desirable, what is possible, and what is wise.

---

[33]Illinois Sex Education Advisory Board, *Policy Statement on Family Life and Sex Education,* Springfield, Illinois: Office of the Superintendent of Public Instruction, Revised.

Figure 8–26. "Hut, Toop, Threep, Forp, Fiivp, Sex, Sevm, Hate, Niieen, Tem! Hut, Toop, Threep . . ." (Courtesy, *Instructor* magazine and Ford Button.)

An early start in the sex and family living area builds a firm foundation of understandings and attitudes before complex emotional problems confront boys and girls in their teens. Thus, Glen Cove, New York kindergarten children discuss the coming of a new baby into the family group. Moreover, the baby was not "got" at the hospital, but grew inside the mother until the doctor helped bring it out.

In numerous elementary schools, programs have been carefully planned to meet local needs. These needs are much the same everywhere. Whether it is Washington, Illinois, or Oregon, the teacher is the key to a good program. No teacher should be forced to teach in an area in which he or she feels uncomfortable. Fortunately, many elementary school teachers are usually "at home" discussing the world of persons and families both formally and informally in their classrooms.

The following selected references are especially useful in building a rationale for teaching sex and family living education early in the grades and for appreciating the need for a sequence of experiences which will contribute to the development of appropriate concepts of sexuality in the later years:

American School Health Association. *Growth Patterns and Sex Education*. Kent, Ohio (revised).

Berstein, A. "How Children Learn About Sex & Birth," *Psychology Today, 9*:31–35, January 1976.

Breiner, S. J. "Psychological Principles of a Sex Education Program for Grades K Through 12," *Journal of School Health, 42*:227–230, April 1972.

Broderick, Carlfred B. "Sexual Behavior Among Pre-Adolescents," *Journal of Social Issues, 22*:6–21, April 1966.

Brower, Linda and Southworth, Warren, H. "A Guideine for Discussion of Sexual Behavior," *Journal of School Health, 39*:715–720, December 1969.

Calderone, Mary A. "Planning for Sex Education: a Community-wide Responsibility." *NEA Journal,* January 1967.

Fitz Mahan, Don L. "Venereal Disease Prevention Education," *Health Education, 8*:13–14, January/February 1977.

Gordon, Sol. "What Place Does Sex Education Have in the Schools?" *Journal of School Health, 45*:186–189, April 1975.

—————————. *Girls are Girls And Boys are Boys: So What's The Difference?* New York: John Day, 1974.

Hawkins, Barbara. "The Family Life Education Program in the Chicago Public Schools." *School Health Review, 2*:33–35, April 1971.

Johnson, Eric W. *Love and Sex and Growing Up*. Philadelphia: Lippincott, (revised), 1973.

Lennon, Mary Louise. "Selection of Family Life Education Materials Used in the Chicago Public Schools." *Journal of School Health, 42*:233–237, April 1972.

Levin, Barbara B., et al. "A Peek at Sex Education in a Midwestern Community," *Journal of School Health, 42*:462–465, October 1972.

Maxeiner, Barbara A., O'Rourke, Thomas W., and Stone, Donald B. "Knowledge, Behavior and Attitudes of Sixth-Grade Students Toward Family Life Education," *Journal of School, 46*:81–85, February 1976.

McNab, Warren L. "Sexual Attitude Development in Children and the Parent's Role," *Journal of School Health, 46*:537–541, November 1976.

Mervis, Rosalyn M. and Watson, Marsha D. "Learning About Sex Education from Children," *Journal of School Health, 46*:229–231, April 1976.

Schiller, Patricia, *Creative Approach to Sex Education and Counseling,* New York: Association Press, 1973.

Simon, William, and Gagnon, John H. 'The Pedagogy of Sex." *Saturday Review,* November 18, 1967, p. 79.

Wiederholt, Kathleen and Hosokawa, M. C. "Away from the Cabbage Patch," *Journal of School Health, 48*:687–691, January 1978.

Woody, J. D. "Contemporary Sex Education: Attitudes and Implications for Childrearing," *Journal of School Health, 43*:241–246, April 1973.

There is a reasonably good amount of experience to draw upon when it comes to structuring a program. The list of communities with effective elementary programs is rather extensive. Well-prepared guides to the curriculum such as the following may be obtained at moderate cost:

Sex Education–a Working Design for Curriculum Development and Implementation, Grades K–12. The Education Council, 131 Mineola Blvd., Mineola, N.Y. 11501.

Curriculum Guide for Family Life and Sex Education, Great Neck Public Schools, Great Neck, N.Y.

Guide to Health and Family Life Education, Grades K–12, San Francisco Unified District, San Francisco, Ca.

Guidelines for Family Life and Sex Education, Grades K–12, Curriculum Bulletin No. 32, State of Minnesota, Dept. of Education, St. Paul, Minn.

Personal and Family Living for the Elementary School, Curriculum Resource Bulletin, Public Schools, District of Columbia, Administration Annex No. 7, North Street, N.W., Washington, D.C. 20007.

Educating For Sexuality: Concepts and Programs For Teaching, 2nd ed., by John J. Burt and Linda A. Meeks, W. B. Saunders Co., Philadelphia, Pa., 1975.

Teaching About Family Relationships, by Richard Klemers and Rebecca Smith, Minneapolis Minn. Burgess Publishing Co., 1975.

Venereal Disease Education: Teachers' Resources, Ohio Department of Education, Columbus, Ohio, 1976.

Interest surveys tend to help teachers structure the curriculum. In the *Teach Us What We Want To Know* study (Connecticut State Department of Education, Hartford, Connecticut) there was tremendous interest among second and third graders relative to babies—"Where do they come from?" "How do they out of the mother's stomach?" "Why can't babies talk and walk?" "Why do they cry?" By the fifth grade the children ask, "Why do only girls have babies?" "Does smoking have anything to do with babies being formed wrong?" and "What makes it a girl or a boy?" Significantly, these questions are asked at an age when straightforward answers are effective and accepted as matter-of-fact.

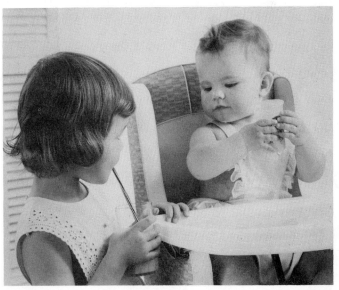

Figure 8–27. Primary grade children like pictures of babies—to view and talk about. (Courtesy Gerber Baby Foods.)

Intermediate graders can ask keen questions calling for detailed answers. Research in Michigan showed that sixth grade students want to know about miscarriage and artificial insemination. They ask: "Why do some girls develop before others?"; "Is something wrong with me? I like sports better than going with girls."; "Sometimes in the movies or on television, a women tells her husband, "We're going to have a baby!', why didn't he know about it?"

After studying a great number of curriculum guides and working with adolescents concerning sex education, Deryek Calderwood concluded that the most common complaint was that their education came too late. Student interest in sexuality is so high at an early age that much sex education comes "after the fact" for young people, rather than preparing them for their psychosexual development and socio-sexual experiences. In short, young people's readiness for effective sex education far exceeds most adults' cautious willingness to provide it. Yet, when it is done well there are deeply felt appreciations. A fifth grade boy in the Chicago program says, "Family life has been the most interesting study I ever had in school. I never realized how wonderful our bodies were." This boy's program received a high rating in a Northwestern University study that covered 54 elementary schools.[34] Some 12,230 children received instruction. Only 43 were withdrawn at the request of parents; 378 classroom teachers were involved. Evaluation by parents was 91 per cent favorable; evaluation by principals was 98 per cent favorable; and there was a solid 100 per cent favorable report by the teachers.

The Program

The finest education relative to sexuality and family living probably takes place in the home itself under the guidance of informed and sympathetic parents. Unfortunately, not all homes function in a way to promote optimum family living. In fact, some of them promote anything but optimum family living. However, prior to initiating a school program, all parents should be oriented to what the school proposes. This important approach is substantiated by several studies that identify a direct relationship between parent and child sex attitudes.[35] The clergy and other leaders in the community should give their support as well. A local elementary school Parent-Teacher Association can be very helpful in the process. It also provides classroom teachers with a little help through an in-service training program. Carefully selected and well-prepared teachers increase support and cooperation of the public in this program.

The question of what to teach and how to teach it is the next consideration. Everyday classroom experiences are suitable for integrating information about the beginning of life and the care of the

---

[34]Hawkins, Barbara. "The Family Life Education Program in the Chicago Schools," *School Health Review*, 2:33–35, April 1971.

[35]See particularly McNab, Warren L. "Sexual Attitude Development in Children and the Parents' Role," *Journal of School Health*, 46:437–441, November 1976; and Woody, J. D. "Contemporary Sex Education: Attitudes and Implications for Childrearing," *Journal of School Health*, 43:241–246, April 1973.

young. At an early, age children are curious about life in all of its many manifestations—how it originates, how it grows, and how it perpetuates itself. Children's questions are generally not difficult to answer, but they do require that the teacher have the ability to answer them honestly, unemotionally, and accurately. Instruction must be conducted with dignity and discretion. Sex is a life function that is normal, clean, respectable, and admirable. Here are some principles to follow.[36]

Sex education in schools should be integrated with the total health education program at all grade levels. It should not be singled out for separate or undue emphasis.

Example on the part of parents and teachers is far more effective than precept.

Sex education should be couched in terms easily understood by children and should make use of examples within their experience.

Sex information should not be forced upon the uninterested child but should be adapted to the maturity level at each stage of growth.

It should be presented in a dignified vocabulary.

It should be taught positively by showing its nobility in terms of creative drive and family happiness rather than negatively through the enumeration of horrible examples of immorality.

Sex anatomy and physiology (upper grades) should be treated as just another body system; due allowance must be made for modesty.

The many relations of sex to all phases of normal, private, and public life must be discussed in an objective manner.

Although the emphasis differs, there is a fair amount of agreement as to primary and intermediate grade content in sex and family living education. This is particularly true when one compares the courses of study that have been periodically revised in the several communities where established programs have been in operation for some time.

Some idea of the scope of the program, kindergarten through sixth grade, can be appreciated by looking over the Sex and Family Living Education outline, set up by concepts and arranged by the author for the Massachusetts health education curriculum guide.

Kindergarten

I am a member of a family.
Families do many things together.
Boys and girls are important in families.
Mothers and fathers are important too.
Children and parents working and playing together help to make home a happy place in which to live.
Family members show love for each other.
I am a member of a school family.
Every person needs to feel wanted at home and at school.
Our bodies are wonderful and there is nothing shameful about any part of the body.

---

[36]Adapted from the Joint Committee, National Education Association and American Medical Association. *Health Education,* (revised) National Education Association, 1201 Sixteenth St., N.W., Washington, D.C. 20036.

There are proper names for the body parts concerned with elimination.
Everyone has a right to privacy at some times.
Each person should respect the privacy of others.
Show caution when dealing with strangers.

Grade One

Animals are members of animal families.
All life comes from life.
All living things grow and reproduce.
Plants grow from seeds.
Some animals hatch from eggs and others develop inside the body of the mother until birth.
Cats have kittens; humans have babies.
In the beginning every child has a mother and father.
Babies come from mothers.
Both animal and human parents try to keep their young safe, fed, happy and healthy.
Girls and boys are alike in some ways and different in some ways.

Grade Two

Different animals need different amounts of time to get ready to be born.
Mice, cats, dogs and cows are born live through a special opening in the mother's body.
Both human and animal parents take care of their children until they are able to take care of themselves.
Animal and human babies need good food in order to grow properly.
Growing older means more responsibility at home.
Helping at home and in the community helps us learn more about ourselves, other people, and the world we live in.

Grade Three

Every living thing grows and reproduces.
An egg cell develops in the mother to become a baby.
The baby is born through a special opening in the mother's body.
Human beings grow in many ways—physically, mentally and socially.
We inherit many of our physical and mental characteristics from our parents.
Living things are alike in many ways—requiring air, light, food, rest, water, etc.

Figure 8–28. Understanding families, children, and love are needs the world over. (Courtesy Gerber Products Company.)

Each parent contributes something to its offspring.
Children are both alike and different from their parents.
Growing older means more than just getting bigger.

Grade Four

Family patterns differ throughout the United States.
Families may have problems, but they can work together to solve them (broken homes, death, physical and mental handicaps, unemployment, etc.)
How life begins is a wondrous miracle.
The mother's egg (ovum) is fertilized by the sperm of the father.
The fertilized ovum divides into many cells which have a special function to perform.
Both parents contribute their own particular characteristics to their offspring.
All living things develop from a single cell.
When the baby has been in the mother nine months it is ready to be born.
As the baby grows certain glands control its growth and development.

Grade Five

Glands which produce hormones help control body growth and development.
Sex glands at puberty bring about certain physical and emotional changes.
There is a time when girls may be taller than boys, but later on the boys usually catch up to the girls in height.
Menstruation occurs as a natural part of a girl's growing up.
Menstruation indicates that a girl is becoming a woman who will be able to conceive and have children.
Seminal (nocturnal) emissions occurs as a natural part of a boy's growing up.
Though nature readies the body for reproduction at puberty, several years more are needed to prepare for marriage and the responsibility of parenthood.
Menstruation does not occur when the ovum has been fertilized by the male sperm.
As the fetus grows inside the mother, the placenta and umbilical cord bring it food and oxygen from the mother, and carry away the waste products to the mother for elimination.
The baby's blood and circulatory system are separate from the mother's.
Through the process of osmosis oxygen and food are exchanged between mother and baby.
Before being born the baby is well protected by the amniotic sac and fluid in the abdomen of the mother.
The uniqueness of boys and girls is expressed in one's sexuality, not only through the reproductive process but within the framework of the family.

Grade Six

Femaleness and maleness refer to biological characteristics unique for each person.
No person is totally male or totally female; there are characteristics of the opposite sex in both males and females.
Understanding the role of men and women in our society is part of becoming a mature person.
Mature boys and girls learn to control their feelings and emotions.
There are proper and improper ways of expressing emotions.
The endocrine glands secrete hormones that prepare the body for many kinds of actions during periods of emotional stress.
Both boys and girls have natural emotional feelings of affection toward the opposite sex.

There are acceptable ways to express these feelings.

Because one has a responsibility for personal relationships, sexual feelings are controlled.

Recreational activities contribute to the development of wholesome boy-girl relationships. They also help family morale.

It is important to learn to make some decisions early in life and accept the consequences.

A further example from an on-going program in Glen Cove, New York follows:

GLEN COVE PUBLIC SCHOOLS, N.Y.
Health Guidance in Sex Education—Aims at Each Level

Kindergarten

1. Know sex differences between girls and boys.
2. Give direction toward male or female role in adult life.
3. Learn correct names for body parts and terms concerned with elimination.
4. Understand that human baby develops inside body of mother.
5. Understand baby gets milk from mother's breast by nursing.
6. Appreciate that there are good body feelings.
7. Learn to recognize signs of love and devotion within family.
8. Develop idea of continuity of living things—incubate eggs.

First Year

1. Understand egg cell is basic to new life.
2. Learn that some animals hatch from eggs and others develop inside body of mother until birth.
3. Appreciate wonder of human body.
4. Develop sense of responsibility for own body.
5. Appreciate efforts of mother and father for family members.
6. Recognize influence of emotions on body health.

Second Year

1. Learn that different animals need different amounts of time to get ready to be born.
2. Understand that the egg cell does not develop into a baby by itself—role of father.
3. Learn that some animals are born live through a special opening in the mother's body.
4. Recognize that growing up brings responsibility.
5. Appreciate importance of mutual love and consideration in family.
6. Understand composition of family does not necessarily determine happiness of family.

Third Year

1. Understand that each person's unique heredity is determined at moment of fertilization.
2. Observe influence of heredity in your family.
3. Know that growing up means more than just getting bigger.
4. Develop increasing sense of responsibility to self and family.
5. Understand relationship between a healthy body and mind.
6. Study life cycles of various animals, including humans.

Fourth Year

1. Learn that certain glands control body growth and development.
2. Recognize importance of protecting vital body parts from injury, i.e., during sports.
3. Appreciate miracle of reproduction and maternal care among various forms of animal life.
4. Appreciate superiority of brain of man over instinct reaction of animals.
5. Learn meaning of responsible behavior in peer and family groups.
6. Study circulatory and digestive systems and realize their functional potential is influenced by habits being developed.

Fifth Year

1. Learn role of sex glands at puberty and emotional changes they bring.
2. Understand menstruation occurs as a natural part of a girl's growing up.
3. Understand seminal emissions occur as a natural part of a boy's growing up.
4. Learn that although nature readies our bodies for reproduction at puberty, several years more are needed to prepare for marriage and responsibility of parenthood.
5. Discuss importance of wholesome life attitudes and values as manifested in responsible behavior.
6. Discuss acceptable and unacceptable ways of showing emotions.

One of the most thorough reports to appear in recent years was prepared by the Committee on Health Guidance in Sex Education of the American School Health Association.[37] An outstanding feature of this extensive publication is that specific concepts and attitudes are set forth for each grade level in a manner readily understood by the teacher.

AMERICAN SCHOOL HEALTH ASSOCIATION

Kindergarten and Grade One

A. **Concepts.** As a product of their experiences in the study of this unit, it would be hoped that some such concepts as these would be formulated by children in kindergarten and the first grade:

1. All living things reproduce. Life comes from life.
2. The creation of new life is one of nature's greatest miracles.
3. Every child has a mother and a father in the beginning.
4. Every person needs to have a feeling of belonging.
5. Each member of a family is an important member. Children and parents working and playing together help to make a home a happy place to live. There are many ways in which children can help to make their homes happy ones.
6. Each member of a family is interested in the well-being of every other member.

---

[37]"Growth Patterns and Sex Education: a Suggested Program K-12." This total in-depth issue of 136 pages is available for a small cost from American School Health Association, 515 E. Main St., Kent, Ohio 44240.

7. Using good manners lets other people know that we like and respect them. Thoughtful boys and girls are courteous to each other, to their mothers and fathers, their brothers and sisters, and to everyone else.
8. Every person desires privacy at some times. Each person has a right to privacy, and each should respect the privacy of others.
9. Each part of the body is an important part of the whole person, and their is nothing shameful about any part of the body.
10. We should be cautious in dealing with strangers. Although some strangers who offer rides or candy to children are trying to be kind, others are not. We should always refuse such offers and should tell our parents and teachers about them.

B. **Attitudes.** As an outcome of this unit, it is to be hoped that the student will form some such favorable attitudes as these toward himself or herself, others, family living, and reproduction:
1. An appreciation for the role of each family member.
2. An appreciation for his or her own importance as a member of the family and a desire to contribute to the family's well-being.
3. A respect for the rights of others.
4. A sense of wonder in regard to reproduction.
5. A wholesome respect for all parts of the body and a desire to learn and to use correct terminology in referring to them.

Grades Two and Three

A. **Concepts.** As a product of their experiences in the study of this unit, it would be hoped that some such concepts as these would be formulated by children in the second and third grades:
1. All living things grow and reproduce.
2. Every child has a mother and a father in the beginning.
3. Parents or guardians take care of their children in many ways until children grow up and are able to take care of themselves.
4. Human babies and children live with their parents or guardians for many years because it takes a long time for them to grow up and to learn how to do for themselves all the things that parents do for them while they are young.
5. Human beings grow in many ways—physically, intellectually, emotionally, socially, spiritually.
6. All living things have basic needs which must be fulfilled for optimal growth.
7. We need many different kinds of food to help us grow.
8. The food we eat is changed and used by our bodies to help us grow.
9. Optimal growth depends in part upon how well we utilize the food we eat.
10. Babies need special foods for optimal growth.
11. Everything we do helps us to learn more about ourselves, other people and the world we live in.
12. We can do our best work and have the most fun when we are happy.
13. Being neat and clean helps to make us feel good about ourselves.
14. Boys and girls enjoy playing and working with other boys and girls who are neat and clean.
15. There are many ways that mothers and fathers and children can show that they love each other.
16. Using good manners is one way we can let members of our families, other grown-ups, and other boys and girls know that we like them.

17. Fathers do many kinds of work in the community, and all of them can help to make the community a better place in which to live.

18. Mothers help the community in many ways—by making the home a healthy and happy place to live, by working at jobs outside the home, or by participating in community activities which they enjoy.

B. **Attitudes.** As an outcome of this unit, it is to be hoped that the student will form favorable attitudes toward himself or herself, others, family living, and reproduction.

1. An appreciation for the roles of each member of the family as an individual and as a contributing member of the family unit.

2. A desire for optimal nutrition.

3. A desire to develop or to continue personal practices which lead to cleanliness and good grooming.

4. An appreciation for clothing that is clean and functional, regardless of its "fashionableness."

5. A respect for other persons as individuals and a desire to show respect for others by treating them courteously.

6. A growing regard for masculine and feminine roles in our society.

7. An appreciation for the ways in which adult men and women contribute to the community and the desire to become future contributing adult members of the community.

8. A sense of wonder concerning the complex nature of the human personality and its development.

9. An appreciation for the effect that a pleasant manner has upon one's relationship with others.

Grade Four

A. **Concepts.** As a product of their experiences in the study of this unit, it would be hoped that some such concepts as these would be formulated by children in the fourth grade:

1. We are made of many cells which have important tasks to do in making it possible for us to live and grow.

2. Blood carries food to the cells and waste products away from the cells to places where they can be collected and excreted.

3. A person's heredity refers to those personal characteristics that have been passed down from parents through genes and chromosomes.

4. Each person receives half of his or her inherited characteristics from each parent.

5. Each person's inherited characteristics are determined at the moment of conception when the father's sperm fertilizes the mother's ovum.

6. A person's heredity influences growth, appearance, and height.

7. What a person becomes is determined by his or her heredity, environment and, to some extent, what he or she wants to be.

8. Each member of a family contributes to the well-being of the whole family and each of its other members.

9. The health of each family member affects the well-being of all family members.

10. There are many activities that all members of a family can participate in and enjoy together. Playing together and working together helps mothers and fathers and children know each other better and strengthens the family as a unit.

11. Having a hobby is one way a person can use leisure time constructively. Hobbies add enjoyment to living. Sometimes the members of a family enjoy sharing the same hobby.

12. A friend is someone who likes you and whom you like. A person

can have many different kinds of friends among people of all ages.

13. One of the best ways to make new friends is to be friendly to other people. Being friendly lets others know that we would like to have them as our friends.

B. **Attitudes.** As an outcome of this unit, it is to be hoped that the student will form favorable attitudes toward himself or herself, others, family living, and reproduction:

1. An appreciation for one's family heritage, both hereditary and environmental.
2. An appreciation for the influences that heredity and environment have upon growth and development.
3. An appreciation for the ability one has to control the direction of his or her own development and a desire to exercise this control to the greatest extent possible.
4. A regard for the effect that the health of each family member has upon that of all other family members and upon the family as a unit.
5. A desire to have one's own health status and practices contribute to rather than detract from family well-being.
6. A willingness to understand and adjust to the health problems of all members of the family.
7. An appreciation for the contribution that children this age can make to the leisure-time activities and fellowship of the family and a desire to help plan and participate in such activities with other members of the family.
8. An appreciation for the values and enjoyment that can be gained from constructive solitary activities.
9. A desire to select and pursue some activities that one can do on one's own.
10. A respect for the desire others have to engage in solitary activities and a regard for their right to do so.
11. An appreciation for the different kinds of friendships one can develop with many different persons of various ages.
12. A desire to be a friend to others.

Grade Five

A. **Concepts.** As a product of their experiences in the study of this unit, it would be hoped that some such concepts as these would be formulated by children in the fifth grade:

1. Although the general pattern of growth and development is the same for everyone, each person follows this pattern at an individual rate.
2. At some times in their lives, girls are taller than boys, but boys catch up later and usually become taller than girls.
3. A person's growth and development are determined by hereditary potential for growth and development and by the influence of the many kinds of experiences in his or her environment.
4. Hormones are responsible for the changes in appearance that occur as boys develop into men and girls develop into women.
5. Hormones influence not only a person's growth and physical development, but also the way one feels and behaves.
6. As boys and girls become men and women, their feelings and actions toward themselves and others change.
7. As people grow older they are able to assume more responsibility for their own care and for the well-being of others.
8. Although most habits are helpful to us, some of the habits people form can interfere with their well-being and ability to get along with others.

9. Seminal emissions are nature's way of releasing stored-up sperm.

10. Menstruation is a normal, healthful function which indicates that a girl is becoming a woman who will be able to conceive and have children.

11. The creation of a new life is one of the most wonderful acts of Nature.

12. Parenthood is a privilege and a responsibility.

13. Each new life begins with the union of a single sperm from the father and a single ovum from the mother.

14. The fertilized ovum divides into many cells which have different structures in order to assume different tasks. Cell division and differentiation begins at the time of conception and continues in order to form a fully developed human being.

15. As a baby lives and grows and develops inside the mother, the placenta and umbilical cord bring it food and oxygen from the mother and carry its waste products to the mother for elimination.

16. The blood of a developing baby is formed in its own body. Its circulatory system is separate from the mother's. Food and oxygen and waste products are exchanged between mother and baby through the process of osmosis.

17. The amniotic sac and fluid create an environment which protects the fetus until it is ready to be born.

18. The best way to assure that one's body will continue to function efficiently and well is to give it the normal care and attention it requires.

19. As a person grows and develops from a child into an adult, his or her changing body requires additional kinds of care in order to keep functioning at its best.

20. Although some children do not grow as rapidly as others, this is not an indication of any abnormality.

B. **Attitudes.** As an outcome of this unit, it is to be hoped that the student will form favorable attitudes toward himself or herself, others, family living, and reproduction:

1. An appreciation for normal individual differences in rates of growth and development and an acceptance of one's own rate.

2. A desire to seek information pertaining to sex and sexuality from reliable sources as replacement for unscientific information and hearsay.

3. A persistent regard for medical services and health consultation from scientific sources.

4. An appreciation for the uniqueness of each individual and for the ways in which all individuals are similar.

5. An appreciation for the contributions that families make to the total development of each person.

6. A desire to contribute to wholesome family living by participating in family activities.

7. An appreciation for the constructive expression of one's sexuality through the reproductive processes and within the framework of the family unit.

8. A desire to respond to increased privilege by displaying a growing sense of responsibility for self and others.

9. A desire to form habits which will contribute to one's well-being and to eliminate or avoid developing habits that may be destructive to optimal growth and development.

10. An appreciation of one's sexuality as a healthful expression of the personality.

11. A wholesome acceptance of oneself as a sexual being and of those physiological processes (e.g., menstruation and seminal emissions) related to this aspect of one's being.

12. A regard for both the privileges and responsibilities attendant upon parenthood.
13. An increasing appreciation for the complexity of the human personality.
14. A persistent regard for the nature of the phenomena involved in the creation of a new life.
15. A respect for one's body as a tool for creative self-expression and the desire to give it the care it requires and deserves as such.

Grade Six

A. **Concepts.** As a product of their experiences in the study of this unit, it would be hoped that some such concepts as these would be formulated by children in the sixth grade:

1. Cells have different kinds of structures which enable each kind to perform its specialized function.
2. A person's emotions affect the way the body functions.
3. The hormones secreted by the endocrine glands regulate many physiological functions. They prepare the body for actions during periods of emotional stress.
4. Emotions are natural human feelings existing in all persons. They are aroused in response to other people and to situations in one's environment.
5. Emotions need to be expressed in some way. There are constructive and destructive ways of expressing emotions.
6. Emotions can be expressed in the most constructive way when their expression is controlled by the use of one's ability to reason.
7. One of the tasks involved in becoming a mature person is that of learning to control the emotions in such a way that their expression helps, rather than hurts, both oneself and other people.
8. Maleness and femaleness refer to biological characteristics unique for each individual.
9. Although boys are mostly male and girls are mostly female, no person is all male or all female. There is some degree of femaleness in all boys and some degree of maleness in all girls.
10. Masculinity and femininity refer to patterns of behavior that are characteristic of males or of females in a particular culture. These patterns of behavior are not present at birth, but are learned through the experiences one has in the family, the school, and community. As boys and girls grow up, they learn how to be masculine or feminine by observing and behaving like the men or women they know and admire.
11. The process of growing and developing from children into adults is very complex and involves many physical, emotional and social changes and adjustments.
12. The growth and development of a baby from one fertilized cell into a complex human being is one of nature's greatest and most miraculous achievements.
13. An appreciation of "maleness" and "femaleness" is an important aspect of becoming an adult.
14. There are such normal variations in physiological activity in each individual that it is important to recognize, understand and accept the many characteristics which may be common to both sexes.

B. **Attitudes.** As an outcome of this unit, it is to be hoped that the student will form favorable attitudes toward himself or herself, others, family living, and reproduction:

1. An appreciation for the integrated nature of man.
2. An acceptance and appreciation of the emotional dimension of

being and of the human quality that emotional expression gives to personality.
3. A desire to express one's emotions in constructive ways.
4. A willingness to explore a variety of alternatives in the attempt to learn how to channel one's emotions into constructive outlets.
5. A growing acceptance of and appreciation for the sexuality of oneself and others.
6. A desire to adopt the behaviors natural to and characteristic of one's assigned sex role in our culture.
7. A sensitivity to, acceptance of, and appreciation for behavioral characteristics which may be exhibited by members of both sexes, which are natural to both sexes, but which may be culturally expected of one sex rather than of the other.
8. An acceptance of and appreciation for the complex physical, emotional, and social changes that one undergoes in the process of growing and developing into an adult.

Here is an outline of five lessons for sixth graders from the San Diego Public School Teaching Monograph. Note how vital the topics are and how they develop:

LESSON 1

How we grow, differences in the growth patterns of boys and girls, responsibilities of growing up, the importance of caution with strangers, how to choose the right friends, your appearance, glands that are responsible for growth and changes in our bodies, good attitudes, and the right names of the body's organs and functions. Questions and answers.

LESSON 2

Films on animal reproduction (The Sunfish, The Snapping Turtle, Snakes Are Interesting). Questions and answers. This is a fine impersonal introduction to human reproduction; it helps boys and girls understand that in most animals a male cell and a female egg must join before a new life can begin.

LESSON 3

Read a short book or monograph on human reproduction.[38] Questions and answers.

LESSON 4

(Girls) Review the sex organs, discuss menstruation, discuss reason for body changes, sex relations, and self-control (a film may be used).

LESSON 5

(Boys) Discuss glandular changes, growth of sex organs, formation of sperm, seminal emissions, masturbation, reasons for body changes, and use of self-control. Questions and answers.

LESSON 6

Show the film Human Growth to review and clarify previous lessons and to set the stage for further discussion of such things as strengthening right attitudes toward sex and growing up, correct terminology, cell division, twins, sex determination, heredity, boy-girl relationships, moral and spiritual values. Question and answer period.

---

[38]One of the most clearly written student references is "Birth and the First Journey" which appears in Current Health, September 1976, pp. 3–14.

Help for the new teacher concerned with teaching sexuality may be found in many places. Well over 100 organizations distribute appropriate films, filmstrips, tapes, and other teaching aids. (See extensive sources in Chapter 11.) Especially well done for primary grade children is *Baby Animals* (McGraw-Hill Text Films), *Farm Babies and Their Mothers* (Film Associates), and *Human and Animal Beginnings* (E. C. Brown Trust Foundation). Intermediate level students will respond to *Boy to Man* (Churchill Films), *Girl to Woman* (Churchill Films), and *The Miracle of Reproduction* (Sid Davis Productions).

There exists in Cleveland, Ohio the now famous Cleveland Health Museum. It is unique among educational agencies in the way it has informed the community about personal and public health. *Sex and family living education is the mainstay of this institution.* The visitors at every age are motivated not by a love of esthetics as in an

Figure 8–29. "Better to learn *facts* in the school room than half-truths in the school yard."

art museum or a curiosity about nature as in a natural history museum but by a strong interest in their own physical and mental well-being. It is in this museum that sex has a unique setting and it is in this area that the museum has made a lasting contribution over the years. Within 50 miles of Cleveland there are a large number of Ohio counties consisting of hundreds of schools that make at least one museum trip a year for a lesson on human reproduction. Elementary schoolchildren study the pictures and incomparably fine models for an experience conducive to a high retention of facts in an atmosphere with a minimum of emotional trauma. So high does interest in these exhibits run, in fact, that one often finds a youngster explaining them to the parents on a Sunday afternoon following the class visit.

The famous birth series models are now available for purchase from the Cleveland Museum. These lightweight, durable polystyrene models present the growth and development of a baby sculptured in three dimensions for teaching purposes.[39] They are a superb teaching aid.

There will be times when it seems necessary to separate boys and girls, particularly in the fifth or sixth grade when a discussion of menstruation arises. As a general rule, sex instruction should be in mixed classes and the materials and methods of instruction adapted to the situation. When a topic is peculiar to a single sex, it might be more convenient to meet the sexes separately. Menstruation, for example, is so full of mystery and misconceptions that both preadolescent boys and girls should know something about it. There should be open classroom discussion regarding superstition, primitive beliefs regarding "uncleanliness" associated with menstruation, and the fear of blood. This topic is a normal part of growing children's lives. Mature attitudes begin early when the need for teaching first occurs. So we teach the life cycle and the menstrual cycle, that menstruation is normal, and we answer the question, "What is happening inside?"

Three very good films for fifth and sixth grade use are:

The Story of Menstruation. Kimberly-Clark Corporation, Neenah, Wis., color, sound, ten minutes. Delightful Disney animated film, showing causes and characteristics of menstruation. The same company distributes (free) the booklet *Growing Up Young* for parents and teachers of the retarded girl. Also, English and Spanish versions of *Very Personally Yours* teacher basic menstrual health. This company distributes, at a modest cost, thought-provoking colored transparencies, *The Me I Want To Be,* and a teacher's guide for elementary school use. It is designed to stimulate open-ended discussion about physical and emotional growth. An extremely attractive booklet from Personal Products Company is *Growing Up and Liking It.* Three girls keep in touch with each other by writing letters, chiefly about growing and menstruation. Braille booklets are also available. The same company has both an English and Spanish translation of the film *It's Wonderful Being a Girl (Es Maravilloso Ser Mujer).*

An especially useful booklet entitled *World of a Girl* is distri-

---

[39]Cleveland Health Museum, 8911 Euclid Avenue, Cleveland, Ohio 44106.

buted (free) by the Scott Paper Company in Philadelphia. It is designed for fifth and sixth grade girls, to enable them to understand and respond wholesomely to the miraculous changes that begin their grownup life. A detailed teacher's guide is available for use with the booklet.

Another highly successful booklet for girls is *Accent on You*, distributed (free) by Tampax, Incorporated, 5 Dakota Drive, Lake Success, New York 11040.

A number of appropriate books for children follow:

Ages 4–9	Ages 10–14
How Babies Are Made by Andrew C. Andry and Steven Schepp, Time-Life Books	*Learning About Sex* by Gary F. Kelly, Barron's Educational Services
The Story of A Baby by Marie Ets, Viking Press, Inc.	*Facts About Sex for Today's Youth* by Sol Gordon, The John Day Company
Did the Sun Shine Before You Were Born? by Sol and Judith Gordon, The Third Press	*Boys and Sex* by Wardell B. Pomeroy, Dell
The Follett Family Life Education Program, six letter, Follett Educational Corporation	*Girls and Sex* by Wardell B. Pomeroy, Dell
How Was I Born? by Lennart Nilsson. Delacorte Press	*Love and Sex and Growing Up* by Eric W. Johnson and Corrine B. Johnson, J. B. Lippincott Co.

Suggested Activities

Primary Level

1. Keep a pet cat with kittens or a dog with young puppies in the classroom for several days for general observation.
2. Discover how many children have a baby brother or sister. To class: What is your favorite way to help with the baby? What are some things your baby can do?
3. Visit the zoo, a health museum, or any place where baby animals may be observed and talked about.
4. Visit a local dairy farmer shortly after the birth of a calf. Children never fail to appreciate such a visit.
5. Keep a pair of canaries and observe the building of the nest and laying and hatching of eggs.
6. Raise guppies. These live-bearing fish are inexpensive and most interesting. The young may be seen inside the female late in pregnancy. Collect tadpoles or grow eggs in the spring.
7. Have pupils describe family vacations and ways of having a good time at home.
8. Build a list of ways that children can help to make home more pleasant. Such a list should be posted with art work to illustrate this type of activity in action. A few examples of items that might appear on the list are:
   Run errands willingly
   Care for younger children

Come on the first call so Mother does not have to raise her
voice or get angry
Help Mother with the cleaning
Hang up our clothes
Pick up our toys
Share good stories with the family

9. Talk about the effect of a happy home at mealtime and at
bedtime. Set up a role-playing situation.
10. Read a pleasant story or poem to the class about family
living and good times.

> We scrub the big potatoes
> That Mother wants to bake
> We pour the milk and water,
> We cut the bread and cake,
> When supper's almost ready,
> We rest a little while,
> And think of something funny
> That will make the family smile.

11. Draw body outlines of children on large pieces of paper. Do
it again toward the end of the school year and note growth
changes.
12. Compare families around the world.
13. Show a picture of a new baby coming home from the
hospital. Ask: "Why do the grown-ups look so excited?
Why are they happy? What do you like best about having a
baby in a family?"
14. Read the story to class: *Laurie's New Brother* by Miriam
Schlein. The joy of the new baby is depicted.

Intermediate Level

1. Raise tropical fish or collect caterpillars for the room ter-
rarium. Watch the development of the cocoon.
2. Show pictures of tiny babies. Discuss special care needed
for small babies. Listen to student experiences. Use the wall
chart, *How A Baby Grows,* available (free) from Johnson &
Johnson. It shows clearly body and hand language and
social development.
3. Examine charts of high-grade animals such as certain
breeds of cows or dogs. Study the characteristics looked for
in breeding these animals. Seek help from a 4-H club
leader.
4. Examine the word "love." Ask: *What is Love?* What does
Ashley Montague mean here?: "Love is the principal de-
veloper of one's capacity for being human, the chief
stimulus for the development of social competence, and the
only thing on earth that can produce that sense of belong-
ingness and relatedness to the world of humanity which is

the best achievement of the healthy human being,[40] (sixth grade).

5. Study the teacher guide on menstruation and menstrual health, *From Fiction to Fact,* published by Tampax, Incorporated, New York. This is filled with excellent teaching suggestions for boys and girls together and separately. See also the booklet, *Accent on You,* published by and distributed free by the same company.

6. Discuss (with fifth and sixth grade girls) the question of good menstrual health as a necessary part of a girl's growth into womanhood. Clear up misconceptions relative to cramps, water taboos, exercise restrictions, and the period itself. (Obtain illustrative materials from Personal Products Corp., Milltown, N.J.; Tampax Incorporated, and Kimberly-Clark Corp.)

7. Set up a question box to be used, especially during the unit on family relations. This encourages the pupils who do not feel free or comfortable enough to ask questions in class (sixth grade).

8. Discuss family vacations. Have the pupils tell what they like about their father's or mother's job. Have them add to this what they would like to do to earn a living in the future.

9. Talk over the relationship of family health to family happiness. Show also how fear, prejudice, outbursts of anger, and other similar items keep a home in a state of unpleasantness. List socially acceptable ways to counteract these feelings.

10. Chart the combination of chromosomes (23 in the ovum and 23 in the sperm). Discuss hereditary influences and bearing on "how we look." Students should bring pictures to class to illustrate differences in height, weight, color, ears, eyes, and other body structure items.

11. Plant a fast-growing green bean seed in fertile soil and water it in class. Put the other on the windowsill. Relate this experiment to nutrition and reproduction.

12. Show film *Growing Into Womanhood/Growing Into Manhood* (Guidance Associates)—a study of male and female reproductive systems relating to puberty. A slightly more advanced film is *Becoming A Woman/Becoming A Man* (Revised).

13. Obtain several copies of Sol Gordon's colorful *Facts About Sex for Today's Youth* (John Day Company). After the class has had a chance to read it, set up a discussion on points raised by class members.

14. Have girls read the colorful booklet of letters, *Growing Up and Liking It* (obtained free from Personal Products Company, Milltown, N.J. 08850). Read and respond to what is said about menstrual cramps and try the exercises in Figure 8–30.

---

[40]Montague, Ashley, in *Age of Aquarius* by K. Jones, L. Shainberg, and C. Byer, New York: Goodyear, 1971.

Dear Donna,

I think you are lucky not to be a kid anymore. Ask your mother for a book about the facts of life. In the meantime, I will tell you some things you should know. You are hardly losing any blood at all....only three or four ounces. That's not very much, especially if you know there are at least 120 ounces in your whole body and your body keeps on making new blood. And anyway, it's not really like when you get a cut. It's much thicker. That's because mentrual flow is a combination of blood and soft tissue from the inside of your uterus. So stop worrying! Most of the girls here don't have cramps but here are some good exercises to make your cramps go away. They're from my sister Janie's booklet she got in high school. You can do them everyday and when you're menstruating (men stroo ate ing). (That's the right way to say it). Now that you've got your period, you better watch out about "odor" -- that's what my mother said.

Love,

Patty

1. Stand with your face directly toward a wall. Your feet should be about 12 to 16 inches away from the wall. Raise both your elbows to the level of your shoulders and cross your arms. Lean forward so both elbows touch the wall and feel comfortable in this position. Next tilt your pelvis forward to touch the wall. While in this position keep your heels on the floor and your knees straight. Hold for one minute and return to original position.

2. Lie on your back with knees bent, feet flat on floor and arms extended straight over head.

Swing your arms forward and at the same time push feet forward and move to sitting position.

Reach forward and try to touch toes with fingers. Return to original position.

Figure 8–30. From the booklet, *Growing Up and Liking It.* (Courtesy Personal Products Company.)

10. ENVIRONMENTAL HEALTH

Behavioral Objectives (Primary Level)

Explains how one person's health practices can affect the health of other people.

Investigates how to keep the school, home, and community environment reasonably clean.

Selects community services having a bearing on the welfare of himself or herself and others in the class.

Relates how fire and police officers protect children, adults, and property.

Identifies ways in which milk is kept clean, fresh, and safe to drink.

Describes briefly how all living things somehow relate to the happiness and health of children as well as adults.

Behavioral Objectives (Intermediate Level)

Investigates the health services in the community with a view toward using them when necessary.

Explains the contributions made by people such as medical and dental personnel, barbers, sanitarians, street cleaners, opticians, public works engineers, conservationists, and others.

Differentiates between public health personnel and other health-related people in the community.

Chooses hospital services as a significant community agency necessary in every part of the country.

Develops some responsibility for promoting health in the total environment through cooperative and independent activities.

Distinguishes between proper and improper food inspection, food storage, and use practices.

Demonstrates how to conserve land to protect water supply and other environmental items such as wildlife and open space.

Identifies with the historical development and present planning of a community for future growth in terms of healthful living.

Comments

INVITATION

I just stopped by to tell you
the lily on the seaward moor has opened.
I was out to watch dawn
wash in on the breakers,
and walking back, I saw—
something a little like leftover dawn,
a shade of shining in the wavy brush.
I was looking upon the lily.
An inward sun rose in me.
The lights I've seen today might well last
for all eternity, the way I feel.
I think the grave is not half so dark
since seeing such color
come out of the earth . . .
But I stopped by to tell you about the lily.
I could not bring it to you
without spoiling it for good.
Let me spoil you forever
by taking you to it.

—John Fandel

The "feeling" for preserving the environment that Fandel writes about is so artful and delicate that it can easily be missed by the bulk of humanity.[41] After all, hasn't the traditional American lifestyle changed over the years from one of general conservatism and careful usage of all materials ("make it do" philosophy) to a technological and consumer appetite which gobbles more than half of the resources consumed in the world each year? It is only now that one asks . . . what can I do? And this, of course, is a difficult question since solutions to environmental problems are multi-disciplinary and often beyond the capacity of any individual. As reflected in the poem, one must become more concerned with the quality of one's life rather than with one's pile of possessions—three fourths of which are thrown away each year.

One cannot deal adequately with the unwelcome by-products of a complex, industrialized society as though they existed outside the total structure of that society. Environmental ills are profoundly and intimately related to our most basic social, philosophical, and religious motivations. They reflect our concept of human purpose, our view of ourselves in relation to the world, and our view of our responsibility to ourselves and the generations that will come after us. Moreover, urban and other problems resulting from an environmental crisis are treatable. And, as Dentler points out, the desirability of environmental protection is enormous; and because environmentalism is linked to human longevity and well-being, there is an increasing amount of cooperative concern demonstrated.[42]

It is for this very reason that school-children at an early age must begin to develop a lasting appreciation for their environment—an environment in which problems did not suddenly emerge, but have resulted from the interaction of many complex forces. These forces—increasing population, technological advances in industry, the inability to satisfactorily absorb waste products, and an attitude of exploitative dominance of life space—have played a part in the current ecological crisis. Complicating education in this area is the sheer magnitude of ecologically oriented materials available to students and teachers, as well as the political and racial overtones of environmental issues.

Further complicating this area of education is the charge that many well-known environmentalists tend to be prophets of doom and have overdramatized the plundering of the planet. How indeed is the schoolteacher to know for certain that ". . . the human race is in danger of suffocating from overbreeding, of poisoning itself with pollution, of undermining its essential character by tampering with heredity, and of weakening the basic structure of society through too much prosperity"?[43] Does alarm provide the best atmosphere for finding rational solutions to worrisome problems? Was Aesop telling

---

[41]Fandel, John, "Invitation," *Commonweal*, September 17, 1971, p. 17.

[42]Dentler, Robert A. *Urban Problems: Perspectives and Solutions.* Chicago: Rand McNally, 1977, p. 118.

[43]Maddox, John, "The Doomsday Syndrome," *Saturday Review*, October 21, 1972, p. 31.

us something with his fable of the shepherd boy who cried wolf too often? How right in their forecasts are people such as Paul Ehrlich (*The Population Bomb*), Rachel Carson (*Silent Spring*), Barry Commoner *(Science and Survival)* and René Dubos *(Reason Awake)?* The answer to this question is that it took imagination, clear writing, an abundance of speechmaking, and staggering prediction figures to shake the average American out of his state and her state of lethargy relative to the environment. Even though Commoner may have been in error when he said in 1963 that Lake Erie was so polluted that it was dead (it yielded 25,000 tons of fish in 1970 and considerably more than this by 1978), his admonitions and challenges to people to do something about pollution should make all Americans grateful to him. The danger now is that any exaggeration to stir people up or to get things done may result in large numbers of people becoming anesthetized by overstatement and the movement to measurably upgrade the environment will suffer a serious setback. It is important for teachers, therefore, to get their facts straight, treat the subject soberly rather than fanatically, and involve students in small community projects with wide appeal.

By employing the phrase "environmental health" carefully, much can be achieved. This may not be easy, because the phrase is somewhat of a misnomer; the problems of environmental health are not those stemming from a health environment. Rather, they are the problems arising from the deteriorating quality of the environment. Furthermore, the problems are not neatly packaged but are involved with the transformation of the natural ecosystem to the human ecosystem.[44] It takes a clever teacher to define and measure health in terms of an adaptive capacity toward environmental circumstances and hazards. With human adaptability the prime issue, health no longer is absence of all disease; instead it ". . . is a process of continuous adaptation to the myriad of microbes, irritants, pressures, and problems which daily challenge man."[45]

To make this topic more meaningful, one must do more than visit the local establishments such as bakeries, water works, and garbage disposal plants. There has to be some extensive thinking and action associated with the project. Very often a problematical situation calling for investigation and preplanning is necessary to arouse the class to see the value of a particular community health issue. Certainly it is hardly a treat in many school systems today to be taken on a field trip to see the local organizations, but a sixth grade visit to a readily accessible mosquito breeding water hole may challenge the class to do something about it. Such was the case in a Georgia community a few years ago. A project planned and initiated by schoolchildren blossomed into an endeavor by the whole community and greatly reduced the mosquito threat in the whole area. Even the pupil with the poorest memory would have trouble forgetting this

---

[44]For an elaboration on this point see Carl E. Willgoose, *Environmental Health: Commitment for Survival,* Philadelphia: W. B. Saunders Company, 1979.

[45]See full review of this concept by Frederick Sargent II, "Man-Environment—Problems for Public Health," *American Journal of Public Health,* 62:628–633, May 1972.

kind of experience. And there are other activities along the same line. The report of a fifth grade committee on the cleanliness of rest rooms in local eating establishments would normally be received with a good amount of interest and enthusiasm, particularly if the report were to be followed up in some way. When it comes to garbage and refuse disposal, clean air, and water pollution, children have a real concern. They know first-hand when the air is odorous and they want safe water for drinking and clean water for their own boating and swimming. Thus, they are capable of getting the facts, telling the story, and influencing others to take action. Many up-to-date and informative teaching pamphlets are available each year from the U.S. Public Health Service, the U.S. Department of the Interior, and the U.S. Environmental Protection Agency.

The Environmental Circle developed in New York State is an excellent teaching device, especially when the objective is to vividly demonstrate the association of land, water, and air pollution (see Figure 8–31). This circle can be enlarged and hung before a class for all to see. Helpful sources of scientific information, coupled with ideas for involving elementary students, may be found in magazines such as *Consumer Reports, Family Health,* and *Instructor.* In most areas there is an Audubon publication which is rich in environmental

ENVIRONMENTAL CIRCLE

SHOWING MANY KINDS OF POLLUTION AND THE EFFECT ON THE TOTAL ENVIRONMENT

Figure 8–31. A proven teaching aid in environmental health. (Courtesy New York State Department of Environmental Conservation.)

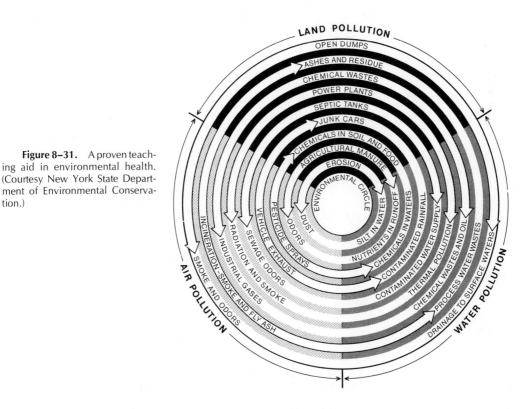

and ecological items of use in the classroom. Now available throughout the country is the *Environmental Newsletter,* published each month by the U.S. Environmental Protection Agency (free). The one from the New England Regional Office has been used widely in schools because it not only reports environmental happenings bearing on health but it also tells what groups of citizens and school children are doing to improve their immediate environment. The U.S. Public Health Service also has many materials. The film *The Endless Chain* (Tribune Films, Inc.) is superb for bringing an intermediate class to face the ecological problems. The filmstrips *Man and his Environment: a New Approach to Environmental Education* (American Association for Health, Physical Education, and Recreation) and *Man's Natural Environment: Crisis Through Abuse* (Guidance Associates) can be very helpful in Grades 3–8. Of the several books dealing with this area, the following should help the teacher put together interesting content and pupil activities:

DeBell, Garrett. *The Environmental Handbook,* New York: Ballantine Books, 1970.
Dubos, René. *Man, Medicine and Environment,* New York: Praeger, 1968.
Environmental Education Instructional Activities, K–6, Albany, New York: The State Education Department (revised).
Mitchell, John. *Ecotactics: The Sierra Handbook for Environment Activities,* New York: Pocket Books, 1970.
Odum, H. T. *Environment, Power and Society,* New York: John Wiley, 1971.
Smolensky, Jack. *Principles of Community Health,* 4th ed. Philadelphia: W. B. Saunders Co., 1977.
Environmental Study Guide, Grades 4–8, *All Around You,* U.S. Government Printing Office, Washington, D.C.
Willgoose, Carl E. *Environmental Health: Commitment for Survival.* Philadelphia: W. B. Saunders Company, 1979.

Ecological thinking, says Russell, ". . . suggests that most health-related issues are not so much problems to solve as relationships to understand—some of which might be changed and others just lived with.[46] By the time a child is nine or ten, he or she can be expected to respond to environmental health issues. This viewpoint seems to tie in fairly well with the writers of the State of New York curriculum guides. The guides are worth reviewing, for they are particularly well organized. Content (topics) for the intermediate level is as follows:

    I. The Environment and Health Status
        A. Explanation of relationship between man, environment, and health
        B. History of environmental control
            1. Past
            2. Present
   II. Man's Environment and Disease
        A. Explanation of the relationship
        B. History of relationship
  III. Water
        A. Need for water
            1. Sources of water

---

[46]Russell, Robert D. "Effects of Ecological Thinking on Health Education," *School Health Review,* 3:3–6, July/August 1972.

2. Uses of water
 B. Management for clean water
  1. Methods of management
  2. Role of government
   a. national
   b. state
   c. local
 C. Pollution of water
  1. Definition of water pollution
  2. Causes of water pollution
   a. communities
   b. industries
   c. improper use of land areas through highway construction, farming, forestry
  3. Effects of Pollution
IV. Air
 A. Composition of air
 B. Need for air
 C. Pollution of air
  1. Definition of air pollution
  2. Causes of air pollution
   a. residential
   b. industrial
   c. automotive
   d. natural
   e. atmosphere conditions
  3. Harmful effects of air pollution
   a. health
   b. agriculture
   c. reduce visibility
 D. Control of air pollution
  1. Need for control
  2. Devices for control
   a. automotive
   b. industrial
  3. Measurements of pollution
   a. Ringelmann chart
   b. Dustfall
  4. Laws and regulations for air pollution control
   a. federal
   b. state
   c. local
V. Food Protection
 A. Importance for health
 B. Food handling
  1. Definition of food handling
  2. Contamination problems
  3. Additive problems
 C. Supervision of food
  1. Agencies—laws
  2. The consumer

VI. Water Treatment
    A. Improvement to health
    B. Sewage (liquid wastes)
    C. Refuse (solid wastes)
VII. Insects and Rodents
    A. Rodents
    B. Insects
    C. Need for control
    D. Methods of control
    E. Responsibility for control
VIII. Maintaining a Healthful Environment
    A. In the home
      1. Purpose
      2. Responsibility
    B. In the community
      1. Purpose
      2. Service responsibility

Whether environmental health is taught indirectly or directly it is a potential contributor to the basic understandings sought through such educational aims as self-realization and civic responsibility. One does not fully realize onself until he or she feels responsible for the welfare of others in the home town. And one does not come of age in this realization until one gains a certain satisfaction from actually participating in community projects.

Suggested Activities

Primary Level
1. Write the following question on the board and ask for suggestions:

HOW CAN I MAKE MY TOWN A MORE PLEASANT PLACE IN WHICH TO LIVE?

Here are some of the expected answers:

Do unto others as you would have them do unto you.

Do not throw paper and other items out the window for someone else to pick up.

Do not leave cans or bottles on the public beach or picnic area.

Stay home when you have a cold.

Use sprays such as DDT to help eliminate flies and other harmful insects.

Help keep the house clean and sanitary.

2. Ask the class to take home the following statement to think about overnight:

HEALTH IN OUR COMMUNITY IS THE RESULT OF THE WORK OF MANY PEOPLE.

Properly carried out, this may involve parents and others in the family and therefore become a far more valuable experience than it may appear to be on the surface (second and third grade).

3. Call upon the local Audubon chapter for special programs and materials. The principles of ecology are well handled by this group; ways of developing observational skills will be brought out.

4. Through committee action, discover how fast the population is increasing or decreasing in the community. Build a simple line graph to cover a 20-year period (third grade).

5. Raise the question: *How can some kinds of pollutants in the air be detected?* Fasten a sheet of white paper inside a shallow pan or spread a piece of glass with a thin coating of petrolatum. Place outside in different areas. Examine the surfaces now and then with a magnifying lens. Or, place white paper tissues outside in different places. Vary the length of time that the tissues are exposed to the air and *observe* their condition. Students will draw conclusions orally.

6. Show a large picture of a lake, reservoir, nearby stream, or river. Ask the class if they think it is safe to drink the water? Safe to swim in? Shortages of clean water affect the life of us all. Show the film, *Bulldozed America* (Carousel Films, Inc.).

7. Dramatize the effects of pollution; dramatization has more impact on children than talking about it. Start with two fish bowls with equal amounts of clean sand, washed pebbles, healthy greens, pure fresh water, four goldfish, and a snail as a garbage-disposal scavenger, in each. Both bowls will receive the same amount of light and warmth. Label one "Clean Environment" and the other "Polluted Environment." One team of students changes water daily, feeds fish, and keeps the "clean" bowl clean. The other team keeps a record of things put into "polluted" bowl: dirty nail, spit, dust, scrap of greasy bag, mud from shoe, dead leaf, cigar ashes, chewing gum, etc. Pupils note developing murky water and odor as well as lethargic fish with poor appetite. Clean "Polluted" bowl before fish die. (Second grade.)*

8. Talk about and illustrate with pictures and stick people drawings the various kinds of occupations in the community and how they have a bearing on one's health.

9. Plan together how elementary schoolchildren can promote good health in town or city. An idea or "think" session with teacher in background.

10. Ask the question: "How is the life of our town affected by the extremes of weather?" Post pictures collected by pupils depicting how the different plants and animals protect themselves against bad weather. Show the effects of unusual weather conditions. How do these things affect the fire departments, police departments, public works, doctors, and nurses?

11. Talk about *trash* and how it is handled in the local community. Enlarge and post the illustration:

12. Visit a large grocery store. Prepare for this by having each pupil bring from home the name of one relatively inexpen-

---

*Activity reported by June Marie Schasre of Buffalo, N.Y., who used it with her second grade class.

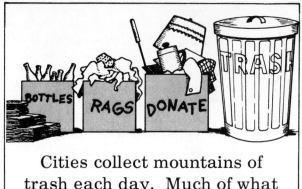

Cities collect mountains of trash each day. Much of what fills up the dumps could be used again; or recycled. Many people now separate these things from their trash.

sive item to be purchased during the class visit. This will work with over 90 per cent of the pupils bringing the necessary money to purchase a particular food product. While at the store, ask the manager to show the class how perishable foods are stored and how cleanliness is practiced.

13. Investigate noise pollution. Experiment with different kinds of sound-absorbing materials. Line some cardboard boxes of the same size with various types of materials and place the same sound source, such as an alarm clock, inside each container in turn. What types of material reduce the sound most? Try acoustical tiles, bricks, cork sheets, fabrics, building insulation, glass plates, sheet metal, etc. Chart comparisons on a line graph. (third grade.)

14. Bring a painted turtle to class. They balance our fresh water economy by having a diet of 65 per cent pond weeds and many insects—and especially mosquito larvae.

15. Have class members collect pictures that depict streams, ponds, lakes, and other bodies of water (similar to Figure 8–32). Consider both the sources and uses of the water shown.

16. Clean up the classroom and follow this with voluntary statements from individual pupils on how they keep their homes and yards clean.

17. Secure copies of *Walter Waterdrop,* a coloring book from U.S. Environmental Protection Agency, Region VII, Kansas City, Mo. 44106 (revised). (First grade.)

Intermediate Level

1. Receive a visitor from the local health department. Let this person tell about all the interesting jobs to be done. (Many people are available for this. In the small city there are only a few workers, but in a city like New York there are some five thousand workers in the health department.)

Figure 8–32. Mountain stream passing over rocks and gravel delivers pollutant-free water. (Courtesy U.S. Forest Service.)

2. Build a series of eight or ten models depicting *What Our Community Should Do to Keep Everyone Healthy.* Assign several pupils to each model. When they are completed, exhibit them in the school library or other appropriate place. Following are some examples of models:
   a. *Maintain health records:* Show a clerk in an office pulling out a file drawer in a file cabinet.
   b. *Collect garbage:* Show a garbage man carrying a garbage can from a house to the truck.
   c. *Promote safety in industry:* Show a group of workers on the job wearing protective helmets, gloves, and so on.
   d. *Inspect restaurants and dairies:* Show a clean restaurant with people sitting and eating at tables or show a scene depicting dishes being washed. A dairy barn scene would also be a good choice.
   e. *Keep drinking water safe:* Show a pumping station or model of a filter system. Or simply attach a real water faucet to a large piece of plywood with a model of a hand holding a glass just below it.
3. Have class *investigate* how much they know about their home sewage system. Where does their sewage go? Does the town or city have a sewage treatment plant? Does raw sewage or treated sewage empty into any stream or body of water? If so, what might the class do about it?
4. Enlarge the U.S. Environmental Protection Agency poster (see Figure 8–33) and discuss water treatment. EPA booklets

Figure 8–33. U.S. Environmental Protection Agency poster.

Needed: Clean Water and *Our Endangered World* are suitable for young children and are available free from EPA regional offices.

5. Write a three paragraph statement on the news of a closed swimming area. What are the implications? (Fourth grade.)

6. Prepare posters for placement in community stores, bus stations, banks, and business establishments. Some titles which suggest a picture are:
   Do Not Jaywalk in (name of town)
   This Community Is What You Make It!
   Treat Others Courteously
   Smile—Be Friendly and Say "Hello"
   Don't Eat at Unclean Eating Places and They Will Be Forced to Clean Up

7. After some work on the topic of community health, ask the pupils to write some statements in support of the sentence:

THE WELFARE OF THE MAJORITY IS RELATED TO THE PRACTICES OF THE MINORITY.

8. Encourage a discovery process in the community with simple bulletin board sketches and instructions to *find out:*

9. Using an appropriate dictionary, look up the meaning of words such as chlorine, fluorine, filter, pasteurized, disinfected, epidemic, swab, septic tank, reservoir, homogenized, bacteriology, abscess.

10. Divide the class into "Health Inspection Committees." Assign committee members according to personal choice. Permit the separate committes to survey the community and report back to class. Topics for survey may include:

    Recreational opportunities for elementary age children
    Cleanliness and handwashing facilities in city eating places
    Cleanliness and handwashing facilities in the school
    Safety hazards in and about the city
    Cleanliness of city streets

WHAT YOU CAN DO

IN YOUR COMMUNITY

❶ FIND OUT

Does your community have pollution control ordinances? For **AIR, WATER, RUBBISH, DUMPING?** Are they <u>enforced</u>?

❷ FIND OUT

Do local **INDUSTRIES, GOVERNMENT,** and **COMMERCIAL** operations have air pollution control **PROGRAMS** and **EQUIPMENT?**

❸ FIND OUT

How your community gets rid of **TRASH, GARBAGE** and other **SOLID WASTES--** (Does it still allow open dumps or open-air burning?)

11. Experiment with clean water and a closed water system, illustrating both evaporation and condensation. Show how temperature, light, and turbidity influence water cycle.

12. Set up water testing stations along a river or stream. Assign pupils to collect water samples. Then test for coliform bac-

ICE CUBES   COOKIE TRAY

CONDENSATION

TEA POT

HOT PLATE   CATCH TRAY

Figure 8-34. A trip to the local dump is an elementary school "must" experience.

teria per 100 ml., pH, NO$_3$, turbidity, and color. (Sixth grade.)

13. Prepare a brochure for the start of a spring clean up campaign. Distribute the brochure.

14. Bring some mosquito wrigglers in water to class. Pour some oil on these and notice the results.

15. Investigate some of the new homes being built in the community. Make a list of the various inspections that a new house must pass and the reasons for these.

16. Investigate noise and hearing loss.[47] If possible, measure noise in decibels about the neighborhood. Indicate also how rock bands and aircraft assault the ear, contributing to hearing loss in 16 million Americans. Excessive noise also contributes to weight loss and fatigue.

17. Search for pollution activities in other lands (especially Europe). Start project by posting Chinese figures:

Everywhere in China these characters appear. They convey the equivalent of Keep America Beautiful, Conserve Resources, Prevent Pollution. Their literal meaning—*Three Wastes, Three Benefits*—alludes to the natural triumvirate of land, water, and air, but to a Chinese person, they are an admonition to recover the wastes in "gas, liquid and residue," thereby turning them into benefits to the environment and, above all, to the economy.

The revolutionary committees in villages and factories devote much attention to how wastes can be utilized. A recent issue of the *Peking Review*

---

[47]Helpful ideas may be found in "Noise—The Challenge of the Future," *Journal of School Health,* 42:172–176, March 1972. Also see *New York Times Magazine* for November 23, 1975.

reports that a complex of factories in Shanghai collectively produced 200 suggestions for utilizing wastes, of which ninety were adopted. As a result, more than 200 tons of raw and other materials were recovered.

18. Enlarge a county map. Appoint groups to fill in rivers, streams, forests, factories, and other environmental items. Conservation districts and flood plain lands may also be added.
19. Post the U.S. Environmental Protection Agency car bumper sticker at the top of the class bulletin board.

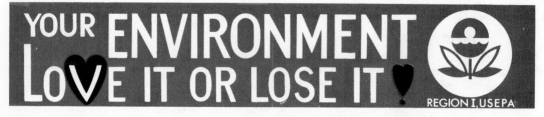

20. Tackle the topic of oil spills and hazardous substances. Up to the middle of 1977, there had been 13,000 oil spills, many of considerable size. (Obtain 1977 copy of *Oil Spills* from regional office of U.S. Environmental Protection Agency.) Discuss Coast Guard involvement (see Figure 8–35).

Figure 8–35. Oil pollution from the sinking *Argo Merchant.* (Courtesy U.S. Coast Guard.)

21. Appoint a *Legislative Experts Committee* to skim periodicals for information on environmental legislation. Particularly useful are periodicals such as *Environmental News* (EPA), *Environmental Action,* and *The Living Wilderness.*

22. Study *noise* and how living things react to it. Compare sounds we like to hear, such as pleasant voices and birds singing, with unpleasant sounds, such as crying, shouting and screeching brakes.

23. Compare energy expenditure for home heating. Compare electricity with fireplace, woodstoves, and oil. Draw a bar graph to show comparisons.

24. Look into occupational respiratory diseases such as black lung, silicosis, byssinosis (caused by the inhalation of cotton dust), asbestos disease, and farmer's lung (caused by the inhalation of vegetable dusts.) Obtain American Lung Association literature, especially *Enemies in the Dust.* Some students could also investigate vinyl chloride and cancer (see *Job Safety and Health* for February 1977; available from U.S. Department of Labor, Washington, D.C. 20402).

---

11. ALCOHOL, TOBACCO, AND DRUGS

Behavioral Objectives (Primary Level)

Describes all medicines as helpful items when illness occurs.
Explains that drugs correctly used help the body fight illness or relieve pain.

Explains that medicines incorrectly used can result in sickness, body damage, and even death.

Demonstrates the dangers related to the home medicine cabinet.

Explains how to recognize glue, paint, and other solvents that can affect health status.

Behavioral Objectives (Intermediate Level)

Explains that tobacco and alcoholic beverages do not contribute to the development of growing boys and girls.

Identifies the factors that point for the need for moderation in adult smoking and drinking practices as one means of preventing heart, respiratory, digestive, and mental illness.

Evaulates the use of sleep promoting and pain killing drugs, and the possible hazards involved.

Develops an explanation of the role of mental health as it bears on things such as excessive smoking, alcoholism, and drug addiction.

Investigates the effects of narcotics in general and the laws governing their sale.

Portray situations in which new drugs are discovered for the treatment of disease.

Comments

The increased visibility and abuse of drugs have spread across the country into all levels of society. Thus, one hears the expression "you are either part of the problem or part of the solution." Far too many educators are a part of the problem, either because of a lack of commitment or an inability to handle this concern. Frequently, there is a lack of understanding of the "real world" of the students, coupled with poor communication. Certainly, if one is to reduce the levels of use of all recreational drugs—from alcohol to phencyclidine—a concerted effort involving both teachers and others must continue to be an objective.

Since everything in the health area cannot be taught before the age of eight, the topics of alcohol, tobacco, and drugs are limited pretty much to the intermediate level where a concentration can be made at what would appear to be the "teachable moment." This does not rule out primary level discussions of helpful medicines, open medicine cabinets, aspirin control, stimulants, glue, paint, aerosol cans, and other items.

In some schools, alcohol and tobacco are scheduled for discussion in the food unit; here they may be considered in terms of the effect on growth and efficiency of the human organism. There is nothing wrong with doing this but there is evidence to indicate that this topic is broad enough to warrant separate consideration. This is more than a growth problem for children; it is something that observing children know much about and it involves people from all walks of life and circumstances.

Actually, education about alcohol, tobacco, coffee, tea, and the like is not new. In 1882 Vermont passed active legislation adding temperance teaching to the public school curriculum with ". . . special prominence to the effects of alcoholic drinks, stimulants, and narcotics upon the human system."[48] Four years later, 18 states and the District of Columbia had essentially the same requirements.

Alcohol and tobacco education have sometimes been labeled as controversial subjects. This is no longer true. Today, there is wide classroom discussion relative to the implications of drinking and smoking.

Alcohol Education. There is an increasing amount of evidence to suggest that alcoholic beverages are a part of the American culture. The government-financed report *Alcohol Problems: A Report to the Nation* (New York: Oxford University Press) recommends that a "deliberate effort" be made to make drinking acceptable—if practiced in moderation—almost anywhere, including at church-sponsored functions. It is known that 75 per cent of all Americans drink and that 40 per cent drink "regularly." Studies from the National Institute on Drug Abuse show that by grade seven, 63 per cent of boys and 54 per cent of girls have tried alcoholic beverages. In a West Coast study, 45 per cent of fourth, fifth, and sixth graders considered themselves users of alcohol. There is little doubt that the increase in youthful drinking may be a reflection of the increase in alcohol consumption within the general public. The problem arises when drinking gets out of hand. One third of all arrests in the United States are for public drunkenness. Thousands of persons with serious drinking problems are committed to mental institutions each year. Over half of the automobile drivers involved in fatal accidents have had high concentrations of alcohol in their systems. Rising death rates from alcoholic disorders (alcoholism, alcoholic psychosis, and alcoholic cirrhosis of the liver) indicate that mortality from alcoholism in the United States is substantial.[49] The true impact of the disease is difficult to measure, however, because of considerable underreporting of alcoholism as a cause of death. It is clear that the alcohol problems are more likely to be reduced through increased educational efforts—through prevention, not abstinence. Thus, the teacher's task is to bring out the factual information regarding excessive drinking and to stress responsible actions, rather than to moralize about the "evils of drink" to children whose parents probably enjoy the cocktail hour every evening. Peter Finn, an education and training analyst, stresses the "enjoyment" dimension:

> Most youngsters know very well that a majority of Americans from the age of 14 on find drinking pleasurable. As a result, when educators fail to discuss this enjoyment at some length, they risk losing a student's confidence in the trustworthiness of what they have to say about alcohol *abuse*. If instructors can cavalierly dismiss the delights of drinking, they are liable with equal glibness to exaggerate the dangers.[50]

[48]As quoted in J. E. Foster, "Scientific Temperance Instruction in the Schools," *Proceedings and Addresses.* National Education Association, 1886, Salem, 1887, p. 83.

[49]Metropolitan Life Insurance Company. "Mortality From Alcoholism," *Statistical Bulletin, 58*:3–5, December 1977.

[50]Finn, Peter. "Alcohol Education and the Pleasures of Drinking," *Health Education, 8*:17–19, January/February 1977.

The secret, of course, is to teach alcohol education at an early age (the maturity of the intermediate level pupil) in such a way that the readily normative drinking models, i.e., television, parents, and friends, are shown to be part of the American scene. Although research shows that the greater the number of drinking models, the more likely youngsters are to drink, it is still possible to point out that some things are saved until one is older—just as driving the family car is saved until later years. In a highly permissive society, of course, it may always be difficult to say just when one is mature enough to learn to drink moderately. Moreover, alcohol research demonstrates again and again that the culture determines the practices—even at an early age. Socioeconomic status and childhood deprivations, therefore, may have more to do with early drinking patterns than what is taught in school.[51] In fact, there is a tendency to expect too much from alcohol education in the school setting. Although school efforts help, the home and peer group influences ultimately will prove very important.

Alcohol education must be acquired in relation to a particular situation; school activity must be related to life outside the school. Swimming can be dangerous, but it is taught in order to survive in the water. Drinking too can be dangerous but it may be possible to teach how to drink safely—with personal and social responsibility. Or, as one educator put it, let us teach "survival in our cocktail culture." In this manner it may be possible in the years ahead to reduce the figure of nearly seven million persons suffering from alcoholism.

The elementary school has a responsibility in this area chiefly because of pupil needs, that is, the "awakening interest." Fifth and sixth graders tend to become very curious about drinking. What does beer taste like? Will whiskey make you feel "funny"? How do people feel? Why do they lose control of their automobiles under the influence of alcohol? Do doctors use brandy or whiskey as a stimulant for sick people? These and a hundred similar questions are being asked today by children of this age level. Stimulants and narcotics are everywhere. Some children have been drinking tea and coffee for years. Many families have beer or wine with the evening meal. Cocktails are served in the home. People drink and drive without giving it more than a passing thought. Moreover, growing boys and girls are extremely observant of these things.

Because so many parents drink, the topic is a difficult one for the teacher to handle satisfactorily. One must not leave the impression that to take a drink is "criminal" or a mark of the "man about town." What is said must lead to abstinence during the growing years and moderation or temperance in the later years. Since a high percentage of adults drink, one should not teach that anything short of total abstinence is reprehensible. Stress the harmful effects but point out that some people use alcohol in moderation and without any complications. For this reason, the best education in this area will be one that encourages young people to develop insight into their feelings

---

[51]Cahalan, Don and Room, Robin, *Problem Drinking Among American Men*, New Brunswick: Rutgers Center for Alcohol Studies, 1973.

Figure 8–36. An attractive teaching aid for alcohol education. (Courtesy Spenco Medical Corporation. P. O. Box 8113, Waco, Texas 76710.)

the Drinking Clock

The DRINKING CLOCK teaches what everyone must know about drinking and driving safety. This audio-visual aid is made from ¼ inch tempered masonite with a steel protected timer and is ideal for driver's education, health classes and law enforcement instruction.

The **classroom model** (17 x 34 inches) is intended for use in front of a room.

After an amount of alcohol is dialed on the clock, the hand points to the blood alcohol level, time required for alcohol to leave the body, minimum wait before driving, and increased risk of accident. The clock then runs down at the same rate at which the body metabolizes alcohol. With practice, a person learns to judge these same factors in any real situation.

about themselves and others and the role that alcohol may play in reducing sensitivity to standards of behavior consistent with their own family or group.

There are a number of fine sources of instructional materials relative to alcohol:

1. *American Medical Association,* 535 Dearborn Street, Chicago, Illinois 60610. (For information and lists of materials available).
2. *National Institute on Alcohol Abuse and Alcoholism,* 5600 Fishers Lane, Rockville, Maryland 20852 (For information and a comprehensive review of audio-visual materials). See "Alcohol: Questions and Answers."

3. *Rutgers Center of Alcohol Studies,* Rutgers—The State University, New Brunswick, New Jersey 08903.
4. *Alcoholics Anonymous,* Information Center, 337 East 33rd Street, New York, New York 10016.
5. *National Council on Alcoholism,* Inc., 2 Park Avenue, New York, New York, 10016. (A list of local affiliates can be provided and a list of materials is available.)
6. *Alcohol and Drug Problems Association of North America* (formerly North American Association of Alcoholism Programs), Education Department, 1130 Seventeenth Street, N.W., Washington, D.C. 20036. (A list of local affiliates can be provided.)
7. *Your State Department of Education.*
8. *Your State Department of Public Health* (or Department of Mental Health). Title of the department varies from state to state.
9. *National Institute of Mental Health,* HEW, Washington, D.C. See *Thinking About Drinking,* pub. no. 1683—Also, *Alcohol and Alcoholism.*
10. *Licensed Beverage Industries, Inc.,* 485 Lexington Ave., New York, New York, 10017. (Free teaching materials for students stressing facts and moderation.)
11. *Al-Anon Family Group Headquarters, Inc.,* "Alateen: Hope for Children of Alcoholics," New York: Al-Anon Family Group, 1973. Addeo, Edmond G. and Reichling, Jovita. *Why Our Children Drink.* New Jersey: Prentice-Hall, Inc., 1975. (Includes various educational programs that have been reported as successful.) Milgram, Gail Gleason. *Alcohol Education Materials: An Annotated Bibliography,* New Brunswick, N.J.: Rutgers Center for Alcohol Studies, 1976.

Smoking Education.   There is no question whether the young people who are now taking up smoking will suffer more illness and die earlier than those who do not. In fact, the earlier one begins to smoke, the greater the danger over a lifetime. According to the extensive research findings of the U.S. Public Health Service, approximately one million children now living in the United States will die prematurely of lung cancer alone.[52] Moreover, there are significant risks from smoking related to chronic bronchopulmonary disease, emphysema, peptic ulcers, cardiovascular disease, pregnancy problems, and skin aging.

The findings of a number of studies are in agreement that children start experimental smoking in the intermediate grades and develop into fairly regular smokers by the eighth or ninth grade. The pupil is more likely to smoke if his or her parents or older brothers and sisters smoke and if his or her friends smoke. If children have low goals, little ability, and little achievement, they tend to smoke earlier.

In a Seattle study of several thousand students, the majority of the boys began smoking cigarettes at age 12 or after, while the majority of the girls started at age 13 or after.[53] An interesting finding, and one of importance to elementary teachers, is that a comparison of those still smoking with those who had given up the practice revealed that those still smoking represent a greater number of boys and girls *who began their smoking habit at the younger ages.* This ties in with Hammond's studies in which he showed that death rates are higher among current cigarette smokers who started at a young age than those who started later in life.

In a society in which cigarettes are advertised, sold, and used everywhere and in which 40 per cent of the adults smoke or use some

---

[52]U.S. Department of Health, Education and Welfare. *The Health Consequences of Smoking,* Public Health Service No. 1696, Washington, D.C., 1964, 1967, 1969, 1972 and 1975.

[53]Harlin, Vivian Krause. "Response of School Children to a Questionnaire About Smoking," *American Journal of Public Health,* 62:566–574, April 1972.

other kind of mood modifier, it is difficult to educate children to the extent that they will not start to smoke. There has been some reduction in adult smoking during the last few years. Concentrated anti-smoking campaigns in Spokane, Washington and other sections of the country were successful. However, there are currently more young people taking up smoking than ever before. In light of such a finding, Seffrin looks at risks, rewards, and values and asks, "Why do people want to smoke so badly?"[54] Are not the consequences of importance?

The primary stumbling block to successful smoking education programs is youth's strong desire to conform and gain social confidence by doing what others do or appear to do. And it depends upon who the "others" are. Having an older sibling who smokes appears to be the most important of all family variables. In the Columbus, Ohio study it was found that if a student has a best friend who smokes, he or she is *nine times* more likely to smoke than are other students.[55] Moreover, where all of one's pals smoke, the probability is three to one that the respondent smokes. Where none of one's pals smoke, the chances are only one in a hundred that the respondent smokes. Of all the variables examined in this study, these two peer smoking behavior variables best differentiate smokers from non-smokers.

Other studies relating smoking to peer group attitudes and behavior point to the need to look beyond the classroom and into the community to observe the associations of youth. In the Indianapolis study of 49,034 schoolchildren, grades five through twelve, dozens of reasons were given for smoking and not smoking.[56] Although there were numerous reasons for smoking, such as "emotional improvement," "imitate adults," "eating substitute," and "to impress others," the big reason given was *peer influence*. This increased through the elementary school grades to a peak at the eighth grade, and declined thereafter to a low in the twelfth grade. This is a significant finding, for it means that somewhere in the 5th through 8th grade period is the prime time to get at the motivating forces and feelings that compel children to follow the gang, to do what they think everybody else does. If *status* is this important, then the teacher had better make arrangements to talk it over and get at the gut-level of feelings through small group discourse and study. The ten year old student is old enough to face this topic. Studies of young children indicate that they have attitudes and have thought quite a bit about smoking. As non-smokers, they are annoyed by second-hand tobacco smoke; but more than this, the attitude they have toward their parent's smoking is generally one of worry and concern for their parents.[57]

---

[54]Seffrin, John R. "Cigarette Smoking: Risks, Rewards, and Values," *Health Values: Achieving High-Level Wellness, 1*:197–199, September/October 1977.

[55]Lanese, Richard R. et al. "Smoking Behavior: a Multivariate Conceptual Approach," *American Journal of Public Health, 62*:807–813, June 1972.

[56]Levitt, Eugene E. "Reasons for Smoking and Not Smoking Given by School Children," *Journal of School Health, 41*:101–107, February 1971.

[57]Cameron, Paul. "Second-Hand Tobacco Smoke: Children's Reactions," *Journal of School Health, 42*:280–284, May 1972.

A number of studies indicate changes in student knowledge and attitudes toward smoking as an outgrowth of smoking education programs.[58] What is missing to date is solid evidence that a particular program or teaching method is definitely effective in changing *behavior* relative to smoking. Multi-method approaches have been ineffective. This has been confirmed by Thompson in an extensive 16-year study of research literature in which she points out that most methods employed with young people have shown little success.[59]

Using older students to work with younger students is helpful. In Honolulu, secondary school pupils visit the fifth and sixth grade classes of elementary schools in the district and help the children become aware of the hazards of cigarette smoking by involving them in laboratory experiments, discussions, and other stimulating activities.[60] *Facts on Smoking* sheets, questionnaires, and a smoke-solution apparatus were prepared. Most of the materials were contributed by the American Cancer Society. The upper-level students were told to use their own words, to take their time, and to relax when carrying on their dialogue. The natural casualness and individual sincerity was delightful to behold and there was evidence that the elementary children were influenced by the older group. This youth to youth method of teaching was tried earlier with over 10,000 fifth and sixth grade pupils in Broome County, New York.[61] All settings were informal as teenagers worked with the elementary students. The reactions reported would encourage greater attention to this method of teaching:

From 5th and 6th Graders

"The high school boys are nearer to our age level and they know what it's like and they told it like it is."

From Principals to Youth

"Thanks for your interest in the boys and girls in our elementary schools."

"You should be aware that these kids really look up to you. You are heroes to them. They are impressed with what you say and do."

From Teenagers

"I quit smoking because I could not stand before the group of 5th and 6th graders and have them ask me if I smoked."

"We want this committee to continue."

---

[58]See Stone, Elaine J. "The Effect of a Fifth Grade Health Education Curriculum Model on Perceived Vulnerability and Smoking Attitudes," *Journal of School Health,* 48:667–671, January 1978.

[59]Thompson, Eva Lynn. "Smoking Education Programs 1960–1976," *American Journal of Public Health,* 68:250–256, March 1978.

[60]Arrigoni, Edward A. "Teenage Anti-Smoking Campaign in the Elementary Schools," *School Health Review,* 3:15–18, March/April 1972.

[61]McRae, Cameron F. and Nelson, Dorothy M. "Youth to Youth Communication on Smoking and Health," *Journal of School Health,* 41:445–449, October 1971.

Throughout the nation a tremendous effort has been made to improve smoking education programs. Practically every state department of education has developed special smoking and health curriculum guides, together with resource material kits. The same can be said for hundreds of large city school systems.

Helpful literature is extensive. Noteworthy curriculum guides may be obtained from states such as California, Pennsylvania, Washington, Oregon, Maryland, New York, Arizona, Rhode Island, and Illinois. A wealth of curriculum materials are available from the American Cancer Society and the U.S. Public Health Service. The Children's Bureau in Washington distributes the pamphlet *Why Nick the Cigarette Is Nobody's Friend* for fourth and fifth graders and *A Light on the Subject of Smoking* for sixth graders. The National Film Board of Canada distributes the Academy Award film *The Drag*—a nine-minute animated film for young audiences. Elementary children seem to love the cartoon spoof film *The Huffless, Puffless Dragon* put out by the American Cancer Society. Their filmstrip *I'll Choose the High Road* is also very good; and the filmstrip and discussion guide of the National Interagency Council on Smoking and Health is of real value to the teacher in this health education area.

A great variety of teaching ideas relative to discussion topics, classroom experiments, and other projects appear in the teaching guide *Smoking and Health Unit* of the Spokane Public Schools. Another source of ideas is the booklet *Classroom-Tested Techniques for Teaching About Smoking* distributed free by the National Clearinghouse for Smoking and Health, U.S. Public Health Service, Center for Disease Control, Bureau of Health Education, Atlanta, Georgia. Also available from the Clearinghouse is *Smoking and Health Experiments, Demonstrations and Exhibits.* Free copies of *What to Tell Your Parents About Smoking* and other publications are available from the American Heart Association.

Drug Education. Early in 1973 a number of school health personnel began to wring their hands in despair over the ineffectiveness of so-called drug education programs. Millions of dollars of local and federal government funds have been spent for teaching materials—from attractive teaching kits with simulated drugs displayed to hundreds of films and filmstrips. Yet, the head of the U.S. Office of Education's drug-education division points out that there is little evidence to support the practice of dispensing information by itself. It may even be counterproductive. In a New York City study there was found to be no evidence of any significant relationship between knowledge about drugs or awareness of the dangers of drugs and their actual use. The same findings have occurred in Harrisburg, Pennsylvania and Dallas, Texas.

What then can the schools do? Because drug abuse is so subtle and multidimensional, so tied up with the "rites of passage" of the young, the "instant gratification" philosophy in the culture, the intrinsic desire to experience the unknown, and peer group activity, it is difficult indeed to be certain that any one teaching technique will be measurably successful. One thing is for sure: the teacher must relate to the students and command their respect. Unfortunately, even in the elementary grades the "lifestyle" of the school as a rigid, conformity-bound institution is an anathema to potential drug abusers. And in many places the school's influence is modest in contrast to home, peers, or neighborhood environment. But, if one will use the latter setting to get at student concerns, feelings, self-doubt, anxiety, loneliness, joy, belonging—the "here now" topics, something productive can emerge. Couple this with a total elementary school approach to the *cultural system* to discover how it fosters or perpetuates drug abuse. This may require institutional changes and be hard to accomplish in many schools. However, peer group programs and peer group efforts can be promoted far beyond anything taking place today. Informational programs researched, developed, and implemented by students, student-assisted counseling programs, student-produced plays, and role-playing are all means of promoting peer group activity. This will call for great classroom and school flexibility but it may lead to some positive student decision making.[62]

The program begins mildly in the primary grades. The concern is more with drug use than drug abuse. By this age children have seen much at home and on television having to do with the drug oriented society. Respect for drugs is taught well before the age at which children might find themselves in a critical decision making position. Youngsters are capable of having a good twenty minute discussion on the role of the physician in assigning drugs to reduce disease, the role of the pharmacist, the importance of understanding information on labels, the safe storage of drugs in the home, how to make phone calls for emergency medical assistance, the effects of certain drugs on the senses and on performance ability, and the history of humanity's discovery of drugs such as aspirin, penicillin, and antibiotics. At an early age one should learn that drugs are good in fighting disease—in preventing infections, in treating illness, in helping cold symptoms, in helping people sleep, in preventing discomfort and pain, and in prolonging life.

The abuse factor is brought in at the intermediate level. The habit-forming tendency of drugs and their poisonous effects are proper emphases. So is the abuse of prescription drugs.

Children should know that alcohol is classified as a narcotic rather than a stimulant. They should appreciate the great need for sleeping pills, aspirin, and pain killing substances. Information about these items should relate to the medical, economic, and social effects when they are used correctly and what is involved from both a personal and community viewpoint when they are misused.

Education pertaining to narcotics is part of the larger problem of health teaching. It relates to values in living, to confidence in oneself, to self-respect, and to the importance of developing personal traits and abilities which one is proud to possess. This is an opportune moment for young people to discover, perhaps anew, that psycholog-

---

[62]For a number of useful teaching ideas, see Girdano, Daniel A. and Girdano, Dorothy Dusek. *Drug Education: Content and Methods,* 2nd ed., Boston: Addison-Wesley Publishing Co., 1976. See also Simon, Robert K. and Moyer, David H. "A Preliminary Assessment of a Cooperative Drug Education Pilot Project in the Middle School," *Journal of School Health,* 46:325–329, June 1976.

CHAPTER 8

ical factors are vital in all health behavior—that happy, secure people have a kind of respect for themselves that does not need building up with narcotics or anything else. In this respect, a humanistic, individualized approach to teaching about people and drugs is appropriate.[63]

Far and away the most helpful and complete manual for the teacher is the American School Health Association publication *Teaching About Drugs: A Curriculum Guide, K–12,* second edition, (revised). (107 South Depeyster Street, Kent, Ohio 44240—Price $4.00.) Almost everything the teacher would want to know is here—colored photographs, descriptions, historical items, pharmaceutical information, glossary of slang terms, ways to identify drug abusers, teaching aids, and fully outlined programs. It is a superb publication with ideas that have been tried and proven. Intermediate grade content is set forth in clear detail with learning activities and resources under eight teaching objectives:

A. To know that drugs come from several sources. To appreciate their long history of use (definitions, sources of drugs, history, ongoing research).

B. To understand the difference between prescription and nonprescription medicines (legal considerations, following directions, destroying left-over prescriptions, types of medicines purchasable on prescription, how to use medicines).

C. To recognize that drugs as medicines have many uses, along with a potential for producing both good and bad effects (drugs as medicines—users, differing effects of medicines).

D. To know that many widely used substances contain drugs (coffee, cola, tobacco, alcohol).

E. To know that misused and abused medicines, drugs, and other agents may have serious effects on the individual (medicines are misused in various ways, dangers of misuse, abuse potential, brain and nervous system reactions, drugs abused for different reasons).

F. To identify common household products and to use them for their intended purposes (essential benefits of products, misused products, consequences of misuse).

G. To assume increasing responsibility for personal health (growing up is to become independent and responsible, early establishment of health practices, ways practices develop, avoiding drug use).

H. To understand and appreciate the relationship of drugs to total health (WHO definition and total health, relationship of medicines to health, potential of medicines).

In view of what has been said previously about the great amount of teaching material available for school use, the following resources have been very carefully reviewed and selected. (Other teaching materials appear in Chapter 10.)

---

[63]Greene, Jerry L. and Huntsinger, Phillip G. develop this view in "A Humanistic–Individualized Approach to Drug Education," *Health Education,* 7:38, July/August 1976.

Drug Education Curriculum Guide Lafayette Elementary School District, 3477 School Street, Lafayette, California 94549 (Price $6.50)

K–6 Drug Education Curriculum Guide Oakland City Unified School District, 1025 Second Avenue, Oakland, California 94606 (Price $2.10)

Values-Oriented Approach to Drug Abuse Prevention Education Orange County Superintendent of Schools, 1104 Civic Center Drive, West, Santa Ana, California 92701 (single copy free)

A Plan for Drug and Narcotics Education for Grades Four Through Twelve Vallejo City Unified School District, 211 Valle Vista, Vallejo, California 94590 (Price $5.00)

Common Sense Lives Here, A Community Guide To Drug Abuse Action National Coordinating Council on Drug Abuse Education and Information, Suite 212, 1211 Connecticut Avenue, N.W., Washington, D.C.

Drug Abuse National Clearinghouse For Drug Abuse Information, P.O. Box 1635, Rockville, Maryland 20852 (no charge)

Facts About Drugs (1972) David C. Cook Publishing Co., Elgin, Illinois 60120 (Manual of lessons to go with sixteen 12¼" × 17" picture cards–See Figure 8–37).

What Will Happen If . . . a programmed instruction course on drugs National Institute of Mental Health, 5600 Fishers Lane, Rockville, Maryland 20852 (50¢)

A Guide to Drug Abuse Education and Information Materials National Institute of Mental Health, 5600 Fishers Lane, Rockville, Maryland 20852 (50¢)

Tips on Drug Abuse Prevention National Institute of Mental Health, 5600 Fishers Lane, Rockville, Maryland 20852

To Parents/About Drugs (Revised) Metropolitan Life Insurance Co., 1 Madison Ave., New York, New York (Free)

The Most Frequently Asked Questions About Drug Abuse Special Action Office for Drug Prevention, P.O. Box 1100, Washington, D.C. 20008 (Free) Also comes with a 3-record set of questions and answers.

Drug Abuse Education Slide Resource Kit National Audiovisual Center (GSA), Washington, D.C. 20409

Me, Myself–and Drugs (Revised) Guidance Associates, 757 Third Ave., New York, New York 10017 (3 part filmstrip)

Drug Information Series, Guidance Associates, 757 Third Ave., New York, New York 10017 (4 sound filmstrips)

Drug Abuse: Everybody's Hangup, National Education Association, 1201 16th St., N.W., Washington, D.C. 20036 (film)

Drugs, Poisons and Little Children (K–3) Educational Activities, Freeport, N.Y. 11520 (a full color filmstrip that complements a larger series of filmstrips related to children)

Drugs: A Primary Film Arthur Barr Productions, Inc., P.O. Box 7–C, Pasadena, California 91104 (A primary grade film which explores the use of drugs by the physician.)

Books

Teaching About Drugs, A Curriculum Guide K–12 (Revised) American School Health Assoc., 107 Depeyster St., Kent, Ohio 44240.

Marihuana 1977 U.S. Dept. of Justice, Bureau of Narcotics and Dangerous Drugs. Washington, D.C.

Drug Education Content and Methods 2nd ed., D. A. Girdano and D. D. Girdano, Reading, Massachusetts: Addison-Wesley Publishing Co., 1976.

Drugs and People by Donald A. Read, Boston: Allyn and Bacon, Inc., 1972.

Drugs, Society and Human Behavior 2nd ed. by Oakley S. Ray, St. Louis: C. V. Mosby, 1977.

Suggested Activities (Intermediate Level)

1. Gather advertisements from magazines and newspapers having to do with the "benefits" of tea, coffee, cigarettes, cigars, pipe tobacco, beer, wine, cola drinks, and headache pills. Secure answers to questions such as:
   a. How much of this advertising is essentially true, and how much appears to be misleading?
2. Over a period of one week, collect newspaper clippings that have to do solely with automobile accidents in which intoxication and drinking are involved. Post these on a

Figure 8–37. Teaching aids poster helps focus attention. (Courtesy David C. Cook Publishing Co., Elgin, Illinois 60120.)

frequently read bulletin board. Ask for questions. Questions will arise somewhat as follows:

a. In how many feet can a driver of an automobile usually stop when traveling at 5 miles per hour (an emergency situation)? How much longer may it take when the driver has had a few drinks?

b. What disposition is generally made of cases of drunken driving in the courts?

c. How many automobile accidents involve intoxication?

3. Discuss the short film *Weed* (Marihuana). This may be obtained on loan from Encyclopaedia Britannica Films. Show also *The Tobacco Problem: What Do You Think?* This is exceptionally provocative.

4. While viewing TV or listening to radio, make a list of the number of times commercials encourage a person to modify (change) feelings or outlook on life through the use of a substance or product. Apply feelings to five ways to respond to smoking (Figure 8–38).

5. Invite a local druggist to appear in class and answer questions regarding habit-forming drugs, drug addiction, and the law on prescriptions. This is also a good time to discuss the sale of sleeping pills. Have the class prepare for such discussion by clipping from the newspaper items pertaining to deaths and near-deaths due to an overdose of sleeping pills.

6. Dramatize the "smoker's cough." Act out three scenes. In scene No. 1, a chain-smoker is seen going about his or her

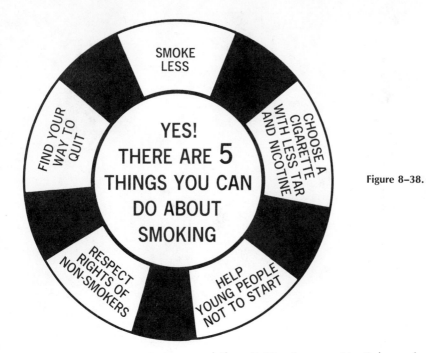

SMOKE
LESS

FIND YOUR WAY TO QUIT

YES!
THERE ARE 5
THINGS YOU CAN
DO ABOUT
SMOKING

CHOOSE A CIGARETTE WITH LESS TAR AND NICOTINE

RESPECT RIGHTS OF NON-SMOKERS

HELP YOUNG PEOPLE NOT TO START

Figure 8–38.

daily activities. In scene No. 2, he or she is observed arising from bed in the morning in a fit of coughing. In scene No. 3, the doctor is warning the chain-smoker to cut down his or her cigarette consumption because of the cough, its effect on appetite and consequent nutrition, its relationship to longevity, its effect on the heart and blood pressure, and its relationship to cancer and the respiratory system. Attract attention to topic by posting *Tar and Nicotine Content* chart. (U.S. Federal Trade Commission) (Figure 8–39).

7. Engage a small panel of community "experts" on the topic of why people smoke. In this case the "experts" may be informed class members. One may be designated as a community physician, another as a parent, and one or two others as active citizens. The panel should meet with the teacher before class in order to have several suggestions each as to why people smoke. (Examples: They enjoy it; they want to do what others do; it gives them something to do while waiting or talking; it is habit forming and they feel a "need" for it; it keeps their weight down.) Moreover, how do you *feel* about the discussion? Would you say one of the following?:

> "SO WHAT?"
> "I DON'T KNOW"
> "I DON'T CARE"

8. Ask the question, "How many students have tried to smoke just for fun?" A few honest hands will be raised. Have these

Tar and Nicotine Content of Cigarettes

Federal Trade Commission, March 1975 — (Ranked from low (1) to high (136))

NF—Non-Filter (All other brands possess filters)
M—Menthol
HP—Hard pack

RANK (tar)	BRAND	TYPE	TAR (mg)	NICOTINE (mg)
27	Alpine	King, M	13	0.8
45	Alpine	100mm, M (HP)	16	0.9
35	Belair	King, M	15	1.0
55	Belair	100mm, M	17	1.2
9	Benson & Hedges	Reg. (HP)	9	0.5
42	Benson & Hedges	King (HP)	16	1.1
57	Benson & Hedges 100's	100mm	17	1.1
54	Benson & Hedges 100's	100mm, M	17	1.1
131	Bull Durham	King	28	1.8
123	Camel	Reg., NF	25	1.6
100	Camel Filters	King	19	1.3
1	Carlton 70's	Reg.	4	0.2
3	Carlton	King	4	0.3
2	Carlton	King, M	4	0.3
119	Chesterfield	Reg., NF	24	1.4
132	Chesterfield	King, NF	29	1.7
82	Chesterfield	King	18	1.2
85	Chesterfield	King, M	18	1.2
104	Chesterfield	101mm	20	1.3
127	Domino	King, NF	26	1.3
116	Domino	King	23	1.2
33	Doral	King	15	1.0
23	Doral	King, M	13	0.9
37	DuMaurier	King (HP)	15	1.0
114	English Ovals	Reg., NF (HP)	22	1.5
133	English Ovals	King, NF (HP)	29	2.2
92	Eve	100mm	19	1.3
90	Eve	100mm, M	19	1.2
130	Fatima	King, NF	28	1.6
36	Galaxy	King	15	1.0
124	Half & Half	King	25	1.8
134	Herbert Tareyton	King, NF	29	1.8
112	Home Run	Reg., NF	21	1.6
8	Iceberg 100's	100mm, M	9	0.6
44	Kent	King	16	1.0
38	Kent	King (HP)	15	0.9
87	Kent	100mm	19	1.2
81	Kent	100mm, M	18	1.2
7	King Sano	King	8	0.3
6	King Sano	King, M	8	0.3
97	Kool	Reg., NF, M	19	1.2
46	Kool	King, M	16	1.2
43	Kool	King, M (HP)	16	1.2
66	Kool	100mm	17	1.4
25	Kool Milds	King, M	13	0.8
83	L & M	King, NF	18	1.2
110	L & M	100mm	20	1.4
94	L & M	100mm, M	19	1.3
77	Lark	King	18	1.2
96	Lark	100mm	19	1.3
129	Lucky Strike	Reg., NF	27	1.6
11	Lucky Ten	King	9	0.6
12	Lucky 100's	100mm	10	0.7
135	Mapleton	Reg., NF	30	1.2
118	Mapleton	King	24	1.2
72	Marlboro	King	17	1.1
67	Marlboro	King (HP)	17	1.1
31	Marlboro	King, M	14	0.8
26	Marlboro	King, M (HP)	13	0.8
73	Marlboro	100mm	18	1.1
60	Marlboro	100mm (HP)	17	1.1
20	Marlboro Lights	King	12	0.8
5	Marvels	King	6	0.2
125	Marvels	King, NF	25	0.9
4	Marvels	King, M	4	0.2
39	Miyako	King	15	0.9
88	Montclair	King, M	19	1.4
70	More	120mm	17	1.4
79	More	120mm, M	18	1.5
21	Multifilter	King	12	0.8
14	Multifilter	King, M	10	0.7
64	Newport	King, M	17	1.2

Tar and Nicotine Content of Cigarettes

Federal Trade Commission, March 1975 — (Ranked from low (1) to high (136))

NF—Non-Filter (All other brands possess filters)
M—Menthol
HP—Hard pack

RANK (tar)	BRAND	TYPE	TAR (mg)	NICOTINE (mg)
71	Newport	King, M (HP)	17	1.2
113	Newport	100mm, M	21	1.5
78	Oasis	King	18	1.2
80	Old Gold Filters	King	18	1.1
52	Old Gold Filters	King (HP)	17	1.2
103	Old Gold Straights	Reg., NF	20	1.2
121	Old Gold Straights	King, NF	24	1.5
117	Old Gold 100's	100mm	23	1.4
128	Pall Mall	King, NF	27	1.7
108	Pall Mall	100mm	20	1.4
68	Pall Mall	100mm, M	17	1.3
13	Pall Mall Extra Mild	King (HP)	10	0.7
10	Pall Mall Extra Mild	King (HP)	9	0.6
34	Parliament	King	15	0.8
32	Parliament	King (HP)	14	0.8
49	Parliament 100's	100mm	17	1.0
107	Philip Morris	Reg., NF	20	1.1
126	Philip Morris Commander	King, NF	25	1.5
56	Philip Morris International	100mm (HP)	17	1.1
65	Philip Morris International	100mm, M (HP)	17	1.0
106	Picayune	Reg., NF	20	1.5
122	Piedmont	Reg., NF	25	1.2
136	Players	Reg., NF (HP)	31	2.1
40	Raleigh	King	16	1.0
120	Raleigh	King, NF	24	1.4
69	Raleigh	100mm	17	1.2
30	Raleigh Extra Mild	King	14	0.9
99	Safari	100mm	19	1.4
62	St. Moritz	100mm, M	18	1.1
84	St. Moritz	100mm, M	18	1.2
89	Salem	King, M	19	1.3
86	Salem	King, M (HP)	19	1.3
74	Salem	100mm, M	19	1.3
115	Salem Extra	King, M	22	1.3
34	Sano	Reg., NF	15	0.8
51	Silva Thins	100mm	17	1.0
48	Silva Thins	100mm, M	16	1.1
111	Spring 100's	100mm, M	20	1.3
59	Super M	100mm, M	20	1.3
109	Tareyton	King	19	1.3
102	Tareyton	100mm	19	1.3
75	Tempo	King	18	0.8
56	Tramps	King	11	1.1
47	Tramps	King, M	16	0.9
16	True	Reg., NF	20	0.6
19	True	King, M	12	0.7
22	True	100mm, M	13	0.7
24	True	100mm, M	13	0.8
53	Twist	100mm (HP)	17	1.2
18	Vantage	King	12	0.8
11	Vantage	King, M	12	0.8
41	Viceroy	King	16	1.0
63	Viceroy	100mm	17	1.1
29	Viceroy Extra Mild	King	14	0.9
50	Viceroy Extra Mild	100mm	17	1.0
61	Virginia Slims	100mm, M	17	1.1
101	Virginia Slims	100mm, M	19	1.3
58	Winchester	King, M	17	1.2
105	Winchester	100mm, M	20	1.4
98	Winston	King (HP)	19	1.3
93	Winston	100mm	19	1.3
95	Winston	100mm, M	19	1.4
28	Winston Lights	King	14	1.0

U.S. DEPARTMENT OF HEALTH, EDUCATION, AND WELFARE / PUBLIC HEALTH SERVICE
Center for Disease Control / Bureau of Health Education / National Clearinghouse for Smoking and Health

DHEW Publication No. (CDC) 75-8703

Figure 8–39

people tell how smoking affected them. It may have made them nauseated, even sick. Explain that medical authorities feel that smoking is of no benefit to anyone but for growing boys and girls it is definitely harmful; one is not at one's best mentally, physically, or socially. In growing people it reduces the effectiveness of the muscle and nervous systems, may cause restlessness, dizziness, nausea, indigestion, increased heart beat, shortness of breath, and loss of appetite for good protein-containing foods.

9. Write to the American Cancer Society for information on the effects of alcohol upon the length of life. Discuss the information received in class. Post information. Use clippings. Distribute American Cancer Society bookmarks (free).

10. Demonstrate the teaching device, The Mechanical Smoker. Available from Spenco Medical Corp., P. O. Box 8113, Waco, Texas, 76710. Let several pupils try it. The bulb draws nicotine from cigarette into plastic lung.

11. Consider alcohol as a beverage and its effect upon the body, mind, and society. Ask the question, "What are the common effects of alcohol on the individual and society?" Permit independent study. Follow up with small group discussion.

12. Call for a variety of words used to describe drunkenness: "high," "tight," "blind," "loaded," "on a binge," "happy," "plastered," "stoned," "tippler," "wino," "derelict," "bum," "common drunk," etc. Discuss how these words make you *feel*. How really comic or tragic?

13. Experiment with water and alcohol, showing that even though the two look alike they affect substances differently. Place such items as raw liver, sugar lump, bread, and egg white in jars of alcohol; and put identical kinds of items in jars of water. Note differences that occur. Live plants can also be used to show how alcohol does not contribute to growth.

14. Talk over whether marihuana is safe to smoke. Obtain copy of National Institute on Drug Abuse report. Point out that new research indicates that being "high" impairs responses in automobile driving and may reduce lung function over a period of time as cigarette smoking does. Note its therapeutic value in treating glaucoma, asthma, and the nausea associated with cancer chemotherapy.

15. Set up and conduct a mock trial, complete with defendant, lawyers, judge, and jury. After searching the law, the pupils should be ready to justify use of a certain drug to judge and jury.

16. Prepare posters that reflect or call attention to the rights of non-smokers. Helpful leaflets are available from the American Cancer Society, American Lung Association, and the National Clearinghouse for Smoking and Health.

17. Look up the story of penicillin (Alexander Fleming). Do the

DRUG ABUSE PRODUCTS REFERENCE CHART

NAME	SLANG NAME	CHEMICAL OR OFFICIAL NAME	SOURCE	PHARMACOLOGIC CLASSIFICATION	MEDICAL USE	HOW TAKEN WHEN ABUSED	USUAL FORM OF PRODUCT	EFFECTS SOUGHT	LONG-TERM POSSIBLE EFFECTS	PHYSICAL DEPENDENCE POTENTIAL	PSYCHOLOGICAL DEPENDENCE POTENTIAL	ORGANIC DAMAGE POTENTIAL
MORPHINE	WHITE STUFF, M.	MORPHINE SULPHATE	NATURAL (FROM OPIUM)	CENTRAL NERVOUS SYSTEM DEPRESSANT	PAIN RELIEF	SWALLOWED OR INJECTED	POWDER (WHITE), TABLET, LIQUID	EUPHORIA; PREVENT WITHDRAWAL DISCOMFORT	ADDICTION, CONSTIPATION, LOSS OF APPETITE	YES	YES	YES, INDIRECTLY
HEROIN	H., HORSE, SCAT, JUNK, SMACK, SCAG STUFF, HARRY	DIACETYL-MORPHINE	SEMI-SYNTHETIC (FROM MORPHINE)	CNS DEPRESSANT	NONE, LEGALLY	INJECTED OR SNIFFED	POWDER (WHITE, GRAY, BROWN)	EUPHORIA; PREVENT WITHDRAWAL DISCOMFORT	ADDICTION, CONSTIPATION, LOSS OF APPETITE	YES	YES	YES, INDIRECTLY
CODEINE	SCHOOLBOY	METHYLMORPHINE	NATURAL (FROM OPIUM), SEMI-SYNTHETIC (FROM MORPHINE)	CNS DEPRESSANT	EASE PAIN & COUGHING	SWALLOWED	TABLET, LIQUID (IN COUGH SYRUP)	EUPHORIA; PREVENT WITHDRAWAL DISCOMFORT	ADDICTION, CONSTIPATION, LOSS OF APPETITE	YES	YES	YES, INDIRECTLY
PAREGORIC		TINCTURE OF CAMPHORATED OPIUM	NATURAL AND SYNTHETIC	CNS DEPRESSANT	SEDATION, COUNTERACT DIARRHEA	SWALLOWED OR INJECTED	LIQUID	EUPHORIA; PREVENT WITHDRAWAL DISCOMFORT	ADDICTION, CONSTIPATION, LOSS OF APPETITE	YES	YES	YES, INDIRECTLY
MEPERIDINE		MEPERIDINE HYDROCHLORIDE	SYNTHETIC (MORPHINE-LIKE)	CNS DEPRESSANT	PAIN RELIEF	SWALLOWED OR INJECTED	TABLET, LIQUID	EUPHORIA; PREVENT WITHDRAWAL DISCOMFORT	ADDICTION, CONSTIPATION, LOSS OF APPETITE	YES	YES	YES, INDIRECTLY
METHADONE	DOLLY	METHADONE HYDROCHLORIDE	SYNTHETIC (MORPHINE-LIKE)	CNS DEPRESSANT	PAIN RELIEF	SWALLOWED OR INJECTED	TABLET, LIQUID	PREVENT WITHDRAWAL DISCOMFORT	ADDICTION, CONSTIPATION, LOSS OF APPETITE	YES	YES	YES, INDIRECTLY
COCAINE	CORRINE, COKE, FLAKE, SNOW, GOLD DUST, STAR DUST, BERNICE	METHYLESTER OF BENZOYLECGONINE	NATURAL (FROM COCA LEAVES)	STIMULANT, LOCAL OR TOPICAL ANESTHETIC	LOCAL OR TOPICAL ANESTHESIA	SNIFFED, INJECTED OR SWALLOWED	POWDER (WHITE), LIQUID	EXCITATION	DEPRESSION, CONVULSIONS	NO	YES	PROBABLE
MARIJUANA	POT, GRASS, TEA	CANNABIS SATIVA	NATURAL	HALLUCINOGEN	NONE	SMOKED OR SWALLOWED	PLANT PARTICLES (DARK GREEN OR BROWN)	EUPHORIA, RELAXATION, INCREASED PERCEPTION	USUALLY NONE, BRONCHITIS, CONJUNCTIVITIS, PSYCHOSIS POSSIBLE	NO	PROBABLE	NOT YET DETERMINED
HASHISH	HASH	CANNABIS SATIVA	NATURAL	HALLUCINOGEN	NONE	SMOKED OR SWALLOWED	SOLID, BROWN TO BLACK, RESIN	RELAXATION, EUPHORIA, INCREASED PERCEPTION	USUALLY NONE, CONJUNCTIVITIS, PSYCHOSIS POSSIBLE	NO	PROBABLE	NOT YET DETERMINED
BARBITURATES	BARBS, RED DEVILS, YELLOW JACKETS, PHENNIES, PEANUTS, BLUE HEAVENS, CANDY	PHENOBARBITAL, PENTOBARBITAL, SECOBARBITAL, AMOBARBITAL	SYNTHETIC	CNS DEPRESSANT	SEDATION, RELIEVE HIGH BLOOD PRESSURE, EPILEPSY	SWALLOWED OR INJECTED	TABLETS OR CAPSULES	ANXIETY REDUCTION, EUPHORIA	SEVERE WITHDRAWAL SYMPTOMS, POSSIBLE CONVULSIONS, TOXIC PSYCHOSIS	YES	YES	YES
AMPHETAMINES	BENNIES, DEXIES, HEARTS, PEP PILLS, SPEED, LD DROPPERS, WAKE-UPS	AMPHETAMINE, DEXTROAMPHETAMINE, METHAMPHETAMINE (DESOXYEPHEDRINE)	SYNTHETIC	CNS STIMULANT	CONTROL APPETITE, NARCOLEPSY, SOME CHILDHOOD BEHAVIORAL DISORDERS	SWALLOWED OR INJECTED	TABLETS, CAPSULES, LIQUID, POWDER (WHITE)	ALERTNESS, ACTIVENESS	LOSS OF APPETITE, DELUSIONS, HALLUCINATIONS, TOXIC PSYCHOSIS	POSSIBLE	YES	PROBABLE
LSD	ACID, BIG D, SUGAR, TRIPS, CUBES	D-LYSERGIC ACID DIETHYLAMIDE	SEMI-SYNTHETIC (FROM ERGOT ALKALOIDS)	HALLUCINOGEN	EXPERIMENTAL RESEARCH ONLY	SWALLOWED	TABLETS, CAPSULES, LIQUID	INSIGHT, DISTORTION OF SENSE, EXHILARATION	MAY INTENSIFY EXISTING PSYCHOSIS, PANIC REACTIONS	NO	POSSIBLE	NOT YET DETERMINED
DOM	STP "SERENITY, TRANQUILITY, PEACE"	4-METHYL-2, 5-DIMETHOXY-ALPHA METHYL, PHENETHYLAMINE	SYNTHETIC	HALLUCINOGEN	NONE	SWALLOWED	TABLETS, CAPSULES, LIQUID	STRONGER THAN LSD EFFECTS	?	NO	POSSIBLE	NOT YET DETERMINED
THC		TETRAHYDROCANNABINOL	NATURAL (FROM CANNABIS SATIVA), SYNTHETIC	HALLUCINOGEN	NONE	SMOKED OR SWALLOWED	IN MARIJUANA OR LIQUID	STRONGER THAN LSD EFFECTS	?	NO	POSSIBLE	NOT YET DETERMINED
DMT	BUSINESSMAN'S SPECIAL	DIMETHYL-TRYPTAMINE	SYNTHETIC	HALLUCINOGEN	NONE	INJECTED	LIQUID	SHORTER TERM THAN LSD EFFECTS	?	NO	POSSIBLE	NOT YET DETERMINED
PCP	HOG, PEACE PILL	PHENCYCLIDINE	SYNTHETIC	HALLUCINOGEN	VETERINARY ANESTHETIC	SWALLOWED	TABLETS, CAPSULES	HARSHER THAN LSD	?	NO	POSSIBLE	NOT YET DETERMINED
MESCALINE	MESC	3,4,5-TRIMETH-OXYPHENETHYLAMINE	NATURAL (FROM PEYOTE CACTUS)	HALLUCINOGEN	NONE	SWALLOWED	TABLET, CAPSULE	SAME AS LSD	?	NO	POSSIBLE	NOT YET DETERMINED
PSILOCYBIN		3(2-DIMETHYL-AMINOETHYL)INDOL-4-OL DIHYDROGEN PHOSPHATE	NATURAL (FROM PSILOCYBE FUNGUS ON A TYPE OF MUSHROOM)	HALLUCINOGEN	NONE	SWALLOWED	TABLET, CAPSULE	SAME AS LSD	?	NO	POSSIBLE	NOT YET DETERMINED
ALCOHOL	BOOZE, JUICE, SAUCE	ETHANOL, ETHYL ALCOHOL	NATURAL (FROM GRAPES, GRAINS)	CNS DEPRESSANT	SOLVENT, ANTISEPTIC, SEDATIVE	SWALLOWED, OR APPLIED TOPICALLY	LIQUID	SENSE ALTERATION, ANXIETY REDUCTION, SOCIABILITY	TOXIC PSYCHOSIS, ADDICTION, NEUROLOGIC DAMAGE	YES	YES	YES
TOBACCO	FAG, COFFIN NAIL	NICOTINA TABACUM	NATURAL	CNS DEPRESSANT (NICOTINE)	EMETIC, ANTISEPTIC (NICOTINE)	SMOKED, SNIFFED, CHEWED	SNUFF, PIPE, CUT PARTICLES, CIGARETTES	CALMNESS, SOCIABILITY	LOSS OF APPETITE, HABITUATION	POSSIBLE	YES	YES
GLUE		AROMATIC HYDRO-CARBONS	SYNTHETIC	CNS DEPRESSANT	NONE	INHALED	PLASTIC CEMENT	INTOXICATION	IMPAIRED PERCEPTION, COORDINATION, JUDGMENT	NO	YES	YES

Figure 8–40. Handy reference chart for teachers and students. (Courtesy American School Health Association and Pharmaceutical Manufacturers Association.)

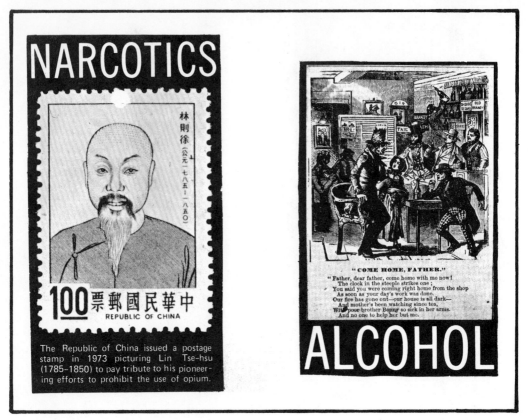

The Republic of China issued a postage stamp in 1973 picturing Lin Tse-hsu (1785-1850) to pay tribute to his pioneering efforts to prohibit the use of opium.

Figure 8–41. Posters to attract attention and raise questions. (Courtesy of U.S. Environmental Protection Agency.)

same for quinine and malaria, and isoniazid and tuberculosis.

18. Role play the troubles an intoxicated person might have climbing the back steps and unlocking a door. Discuss what is incapacitating this person.

19. Invite into class an athletic coach to talk about the relationship of smoking to athletic performance.

20. Visit the back of the drugstore and watch a registered pharmacist prepare a prescription. Note dangers and penalties of misusing potentially harmful substances.

21. Suggest several ways in which to face disappointments, stress, and unhappiness. How do *feelings* relate to behavior?

22. Collect interesting posters such as those in Figure 8–41.

23. Discover and write out the meaning of a peer group. How does it bind a person? How does it relate to smoking? How do *you* feel about peer pressure?

24. Make up a display of such items as model airplane glue, paint thinner, and carbon tetrachloride. Permit everyone to take a light sniff and read the labels. Then discuss ''gluesniffing'' and its relationship to death and permanent brain damage.

12. CONSUMER HEALTH

Behavioral Objectives (Intermediate Level)

Describes the individual role of the consumer of healthful goods and materials.

Explains how truths must be separated from half truths in order to judge whether or not to purchase a health product.

Investigates the extent that superstitions and gullibility frequently prevent people from acting wisely in the selection and use of health products.

Relates how items such as clothing, food, and medical service vary in kind and quality and that the informed consumer, by his or her knowledge and actions, helps keep undesirable and unscientific products out of circulation.

Demonstrates how a careful consumer eventually helps to make a careful producer or manufacturer.

Appraises advertised health products: dentifrices, sports equipment, pain killers, cold tablets, cosmetics, vitamin pills, etc.

Supports the view that there is danger in self-treatment when ill—need to seek top professional care.

Comments

We cannot shield our children from the marketplace. We must prepare them for it. . . . Producers of toys, breakfast cereals, and other foods appeal to children . . . to pressure their parents into buying the advertiser's product . . . no consumer is fully protected unless he can recognize a charlatan when he sees one, unless he can discern the difference between puffery and fact in an advertisement, and unless he can use the information he is given to make the best buying decision for his needs.

Virginia Knauer, former
Presidential Assistant for
Consumer Affairs

If this is the age of the consumer, as Virginia Knauer says it is, then the health teacher has a big job indeed. There is much to cover, from prescription drugs and medicines to foods and cosmetics. Almost every product has a health relationship. Over two million people are burned each year, many of them from flammable fabrics not satisfactorily regulated by government and industry. Worthless health products and remedies cost $1 billion a year. A quarter of a billion dollars is spent by arthritic sufferers alone; and some $75 million a year is taken from cancer patients and their families. So called "consumer steal" takes place daily because of misconceptions, misinformation, and outright superstitions pertaining to diet, weight control programs, toothpaste, hair preparations, deodorants, germ killers, etc. Perhaps it is not strange that in a $6 billion a year cosmetic industry, some 60,000 women develop reactions to cosmetics serious enough to consult skin specialists and many more treat themselves.

In a society accustomed to seeking pleasure and relief through the use of drugs and other related products, it appears normal to be cajoled into popping a couple of pills into the mouth to get "fast, fast relief," "freedom," "pleasure," "sleep," "comfort," "relaxation," and "regularity." Through uncounted advertisements, children and adults are persuaded and conditioned not to accept any minor discomfort. And speed appears to be highly desirable as *Bufferin* is advertised to be "twice as fast as aspirin," *Anacin* goes to work "in 22 seconds after entering your bloodstream," and *Excedrin* would seem to rise above them all by being "an antidepressant to help restore your spirits."[64]

A thorough understanding of how advertising works is necessary. A substantiating campaign involves bringing ads to class, taping radio and TV ads, and doing some price comparison research, particularly of perishable goods, cosmetics, and food sold in a health food store.[65] Consider also slogans, testimonials, and the aesthetic appeal of goods through advertising. Pigg calls attention to the suggestibility factor in many ads that calls for analytical skills necessary to separate fact from assumption.[66]

One frequently realizes that people hear only what other people want them to hear. Thus "educated" citizens are often ignorant. For example, in several communities in which the majority of the voters are college graduates, the issue of fluoridation of the drinking water was voted down, yet fluoridation is by far the most effective means known for reducing tooth decay to a significant extent.

Misconceptions abound everywhere, particularly among children and youth. Here are just a few that fifth and sixth grade schoolchildren subscribe to:

Persons who have pimples usually have bad blood.
Taking vitamin pills will guarantee good health.
Hot food is more nutritious than cold food.
Most fat people are very healthy.
Tooth powders or pastes will always cure a person's bad breath.
It is all right to use sleeping pills without a doctor's advice.
Certain medicines will prevent the common cold.
The best doctors always promise to make people healthy.
Cutting a person's hair makes it grow faster.
If you have any disease you'll always feel some pain.

A prospective mother can make the child more musical if she listens to good music.

According to the Federal Food and Drug Administration's bureau of enforcement, the most effective tool in combating quacks is publicity, particularly exposure in courts. Collecting newspaper

---

[64]See especially the illuminating report, "Aspirin and Its Competitors," *Consumer Reports*, August 1972, p. 540.

[65]For learning suggestions see McFarland, Tom. "A Healthy Consumer Health Class," *Health Education*, 7:36–37, July/August 1976.

[66]Pigg, R. Morgan. "Analysis of Health Advertising," *Health Education*, 6:22–24, November/December 1975.

clippings exposing quacks and false health claims is a practical project for consumer health classes. The class should know that any time the federal government is aware that the consumer is being misled into believing that certain foods and products will prevent a disease that is difficult to treat, they will take regulatory action.

Government regulations, a conscience in the manufacturing world, and such things as better labelling practices all help the consumer, but ultimately the most effective means of creating a more enlightened consumer is an education that starts early to deal with scientific inquiry, discovery, and a sophisticated concern for what is being purchased.

At what age do children become aware of the truths and half-truths in the world in which they live? When is the "teachable moment" for discussing the validity of a multitude of health claims—claims made by the wise and honest as well as the charlatans and quacks? How can we help the student learn that consumer health means to buy wisely from the standpoint of health and safety? This kind of education begins with observant eyes and ears, awakening minds, and the simple but sharp questions of nine and ten year olds. They read the ads, hear the radio and television commercials, and wonder whether one health product really *is* better than another. Moreover, those students who *inquire* during the early years are more apt to be the ones demanding evidence in their later school years. Such inquiry can be nurtured through the presentation of relevant learning experiences. In the final analysis, relevance is one's personal answer to the question "So what?"

According to the American Medical Association, by the time a pupil graduates from the elementary school, he or she should be able to defend at least five concepts:[67]

1. Self-medication should be avoided.
2. It is important to seek sound advice concerning health care.
3. There are no special health foods.
4. There are many kinds of "doctors" who will treat us when we are ill, but some who claim to be able to treat us are not qualified or adequately prepared.
5. Diagnosis of health problems should be made by a medically trained physician and medication should be taken under the direction of a physician.

Concepts and activities go together. For planning purposes, here are a few possibilities for the upper elementary grades:

1. *Consumers influence the price and quality of health products.*
   Both tooth powder and toothpaste used to be widely available. Consumers preferred pastes, so many tooth powders disappeared from the market. Consult newspapers for comparative prices of dentifrices. Do the same for soaps and mouthwashes.
2. *Consumers face individual health problems. Choosing a physician and having an examination are two examples.*

---

[67]*Defenses Against Quackery:* A Resource for Teacher Concepts and a Sample Teaching Unit for the Elementary School (1–6), Dept. of Health Education, American Medical Association.

Have the school nurse discuss physical examinations and the danger of self-treatment. Discuss the qualifications of a physician.

3. *Superstitions may influence what a person buys and does.*

Build a list of health superstitions and misconceptions. Examples: "An apple a day keeps the doctor away." "Carry a horse chestnut to ward off rheumatism."

4. *Not all doctors are physicians.*

Formulate a list of the various kinds of doctors and indicate the specialty of each.

5. *Changes in medicine are happening so rapidly that it is impossible for most people to be aware of the latest happenings.*

Ask each student to name a remarkable medical breakthrough in the past several years.

6. *Prescription medicines are those used safely and effectively only under a physician's or dentist's supervision.*

Examine some prescription labels. Note date and directions.

7. *The main purpose of health advertising is to sell products and services.*

Discuss the meaning of the word *ethical*. What does "fairness in advertising" mean to students?

8. *Advertising labels should be correct; they must not be false or misleading.*

Examine ads and labels. Do the names of famous people influence persons to buy a product?

9. *Advertisements sometimes encourage the consumer to buy things he or she doesn't really need.*

What is "emotional buying"? What is the influence of expressions such as *low calorie, less tar?*

10. *The Underwriters Laboratories (UL) examine and test devices, materials, and apparatus used by the public.*

Compile a list of electrical devices that show the UL label.

11. *The Department of Agriculture inspects and grades meats and poultry.*

Interview some butchers to discover how they aid in safeguarding meat.

12. *Quacks invent nonscientific machines to exploit the gullibility of people.*

Discuss vibrators, spot reducers to remove weight, cancer-cure machines.

The long list of "watchdog" duties carried on by such consumer protection agencies as the Food and Drug Administration, the Federal Trade Commission, and the U.S. Post Office Department can be brought to the attention of schoolchildren by obtaining excellent literature from these respective Washington agencies. Extensive lists of consumer health publications are available. Every topic has been explored. For example, if questions arise relative to cosmetics, then *Cosmetics Facts for Consumers* (FDA Publication No. 26) is most appropriate.

The FDA has *Consumer Protection* packets consisting of booklets, leaflets, and teaching suggestions suitable for use in health, science, and home economics classes. These packets (Packet A:

Foods; Packet B: *Drugs and Cosmetics*) may be obtained from the U.S. Government Printing Office.

A principal reference source is the *Suggested Guidelines for Consumer Education, Kindergarten through Twelfth Grades,* developed by the President's Committee on Consumer Interests and available from the Superintendent of Documents. It contains a general section on methods of implementation including discussions of the individual teacher approach, the team approach, the interdisciplinary approach, and the systems approach.

The following are sources of information for classroom use:

Consumer Information Index, Consumer Information, Public Documents Distribution Center, Pueblo, Colorado 81009.
Consumer Reports, Consumer Union of United States, Inc., Mount Vernon, N.Y. 10550.
Consumer Bulletin, Consumer Research, Inc., Washington, N.J. 07882.
Consumer Power: Whistleblowing, J. Gary Mitchell Films (Film).
In Critical Condition, Edward M. Kennedy, New York: Pocket Books, Inc., 1973.
The Dark Side of the Marketplace, W. G. Magnuson and J. Carper, Englewood Cliffs: Prentice-Hall, Inc., 1972.

Suggested Activities

1. Identify physicians who take care of special health problems such as eyes, feet, and teeth; also, medical specialists such as pediatricians, obstetricians, and psychiatrists. Why are there so many different kinds of specialists?
2. Americans spend many billions of dollars for medical care each year. The hospitals' share of this figure has more than doubled since 1929. Appoint class committees to find out why.
3. Give an overnight assignment requesting the class to make up a list of superstitions about health and disease. Suggest that they check with their parents and others in their neighborhood so that their list will be as long as possible. Make a combined list of these findings the next day. Add to the list a number of superstitions such as the following:
   Onions worn around the neck prevent disease.
   Aluminum cooking utensils cause cancer.
   Wearing an iron ring prevents backache (rheumatism too).
   Toads cause warts.
   Wearing rubbers indoors will injure the eyes.
   An apple a day keeps the doctor away.
   People were healthier in the "good old days."
   When your time comes you will die, no matter how you live.
4. Collect a variety of labels from cans and bottles and advertisements from the newspapers and magazines for class discussion. Post some of them.
5. Post a blank piece of paper under a bulletin board with the heading "The Marketplace." Add *headline* clippings from newspapers and magazines by sticking them on with paste or tape.

6. Post on the classroom bulletin board a list of community sources where reliable health information may be obtained. Follow this up with a committee visit to each of the sources. This will involve most of the class if properly organized.
7. Bring in an outside speaker to show how the consumer is being protected (a county health agent, local physician or health officer, or Food and Drug Administration official). Prepare questions ahead of time to ask the visitor.

the marketplace

8. At one time the Federal Trade Commission had complaints pending against the manufacturers of eight over-the-counter analgesics: *Bayer Aspirin, Bufferin, Anacin, Arthritis Pain Formula, Excedrin, Excedrin P.M., Cope,* and *Vanquish* for false or misleading advertising. Discover why. (At least one source is *Consumer Reports* for August, 1972.)
9. Look into self-medication. Consider the hazards involved and the delay in seeking proper care. Identify reliable health care—medical, dental, nursing, physical therapy, counseling and so on.
10. Identify methods used to sell goods and services; promotion gimmicks, trading stamps, coupons. Discriminate between informational and motivational advertising. Collect leaflets and labels.

QUESTIONS FOR DISCUSSION

1. Because there are so many major health topics and subtopics to cover in twelve years of school, several school systems have set about programming the health instruction by employing cycle plans and integration with other subject areas. To insure that only significant activities are taught, what might a teacher use as his or her guide?

2. What seem to be the two or three significant differences between health emphasis in the primary grades and health emphasis in the intermediate grades?

3. How can proper progression in a health topic between grades be assured? Especially in a school where there is no supervisor or health consultant?

4. Since the word *implementation* is associated with fulfillment and accomplishment and relates ultimately to attainment of educational goals,

how might you build into the various health topic programs a way of evaluation?

SUGGESTED ACTIVITIES

1. Examine the health curriculum materials used in a particular elementary school. *How* are they employed? *How involved* are students? Suggest examples of both good and poor teaching practices, if possible, to fairly appraise a local situation. Also, comment on the difficulty of doing a good evaluation here.

2. Carefully examine several curriculum guides pertaining to elementary school health education. (These are generally found in the college or university library with other professional education materials). How are the specific objectives or purposes set up? Are they arranged in terms of concepts? Competencies? Outcomes? Goals? Behavioral objectives? See if you can discover the rationale behind the terms used.

3. Review the research relative to smoking education. Write a short paper setting forth some of the evidences of success and failure in the smoking education programs nationally. Be particularly concerned with evidences of behavior change.

4. In a sense, Consumer Health embraces all major health teaching topics. After briefly reviewing each of these topics, formulate a list of what might be called "common abuses," that is, a listing of ways in which the consumer may be put at a disadvantage through half-truth advertising and questionable products.

5. Prepare teaching *outlines* for the study of health topics, using suggested teaching activities other than those appearing in this chapter.

SELECTED REFERENCES

Ast, David B. "Prevention and the Power of Consumers," *American Journal of Public Health,* 65:15–16, January 1978.

Barnes, S. Eugene. "The Smoking Classroom," *Health Education,* 7:37–38, March/April 1976.

Barrett, Morris. *Health Education Guide: A Design for Teaching.* 2nd ed., Philadelphia: Lea & Febiger, 1974.

Buhl, Jeanne M., et al. "Smokers versus Nonsmokers," *Health Education,* 8:11–13, January/February 1977.

Cosper, Barbara A., et al. "The Effect of Nutrition Education on Dietary Habits of Fifth Graders," *Journal of School Health,* 47:474–477, October 1977.

Dentler, Robert A., *Urban Problems: Perspectives and Solutions.* Chicago: Rand McNally, 1977.

Engs, Ruth C., Barnes, S. Eugene, and Wantz, Molly. *Health Games Students Play.* Dubuque: Kendall/Hunt Publishing Co., 1975.

Ensor, Phyllis G. and Means, Richard K. *Instructor's Resource and Methods Handbook for Health Education,* 2nd ed., Boston: Allyn and Bacon, Inc., 1977.

Fait, Hollis F., *Experiences in Movement: Physical Education for the Elementary School Child,* 3rd ed., Philadelphia: W. B. Saunders Co., 1976.

Fulton, Gere B. and Fassbender, William V. *Health Education in the Elementary School.* Pacific Palisades, California: Goodyear Publishing Co., 1972.

Girdano, Daniel A. and Girdano, Dorothy D. *Drug Education: Content and Methods,* 2nd ed., Boston: Addison-Wesley Publishing Co., 1976.

Greenberg, Jerrold S. "Teaching Strategies for Mental Health," *Health Education,* 7:38, November/December 1976.

Greene, Walter H., Jenne, Frank H., and Legos, Patricia M. *Health Education in the Elementary School.* New York: Macmillan Publishing Co., 1978.

Hart, Edward J. "Death Education and Mental Health," *Journal of School Health,* 46:407–410, September 1976.

Lee, Essie E. "Female Adolescent Drinking Behavior: Potential Hazards," *Journal of School Health, 48*:151–156, March 1978.

Martin, Ethel A. *Roberts' Nutrition Work with Children.* Chicago: University of Chicago Press, 1972.

Maxeiner, Barbara A., et al. "Knowledge, Behavior and Attitudes of Sixth Grade Students Toward Family Life Education," *Journal of School Health, 46*:81–85, February 1976.

Nelson, Leslie W. and Lorbeer, George C. *Science Activities for Elementary Children.* Dubuque: William C. Brown Publishing Co., 1972.

Parcel, Guy S. *First Aid in Emergency Care,* St. Louis: C. V. Mosby Co., 1977.

Poolton, Martha Anne. "What Can We Do About Food Habits?" *Journal of School Health, 48*:646–648, January 1978.

Ray, O. S. *Drugs, Society and Human Behavior,* 2nd ed., St. Louis: C. V. Mosby Co., 1978.

Schaller, Warren E. and Carroll, Charles R. *Health Quackery and the Consumer.* Philadelphia: W. B. Saunders Co., 1976.

Schurr, Evelyn L. *Movement Experiences for Children.* 2nd ed., Englewood Cliffs, N.J.: Prentice-Hall, Inc., 1975, Part 4.

Sinacore, John S. and Harrison, Gail. "The Place of Nutrition in the Health Education Curriculum," *American Journal of Public Health,* 61:2282, November 1971.

Sorochan, Walter D. and Bender, Stephen J. *Teaching Elementary Health Science,* Boston: Addison-Wesley Publishing Co., 1975.

Swisher, John D. "Mental Health—The Core of Preventive Health Education," *Journal of School Health,* 46:386–389, September 1976.

Wadsworth, Barry J. *Piaget for the Classroom Teacher.* New York: Longman, Inc., 1978, Part 3.

Walton, Elizabeth G. and Russell, Robert D. "Effective Mental Health Education with Sight and Sound Experiences," *Journal of School Health, 48*:661–666, January 1978.

White, Phillip. *Let's Talk About Food.* Chicago: Follett Publishing Co., 1975.

Willgoose, Carl E. *Environmental Health: Commitment for Survival,* Philadelphia: W. B. Saunders Company, 1979.

————————. "Mental Health at an Early Age," *Instructor,* 81:58–59, October 1971.

Zaichkowsky, L. B., Zaichkowsky, L. D. and Martinek, T. S. "Self Concept and Attitudinal Differences in Elementary Age School Children After Participation in a Physical Activity Program," *Mouvement,* October 1975.

Methods and
Teaching Aids in
Health Instruction

9

When a student has approached his concentration from different angles—when he begins to think—that's the liberating influence; that's when he becomes free.

—Samuel Beer[1]

Prior to the making of individual decisions regarding health practices and lifestyle is the need to be motivated to think. Seeking the item, process, or situation that "turns on" the learner is an essential teacher mission.

One reason why courses taught by Harvard University's Samuel Beer are in such great student demand is that they are spirited occasions at which facts are not simply transferred from teacher to student but become very much *alive*. Indeed, they are alive and "liberating" simply because students think broadly as they explore a topic from a number of dimensions instead of concentrating on one or two. They support Pascal's view that it is better to know something about everything connected with a topic than to know everything about one thing. The varied dimensions lend feeling and meaning to the intense study of a single subject. The study of health science, therefore, can usually be made more effective when teachers employ a methodology that seriously considers motivation and explores each of the major health areas from a variety of approaches so that the association between thinking and freedom that Beer refers to become a reality.

The schools, of course, cannot work entirely on their own. Although they may strive in a number of ways to help students get beyond cognitive learning to appropriate actions and to reinforce the values of the culture around them, they will always be faced with a community setting that may not be supportive and cooperative. Or there may be socioeconomic inequality, disadvantaged and dehumanized families, and other shortcomings that are counterproductive for advancing health practices. In short, any discussion of teaching methods and aids must acknowledge that both the school and the immediate environment have to be attractive to children if appropri-

---

[1]Schiefelbein, Susan. "Confusion At Harvard: What Makes An Educated Man?" *Saturday Review*, April 1, 1978, p. 12.

ate decision making is to occur. Fortunately, making the most of unattractive settings is a practice upon which some teachers thrive.

THE MEANING OF METHOD

The word "method" has a number of implications in education. In a sense, it is the very body of educational endeavor, for it involves more than objectives and curriculum. It involves the effectiveness of the program—a program in which curriculum and method cannot be divorced.

Familiarity with methodology makes the teacher an educationalist, rather than simply a specialist in sociology, biology, or mathematics. In fact, sound methodology coupled with an understanding of subject matter and children makes the well-rounded instructor.

Historically, teaching has always been considered an art. Art and science are different and their methods contrast. Science is analytical; it breaks things up, seeks detail, and looks for causes. Art, on the other hand, is engaged in giving *meaning to experience;* it puts things together—it involves synthesis rather than analysis. Fauré in his monumental history of art reminds us that, "Science relates fact

Figure 9–1. Motivation is advanced by a variety of methods. (Courtesy American Alliance for Health, Physical Education, and Recreation.)

to fact; art relates fact to life." Both science and art are regularly employed by the instructor who knows what to teach and how to teach it. The *how* is important. It is the means selected to achieve objectives.

All methods need examination because what works with one child or group may not work as well with another child or group as long as there are bona fide individual differences; "what is one man's meat is another man's poison." Sometimes formal methods operate for the welfare of the pupils; at other times informal methods seem better. There are so many specific and worthwhile objectives in elementary school health education that it is reasonable to expect a number of methods to prove successful, depending on the local situation.

METHODOLOGY AND TEACHING AIDS

Within the limits of their capacities, children can be motivated to learn. Obviously, whatever holds and attracts attention is going to determine action; William James said as much decades ago. Whether attention is held by a particular teaching procedure, such as a warm discussion, or an aid to instruction, such as a model or filmstrip, makes little difference. Both the method and the teaching aid get at the *how* of teaching, the concern of this chapter. Therefore, in this book methods are not divorced from materials, with one chapter following the other as though the topics were somehow disconnected. Methodology—the way instructional materials are used—will be discussed later on. If the teaching aid is employed in such a way that it does what Jean Piaget would have it do—namely, help the student to become the principal agent of his or her own education—then it is a most effective addition to methods employed.

THE FOUNDATION OF METHOD

The chief concern of methods in education is to *involve* children in the learning process. Where such involvement is missing, the school is as Silberman described it—a grim, joyless place where there is little pleasure in creating and little sense of self. In too many schools there is no fun and individual spontaneity is so low that few pupils ask *why* about what they are doing. Paul Tillich defines this pedagogical fault: "To throw answers like stones at the heads of those who have not yet asked questions." Erik Erikson labelled such a condition very well when he said that ". . . the most deadly of all possible sins is the mutilation of a child's spirit." However, lest one become pessimistic and depressed, it should be pointed out that schools *can* and *are* organized to facilitate spirited learning. Increasingly, schools are being organized to encourage students to be creative, to question, and to express their feelings. Teaching schedules have been made flexible; the staff has been differentiated and team teaching practices have been implemented so that teachers with particular strengths can be used efficiently; children are free to move about and talk quietly about what they are doing; instruction is individually prescribed; and numerous ideas are being tried in and around the classroom that were never considered in the past. Years ago John Gardner called for a change in teaching emphasis: "All too often we are giving young people cut flowers when we should be teaching them to grow their own plants. We are stuffing their heads with products of earlier innovation rather than teaching them to innovate."[2]

Perhaps more important than anything else in recent years has been the wholesome attention given to the affective and action domains. The goal is to help students learn and accept relevant facts and ideas which will lead to rational decisions and help modify their behavior in line with such decisions. As Godfrey Hochbaum points out, this behavior change or modification is a process—not merely a teaching method, but something that takes place *within* the individual;[3] it is not something done to the individual. Behavior modification occurs when an individual reaches an intellectual and "gut-level" state where he or she is knowingly dissatisfied with present behavior and searches for and finds a new behavior that appears to be more satisfying. The big teaching job is to bring pupils to the state of dissatisfaction where they are aware of their condition.

EFFECTIVE HEALTH TEACHING

Research demonstrates that uniqueness and individuality are characteristics of good teachers. This, says Read, is a "demonstration that *a good teacher is first and foremost a person.*"[4] It is the personality that counts. Carkhuff's research indicates that teachers who rank high on empathy, respect, and genuineness are more likely to facilitate cognitive and affective growth in their students than are teachers who rank low.[5] These conditions, essential for communication, improve interpersonal functioning.

Many who have taught in the elementary and middle schools for a long period of time have found that health and health-related subjects can be made very interesting. Bensley finds that effective health instruction requires four conditions:[6]

One: *Learning must be enjoyable.*
Two: *Students must become emotionally involved in the learning process.*
Three: *Students should be granted a degree of academic freedom to explore their own health needs and interests.*

---

[2]Gardner, John. *Self-Renewal.* New York: Harper and Row, 1965, p. 21.

[3]Hochbaum, Godfrey. "Behavior Modification," *School Health Review,* 2:5–10, September 1971.

[4]Read, Donald A. "The Search for the Person in the Teacher," *Health Values: Achieving High-Level Wellness,* 1:149–154, July/August 1977.

[5]Carkhuff, R. R. *Helping and Human Relations.* New York: Holt, Rinehart & Winston, 1969, p. 315.

[6]Bensley, Loren B. "Ideas for Successful Health Teaching," *School Health Review,* 3:37–38, May/June 1972.

Four: *The teacher needs to know his or her students.*

In health teaching, the method selected should concentrate more on the *why* than on the how. This will get one away from what J. B. Priestly calls "a narrow world of how-the-trick-is-done" to a thoughtful understanding of relationships. In this connection, good teaching brings at least nine variables together so that they bear on one another:

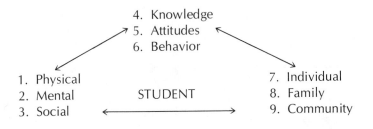

One reason certain health topics have been considered by many pupils to be dull and boring is that they have not been related to the day-to-day experiences of the class. Taught on a strictly cognitive level, the story of human blood could be dry indeed. But related to the social consequences in the larger community it can come alive. Blood is quite different when considered as part of an automobile accident—with the police department, curious onlookers, ambulance service, emergency hospital activity, and the family feelings for the victim all brought to bear on the situation.

The work of Mager in *Developing Attitudes Toward Learning* and Krathwohl and Bloom in the *Taxonomy of Educational Objectives* has been most helpful in focusing attention on student experiences as a way of improving teaching methods. By getting at the development and measurement of behavioral objectives, they demonstrated the need to alter methodology. In short, one cannot expect to reach the behavior/action domain without involvement to a greater or lesser degree with cognitive and affective learning. This was noted in the previous chapter in the discussion of drug education when it was pointed out that "lifestyle" talk and "here-now" views had to be aired and felt in the peer group setting if any behavior change was contemplated. If peer influence and a pupil's idea of status are important in the smoking program, for instance, and call for understanding and appreciation, then they are just as important in other major health areas as a prerequisite to learning and decision making.

As health teaching activities are organized and developed, it makes sense to couple expected behavior outcomes with specific methods and teaching aids. If the objective is to have third grade pupils brush their teeth in a proper and effective fashion, then the question of which method to choose arises. Talking about the subject does little good. Showing a film seldom causes more than a brief pause to think about brushing in a particular way. Even a teacher demonstration appears futile. On the other hand, a classroom toothbrushing drill with real materials, including mouth mirrors to see the teeth, is novel and practical enough to have some carry-over value—particularly if there is less drill and more fun involved. The behavioral statements, of varying degrees of specificity, shown below, are used to clarify objectives but might be achieved by employing one method rather than another.

It is easy to see that effective health teaching in any one health area may well involve several methods, particularly in a school that encourages creativity, has a flexible attitude toward instruction, and has on hand a number of teaching aids. Different children can work on different aspects of the health topic and use different methods.

Behavioral Statement	*Possible Method of Achievement*
1. Administer artificial respiration in an effective manner	Slow motion loop film review coupled with paired teams for practice
2. Read an oral thermometer correctly to the nearest tenth of a degree	Experiment or demonstration
3. Run a fifty yard dash in eight seconds	Experiment or discovery approach
4. Analyze the labels from several cereal packages in terms of nutritive value	Small group investigation
5. Illustrate several ways in which sources of drinking water become polluted	Field trip
6. Demonstrate safety on the playground	Role playing or group demonstration
7. Construct a diagram illustrating the effect of tobacco smoke, tar, and nicotine on human lung tissue	Contract or problem-solving
8. Prepare twenty true-false questions relative to the use of prescription drugs	Library or independent study

Variety bolsters interest and acts as a motivating technique. When all health topics are taught in a similar manner, it is difficult to maintain the interest of the class, for the element of surprise and anticipation is missing. Even a little bit of that which one pupil loves the most continues to remain high in his or her esteem when it is used sparingly.

Experimentation in method is to be encouraged. Varying the health teaching method is an effective way of determining how the class responds to a number of approaches. From this kind of experimentation, successful methods are developed for the teaching of a particular health topic. One can begin to answer specific questions such as, How best to teach alcohol and narcotics? Will a white rat experiment actually put over the true meaning of vitamins? Shall I plan a demonstration? What can my pupils discover?

The versatile teacher who has several ways of approaching health topics does more than successfully teach the topic; he or she actually promotes a mentally hygienic situation in the classroom, for children appreciate something different and they tend to show more real enthusiasm and genuine happiness when their teacher is flexible.

EXAMPLE AS METHOD

In addition to the specific methods employed by the teacher, the very example set by him or her is in itself an educational method.

I

I'd rather see a sermon
  Than hear one any day;
I'd rather one should walk with me
  Than merely show the way.
The eye's a better pupil,
  And more willing than the ear;
Fine counsel is confusing,
  But example's always clear.

II

I soon can learn to do it,
  If you'll let me see it done;
I can see your hands in action,
  But your tongue too fast may run.
And the lectures you deliver
  May be very fine and true,
But I'd rather get my lesson
  By observing what you do.
For I may misunderstand you
  And the high advice you give,
But there's no misunderstanding
  How you act and how you live!

—Anonymous

Those who work with youth do not need superagencies and complicated programs; needed is reemphasis of the simple truth that the kind of people we are is infinitely more important than programs. If we give youth an example of fit living, they will want to be fit themselves. Here is the challenge:

He who would kindle another must himself be aglow.

—Drinkwater

PARTICIPATION AND INTERACTION

It is safe to say that where participation is the fullest and mere spectatorship is at a minimum, effective learning tends to be at its best. Will Durant sums this viewpoint up very nicely when he says, "The wisest of our children will not be those who merely enjoy the spectacle; it will be those who climb out of the pit upon the stage and lose themselves in action.' To lose oneself in action has powerful implications. It means that the activity is total and the individual is completely wrapped up in the subject. It is a rare state, indeed, and one that most teachers hope to witness more often in their teaching careers. It is not a strange state because one cannot set a limit to which children will go to pursue the things they are truly interested in. Methods that promote experiences which fire the curiosity of youth are priceless. For curiosity, says Alexis Carrel, "is a necessity of nature, a blind impulse that obeys no rule."

The "*interaction* of maturation, environmental experience, social experience, and equilibrium" is important, according to Piaget.[7] It is what Ned Flanders appraises through interaction analysis on the verbal level and John Cheffers does on the non-verbal level (Cheffers Adaptation of the Flanders Interaction Analysis System—CAFIAs).[8] Moreover, says Piaget, it is through interaction that minds are formed which can be critical, can verify, and can evaluate everything that is offered. Furthermore:

"We have to be able to resist individually, to criticize, to distinguish between what is proven and what is not. So we need pupils who are active, who learn early to find out by themselves, partly by their own spontaneous activity and partly through materials we set up for them; who learn early to tell what is verifiable and what is simply the first idea to come to them."[9]

UNDERSTANDING AND DISCOVERY

Teaching invariably concerns itself with conceptual understanding. In fact, thinking actually is the process of organizing and storing concepts. In this respect, Bruner has pointed out the importance of establishing these "structures" of knowledge so that the student can find *meaningful relationships* among comprehensive ideas, rather than having to struggle with countless facts in isolation.

Significantly, it is the *experience* itself which seems to count as the greatest single factor in conceptual learning, far outweighing mental age or vocabulary strength. It is at this very point that the discovery idea becomes germane. Concepts are more easily formed when the student's learning is a product of his or her own curiosity and thinking and of the manipulation of basic facts. What the person alone discovers means something.

Brecht the playwright substantiates this method in *Galileo*. In the opening scene, he shows the great Italian scientist Galileo Galilei in the early 1600's teaching a young boy the particulars of the movement of the earth about the sun. As he initiates the lesson, there is no lecturing and no explanation; instead, Galileo asks the lad to exam-

---

[7]Wadsworth, Barry J. *Piaget for the Classroom Teacher.* New York: Longman, 1978, p. 6.

[8]For details see Crispin, David B. "The Technology of Interaction Analysis," *Educational Technology,* 10:14–20, July 1970. See also Cheffers, John T. F., et al. *Interaction Analysis: An Application to Nonverbal Activity.* 2nd ed., Minneapolis: Association for Productive Teaching, 1979.

[9]Piaget, J. "Development and Learning." In *Piaget Rediscovered,* Ripple, R. and Rockcastle, V. (Eds.), Ithaca, N.Y.: Cornell University Press, 1964, p. 5.

ine his device for showing the way the planets move about the sun. "What do you see?" says the great man. "Count the bands. How many are there?" When doubting Thomases and scientists came to visit him, he taught the same way. When each would gaze into the crude telescope, Galileo would ask, "What do you see? Describe to me what you see." This not only awakened interest, but it tied the observer securely to the topic because his own *trusted senses* were involved. What he saw was real to him; it was not something someone described in mere words and phrases. It became a part of him and was not lightly considered and soon forgotten.

To improve understanding through discovery, there are a number of activities that can be performed. Gray and Gerrand list them as thinking skills:[10]

Observing	Synthesizing
Comparing	Creative Thinking
Comprehending	Critical Thinking
Interpreting	Looking for Assumptions
Summarizing	Imaging
Categorizing	Collecting and Organizing Data
Classifying	Hypothesizing
Analyzing	Decision Making

[10]Gray, William A. III and Gerrard, Brian A. *Learning By Doing: Developing Teaching Skills,* Boston: Addison Wesley Publishing Co., 1977, p. 259.

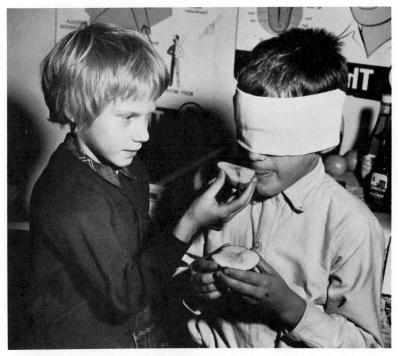

Figure 9–2. The discovery method leads to concept formation. (Courtesy Mrs. R. G. Holmes, Greenacres School, Scarsdale, N.Y.)

VALUE CLARIFICATION AND HEALTH TEACHING

Every course of health action taken is based on consciously or unconsciously held beliefs, attitudes, and values. Carl Rogers views valuing as a process that is more emotional than rational and he shows a relationship between the child's developing values and self-concept.[11]

Believing that lasting decisions can be achieved when individuals are aware of their values, Raths, Harmin, and Simon set out to make the study of human values a practical activity and one that would advance educational methodology.[12] They considered the ways in which values can be transmitted and came to the conclusion that thoughts and accomplishments must somehow be linked together.

In the clarifying approach to values, it is acknowledged that the values held by an individual at any time are relative, personal, and situational. Also, there is no attempt to transmit the "right" values. Instead, an attempt is made to assist a student in the clarification of his or her own values so that he or she can adjust to the world and play an intelligent role in influencing it.

In addition to teaching in such a way that the students will discover values, there is the task of helping them learn skills to enable them to continue the clarifying value approach throughout their lives—values that can be applied personally and socially.The methodology for this approach to learning involves working with children to sensitize them to value issues, to give them experiences in thinking critically, to share perceptions with others, to learn cooperative problem-solving skills, and to help them learn to apply value skills in their own lives.

The broad value skills that can be advanced through classroom techniques are shown on top of the following page.[13]

Note that these seven skills are *progressive*. Activity begins with appraising the situation and noting alternatives. From this develops an affirmation of choice. The decision has been made and from this evolves the behavior change—a change that one is committed to and makes room for a style of living.

Some time ago Albert Einstein characterized this age as "a perfection of means and a confusion of goals." This might well apply to

---

[11]Rogers, Carl R. *Freedom to Learn.* Columbus, Ohio: Charles E. Merrill Publishing Co., 1969. See also Hash, Virginia. *Values: Awareness, Significance, and Action.* Dubuque: William C. Brown Co., Publishers, 1975.

[12]Raths, Louis E., Harmin, Merrill, and Simon, Sidney B. *Values and Teaching: Working with Values in the Classroom.* Columbus, Ohio: Charles E. Merrill Publishing Co., 1966. See also the later work by Raths, *Teaching for Learning.* Columbus, Ohio: Charles E. Merrill Publishing Co., 1967. Also, see the chapter on values by Harmin and Simon in Allen, Dwight W. and Seifman, Eli (Eds.). *The Teacher's Handbook,* Glenview, Illinois: Scott, Foresman and Co., 1971. See also Read, D. A. and Simon, S. *Humanistic Education Sourcebook,* Englewood Cliffs, N.J.: Prentice-Hall, Inc., 1976.

[13]Raths, Louis E. *Teaching for Learning.* Columbus, Ohio: Charles E. Merrill Publishing Co., 1967.

	1. Seeking alternatives when faced with a choice
Choosing	2. Looking ahead to probable consequences before choosing
	3. Making choices on one's own, without depending on others
Prizing	4. Being aware of one's own preferences and valuations
	5. Being willing to affirm one's choices and preferences publicly
Acting	6. Acting in ways that are consistent with choices and preferences
	7. Acting in those ways repeatedly with a pattern to one's life

many children who are not at all clear about what their lives are for. Many have never explored alternatives to any degree. Thus children are seen at times in many expressions of weakness—apathetic, flighty, inconsistent, or uncertain—or as drifters, over-conformers, overdissenters, or role players. One thing uniting them all is that they have not found themselves. To expect them to enter the game of living and find health practices vital is a great deal to expect. But there is hope if the teacher can present alternative health situations and encourage children to make choices and to make them freely. This is where the valuing process begins.

Arriving at values through traditional means is not without useful effect. Thus, the employment of logical arguments, persuasion, setting an example, establishing regulations, and appealing to conscience are all useful approaches. Where value clarifying differs is in the *method of responding to things a student says or does*. If, for example, in a lesson on vision, a fifth grade boy were to say, "I'm getting some eyeglasses this weekend," how might a teacher respond? Possibly, "Isn't that wonderful," or "I hope you'll like them."

From these responses it is not likely that there will be very much clarifying thought by the student. If the teacher had responded by saying, "Getting some glasses are you? Do you think you'll like them?" Opportunity for a clarifying response is now possible. The student might say, "No, now that you ask, I'm not too happy about wearing glasses. I know a boy who has to wear them and some kids laugh at him." If there is time to pursue this issue further, more clarification should occur and it is likely the student will develop an alternative feeling about wearing glasses—particularly if the total discussion has been open, non-threatening, and avoids moralizing. In short, teaching health in a way that relates to student feelings, attitudes, aspirations, beliefs, and worries is a method with potential for reaching every child. Questions, of course, have to be phrased in keeping with the Raths-Harmin-Simon seven essential and progressive value skills. For example, in advancing the values of non-smoking in an intermediate level class where several children have tried smoking, questions might develop. See chart.

1. Choosing freely
   a. Do your parents know that you have tried smoking?
   b. Where did you first get the idea that smoking might be fun?
   c. Do your friends feel the way you do?
2. Choosing from alternatives
   a. Was there more than one reason for starting to smoke?
   b. Did anyone help you with your decision?
   c. Did you consider not trying a cigarette? What went into your final decision?
3. Choosing thoughtfully and reflectively
   a. Have you thought about the Surgeon General's Report on the consequences of smoking cigarettes? Does it bother you that people who smoke have more heart and lung difficulties?
   b. Can you explain how you might grow up smoking more than you do now and not suffer any illness from smoking?
   c. Where will your choice to smoke take you? Do you have some feelings about having made this choice?
4. Prizing and Cherishing
   a. Would your life be different *without* tobacco? Would it be different *with it*?
   b. Are you glad you smoke? Do you feel bad about it sometimes? Do you really prize cigarettes?
   c. Would you want your good friends or your younger brother or sister to start to smoke?
5. Affirming
   a. Would you be willing to give a short talk to a class of third grade children about the hazards of tobacco smoking?
   b. How do you think you can go about telling others that smoking leads to all kinds of health difficulties?
6. Acting upon choices
   a. What will you do first to help others not to start smoking?
   b. What will some of your friends say if you try to get others to give up cigarettes? Have you thought about this? Have you done much reading on this topic?
   c. Are you making plans to meet with younger children who might take up cigarettes for fun or experimentation?
7. Repeating
   a. What have you done so far to help others? How often?
   b. Have you plans for getting some of your good pals involved in helping you with younger children in your neighborhood?
   c. Are you glad you gave up smoking and are helping others to do the same? Would you do it again?

Since it is frequently difficult in the large classes to work efficiently with individuals, Raths, Harmin, and Simon suggest that the teacher prepare a *value sheet* to be used with groups. This may consist of a provocative statement followed by a number of questions and duplicated on a sheet of paper so that all class members have a copy. In this fashion, a particular health issue may be raised that has value implications for the students. Following a brief period of thinking about the statement, the students may enter into discussion, or each may prepare answers to the questions. The value sheets can have statements that are controversial, dealing with such topics as the legalization of marihuana, lowering the drinking age, the use of shoulder straps as well as seat belts, etc. Or, they can be simple and deal with four or five questions such as shown in the area of mental health:

Value Sheet for Mental Health

Fair Play

1. Does fair play mean anything to you? Explain.
2. When you play a game with your friends, what is it that you do that is an indication of fair play?
3. Just what is sportsmanship? How would you describe it?
4. Is sportsmanship necessary in games and sports? What have you read or heard about justice, equality, and fair play? Is there fair play in the world of business? In sports?
5. How do you feel when you are fair with people? Are people who treat others fairly in a good state of mental health?
6. Do you plan to make any changes in your manner of working with people? If not, write "no changes."

Although there are numerous ways of provoking a discussion of health values, Simon likes the method of getting at value clarification through *weekly reaction sheets*. Each week for four or five weeks, the student is confronted with a series of questions for which he or she must write out answers. Basically the sheets ask the point blank question: did you act on any of your values this week? What did you do? Looking at how people live their lives in a systematic, non-moralizing fashion works to bring health issues to the forefront. Simon asks soul-searching questions. They can be applied to any intermediate and middle school health topic. Note how they progress to the action level:

1. What was the highpoint of your week?
2. With whom were you in emphatic disagreement or agreement this week?
3. Do you have any gripes about your educational program?
4. Did you work on any plans this week for some future adventure you are planning to have?
5. In what way could the week have been better?
6. Did you make any changes in your life this week?
7. What did you procrastinate about? Do you know?
8. Did you *act* on any of your values this week?

Answers to these questions serve to focus both student and teacher attention on value indicators such as purposes, aspirations, attitudes, interests, feelings, beliefs, problems, and obstacles that can be related to most health topics.

Donald Read has developed an interesting workbook suitable for upper elementary and middle school students that provides page after page of opportunities for students to respond to a number of health value situations.[14] His value clarification exercises and feedback schemes are especially worthwhile for classroom use.

ENRICHING HEALTH INSTRUCTION

Method continues to make a difference when some of the following points are kept in mind:

1. *Present day concepts of method are far removed from the days of the teacher-dominated classroom.* The emphasis upon the teaching of health facts and memorization of body parts has given way to an emphasis upon understandings which will improve living. Says Allan Cohen, a clinical psychologist from the University of California, "Treat kids as humans in discussion groups." Present objective evidence, and not just from textbooks. Focus on the person. Discuss social responsibility for youth by youth. Moreover, teach children to accept themselves for what they are and for what they can be. They need high expectations from others which will inspire them to be the best they can be. Said Goethe:

   If you treat an individual as he is, he will remain as he is, but if you treat him as if he were what he ought to be and could be, he will become what he ought to be and could be.

2. *Cooperative planning of the health lesson is time-consuming but it is well worth the effort.* Even in the kindergarten the children can and should begin to plan some of their activities. Cooperative planning for projects, units of work, parties, trips, and other classroom activities helps develop a sense of social responsibility, for children are concerned with the success of those activities which they themselves have planned.

3. *Health instruction lends itself most favorably to creative activity on the part of elementary school pupils.* There is hardly anything more personal than one's creative activity, but to be creative requires a definite setting, an atmosphere within the classroom conducive to freedom of expression. Practically all courses of study that border on some form of science present a number of opportunities for creativity. Health is no exception.

   Children are creative in different degrees in different media. They may paint, draw, engage in dramatic play, ex-

---

[14]Read, Donald A. *Looking In: Exploring One's Personal Health Values.* Englewood Cliffs, N.J.: Prentice-Hall, Inc., 1977.

press themselves through pantomime or impersonation or with puppets or other dramatic forms, may develop rhythms or dances, write music to be sung or played, make a simple musical instrument, model with clay, weave, cook, sew, build with blocks, and write stories or poems. These and many other related forms of expression are natural to children. A number of these experiences, when carried on during health instruction, may be drawn together in such a way as to supplement each other and enrich the whole school program.

4. *Health is taught accurately and from a positive viewpoint.* Well-being is emphasized rather than ill health. Health is associated with happy people and more productive living.

5. *In teaching health, certain learning practices and experiences are to be avoided.* Not ony are some activities ineffective but they also may be actually harmful. Avoid such things as the following:

Awarding artificial prizes for good habits of attendance in school or promoting "healthiest child" contests.

Scheduling health education on rainy days as a substitute for physical activity, thereby punishing the pupils because it rained.

Making children overly health conscious. There are already too many neurotic adults filled with fears and worries about their health.

Using one pupil in the class as an example of a defect.

Over-using parodies or nursery rhymes and songs.

Preaching good health and promising a long life. It is better to practice healthful living oneself and be the example of the moment.

6. *In health teaching, the wise teacher uses the classroom only as a useful adjunct or tool in learning.* Simply stated, the classroom has its limitations. It might at times be referred to as an educational roadblock, because it often places a barrier between student and teacher and frequently removes the world of books, ideas, and words from the real world. Fortunately, in many places, classrooms have changed. Freedom to learn is reflected in flexibility of various kinds of "furniture." Differentiated staffing benefits children by the variety of adults with whom they come in contact. And the library where children relax and read in attractive surroundings is seen more often.

Most children live in communities large enough to provide an excellent laboratory setting in which to seek the solutions to problems initiated in the classroom. The manner in which one seeks the solution is the meat of the experience. Cantril says that the very process of seeking the solution may be more satisfying than the end goal achieved.[15] He is referring here to the value placed on the process of seeking and

---

[15]Cantril, Hadley. *The Why of Man's Experience.* New York: The Macmillan Co., 1950, p. 202.

striving and the satisfactions derived from trying to determine direction or achieve a solution. It is what children mean when they exclaim, "Golly, that was fun!" or "I certainly enjoyed that game," and secretly regret that the game is over, no matter who won.

7. *Instruction in anatomy and physiology as a means of health education has its limitations.* The emphasis is controlled, for there is a tendency for pupils who have been taught with a maximum stress on anatomy and physiology to have less of an understanding of the basic health concepts than pupils taught with a minimum emphasis on these two helping sciences. This is not to say that one should omit reference to body structure and function. It is just a word of caution to those teachers who may find themselves teaching the names of bones and organs, and other similar facts and figures, without proper concern for the use of such knowledge by the students. Several pupil-interest surveys have revealed that some of the health studies of body functions have been "dry" indeed. And one of the dryest is the lesson on the circulation of the blood. With a little preplanning by teachers and pupils, such a topic may be taught in a way to satisfy the inherent curiosity of most of the class.

8. *Health facts brought out in the various methods of teaching are related to life situations.* This is a rewording of the old statement that knowledge is power but it is not necessarily so without understanding. Facts are facts, and they may be learned as such, but attitudes and habits do not change

Figure 9–3. Good teaching promotes involvement with fun. (Courtesy Society for Visual Education, Inc. Print SP 178 from picture-story print set.)

unless teaching methods provide for changes. Edna St. Vincent Millay wrote a poem, *Huntsman, What Quarry?* It clearly expresses the need for something more than facts.

Upon this gifted age, in its dark hours, rains from the sky a meteoric shower of facts . . . they lie unquestioned, uncombined. Wisdom enough to leech us of our ill is daily spun, but there exists no loom to weave it into fabric.

9. *Materials strengthen methods.* Teaching aids exist to facilitate the method. Because of them the method should be more meaningful. In the large 15″ × 20″ study print (Figure 9–3), the teacher employs this display aid to focus on germs. Cleaning tools are brought to class and demonstrated. A "mess" is made in one part of the classroom. Volunteers clean it up. Then drawings are shown of germs, rats, flies, and other things that thrive on dirt. The concept that germs live in dirt is put across.

A CLOSER LOOK AT PRACTICES

In the health teaching area, one responds to the answers from three questions:
1. What can students learn largely by themselves?
2. What can students learn from explanation largely by others?
3. What learning requires personal interaction among students and teacher?

The clever teacher may be able to apply almost any teaching method to health instruction. The following paragraphs explain the more common teaching techniques or practices with some comments relative to suitability for health teaching.

Lecture. Despite the admonitions of some people, there is little cause to condemn the lecture method. Properly applied in the grades, it can be used to bring basic health facts to the pupils, a necessary foundation for more work to follow. It need not be dry,

Figure 9–4. When interest is high the method is sound. (Courtesy National Education Association and Joe DiDio.)

authoritative, uninteresting, and unstimulating—criticisms sometimes launched by students.

With the short span of interest evidenced at the elementary level, the lecture by the teacher should probably be given in the form of a chat or story, informal and yet precise. Frequent repetition can produce hostility toward the communicator, greater rigidity in existing attitudes, and forgetting or distortion of previously received information.

The health lecture must be arranged carefully with the teacher using appropriate instructional aids to put across significant points. Facts about vitamins or the physiological effects of alcohol on the body may be given orally but they will probably be better retained and recalled if they evolve from student explorations and questioning.

Class Discussion.   A short lecture followed by preplanned discussion can be very effective in initiating a health unit. Discussing health information previously presented by the teacher gives meaning to the facts. Ideas are spread about through conversation. Conversation connotes reciprocity, not monopoly. "Discourse," says Pope, "is the sweeter banquet of the mind."

While there are many areas of the truth curriculum which require careful planning and preparation, it is nevertheless possible for a planned unit to have an unplanned beginning. The following lesson was the introduction for a unit on poison prevention in the first grade class of Anne Cornetta of Woburn, Massachusetts:

"We were discussing possible ways of helping mother around the house, with the hopes of deciding a few practical tasks which would be feasible for six-year-olds to carry out. One child announced that he could wash and wax the floors because he knew just where mother kept all her cleaning supplies—in the cabinets under the sink. A few others chimed in that they could do this, too, but some could not—their mothers kept these things on a high shelf where they could not reach them. It seemed best to abandon the discussion of helping mother, since the children seemed much more concerned with the reasons why cleaning fluids etc., should be out of reach; that even though they themselves were old enough to know better, little brother or sister or a visiting baby might get into them. The high interest expressed by the children prompted the development of a unit on this subject. To maintain this interest the following home assignment was given, watch the baby to see what he does when he is handed a small object (or almost anything). The next day someone had a report—he put it in his mouth! We then went on to name and list various things we must be careful of, illustrate and cut them out for display on the bulletin board. . . ."

There are a number of techniques which may be used to make the discussion more effective:

1. An overnight assignment, which requires some study or searching for ideas at home, will provoke a number of good questions the next day in class.

2. A list of questions, raised in earlier sessions and distributed prior to the discussion, helps the student who is a poor thinker. In studying teeth in the third grade, for example, questions such as these tend to generate personal curiosity: How many teeth do I have?

When will I have all of my permanent teeth?

Will baking soda and salt clean my teeth?

3. A cloister discussion or "buzz session" where the class is divided into small groups is often productive.

4. The "show and tell" technique promotes wide discussion, especially when "show" items are carefully chosen (see Figure 9–5).

The discussion also provides a chance for pupils to share their problems in class. Some things are elicited in discussion which may be the basis for trouble in later life. Children will often talk about their fear of the dark, the problems they have with younger brothers or sisters, or the fact that someone does not like them.

Psychologist Kurt Lewin has experimented with group discussion as a decision technique in influencing attitudes and behavior. In essence it allows no one to tell a group what to do; a trained person leads discussions so that decisions come from the group itself. Similarly, in health, individuals may be influenced more by their own decision than by one they are asked or forced to accept.

In one elementary school, the intermediate level of health instruction was measurably enriched and improved through the addition of the *Fishbowl* Technique:

1. Divide class by having them count off in 4's.

2. Arrange 1's and 2's in one part of the room; 3's and 4's should be in another part of the room.

3. Assign a leader and health subject. The 1's are talkers; 2's are observers.

4. *Observers* are not permitted to participate in discussion.

Figure 9–5. Studying cereals in class. The "show and tell" technique continues to hold interest. (Courtesy Cereal Institute, Inc.)

They watch to see that talkers are adding to group and not fooling around.
5. *Talkers* explore the subject together.
6. *Leaders* assume responsibility for getting everyone to talk—or listen.
7. After a set period the roles of talkers and observers are reversed.
8. Following the discussion, talkers and observers each tell the other "how he or she did" when he or she was the talker.
9. Class unites to have a larger discussion with all information reinforced by the teacher.

Fishbowl set up, an inner and outer group:

O = observer
X = talker

```
        O
      OXO
       XX
     OX  XO
     OXXO
        X
        O
```

10. An example of a Fishbowl discussion topic:

Your older brother (eighth grade) smokes. He brags to you how good it is and how all his friends smoke too. How does this affect you? What do you do?

Textbooks. Textbooks may be used so that they are classified as aids in the health instruction program. They may also be used as an effective method of health teaching.

Children cannot learn everything by experimenting or by first-hand experiences. Much is learned from reading textbooks, supplementary books, bulletins, magazines, and newspapers. Reading is sometimes condemned as a poor way to learn about health. It is often used so much that the health course degenerates into a course of reading about health. This criticism is leveled not against textbooks and reading as a method of learning but against the *way* in which reading is used. It must not be a cut and dried approach where the teacher says, "Today we are going to study hearing. Open your books to page 36, read the first four pages, and tell me what you have read." It is this kind of procedure that makes children dislike health education.

In the small elementary school where the teacher may not have enough time to prepare all of his or her own study materials, the textbook can be quite helpful. It should not be a crutch on the one hand or the Bible of the health class on the other. It is simply used as a common tool for all children. In the case of the example of a class about to study hearing, it would be better to engage in some exploratory activity before using the textbook. Children might be asked to bring things to class which make a sound. The next day all kinds of sounds could be demonstrated in class. A violin, a flute, a drum, a ticking watch, a whisper, all stimulate interest in how the ear actually hears sounds. Someone may say, "When I had a cold I couldn't hear very well. Why didn't the sound get into my ear?" This may be the oportune time to delve into the textbook, especially if it has a particularly good picture of the ear structure.

Textbooks, therefore, are useful as guides, and reading is an important tool in learning about health. The reading is done with a specific purpose—to solve a problem, to secure more information, to learn how to do an experiment, or to answer a question. Moreover, health stories can provide informational material which will arouse pupil interest in studying a topic. Most textbook publishers today think of the textbook as a focal point for learning and make available with it a number of other learning materials.

For a discussion of criteria for selecting textbooks and other printed materials, see page

Library. Because reading is more effective when it is done from several sources, the library method of teaching health holds considerable merit. Sources which supplement one another provide more information and present different points of view. It cannot be overstressed that the study of health should develop a scientific attitude in children. This means that pupils need to be open-minded, seek reliable sources for evidence, be curious, and know that there is a cause for everything. It means that pupils need a chance to appraise many health situations by experimenting and reading widely.

The library is well suited for note taking which can be a part of health research needed in problem-solving, independent study, and other learning practices. With the help of the librarian, properly selected reading materials are made available and pupils find things

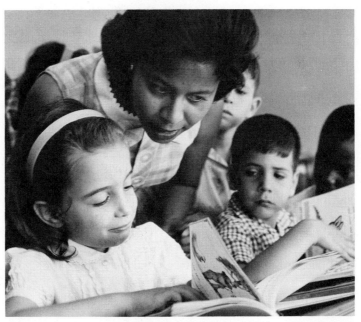

Figure 9–6. Quality textbooks present essential information. (Courtesy *Teach Me!* National Education Association.)

from books that simply cannot be discovered through observing, interviewing, and experimenting.

The elementary school library plays an important role in the entire school health program. Children need to be able to use it freely as a source of books, pamphlets, magazines, recordings, films, slides, maps, globes, reference books, atlases, dictionaries, and audio-visual projectors. The attitude of the classroom teacher toward the library usually determines how functional the library method of teaching about health becomes. The cooperative efforts of the teacher and librarian in setting up a health exhibit in the library or classroom often produce considerable pupil interest.

Problem Solving.   No pupil ever becomes an improved problem solver by filling in the blanks in a workbook, by looking up the definition of something, or by just living in the same room with a cage full of white rats and a set of health textbooks. Here the ancient laws of use and disuse apply. Pupils are better able to solve problems when they have solved previous problems—problems which mean something to them.

The older approach to teaching was to get students to master subject matter by relating it to real external life, thus demonstrating its utility. It was direct teaching. Now, children are encouraged to solve problems in their preferred ways, to use their best abilities, and to employ what they have already learned as tools in their problem-solving.

Solving problems is not something that takes place easily. Children have to want to find answers. They have to *discover* the problem first. They have to be disturbed, even frustrated, before they have the urge to set forth in search of health information. Motivation is involved here. In one school class the children, as they approached the end of the school day, were talking about eyesight. One boy asked the teacher to tell him how many people wear eyeglasses. Someone else wondered how many schoolchildren wore them. An overnight assignment was then made; the children were charged with "counting noses" and finding out how many people wore eyeglasses in their neighborhoods. Such near-at-hand problem-solving activity did much to provoke class discussion the following day.

In a more structured sense, Dacey views the inquiry and problem-solving process in six phases: (1) formulating an inquirable question, (2) formulating researchable questions, (3) developing a plan, (4) organizing and analyzing collected data, (5) evaluating the data, and (6) formulating an answer.[16]

In a southern school the dietitian was invited to tell about her duties to a fourth grade class. She indicated that she was distressed at the amount of food being left on the children's plates following the noon-hour lunch period. After some discussion, the class agreed that this was a problem and that they would accept the challenge to solve it. They formulated a plan of attack, divided into small groups, and made an on-the-spot survey of the school lunchroom during the

---

[16]Dacey, John S. *New Ways to Learn*. Stamford, Conn., Greylock Publishers, 1976, p. 171.

eating period. Upon returning to class and talking over the problem, it was decided that one way to solve the problem might be to organize a "Clean Plate Club." The dietitian decided to give it a try. She had buttons made, such as political candidates use, bearing the words CLEAN PLATE CLUB. All elementary teachers were given the number of buttons needed each day. Each day some buttons were recalled as occasions arose. Most teachers ate with their children and found it easy to observe the plate of each child. The pupils were so eager to wear the buttons that they made a real effort to eat all their food, even the food that they normally disliked. The original fourth grade problem solvers appraised the button situation and concluded, along with the dietitian, that they had successfully solved the problem. They had exercised the strength to act. This strength is what Rollo May calls "the power to do the valuing"—the courage to decide and act for oneself, which is the moving force of human growth. Kierkegaard calls it "the alarming possibility of being able." It can only come from within the person. The "too active" teacher, says Russell, is the one who is so structured that little is left to the students—it is a case of "teacher says," "teacher assigns," "teacher shows," "teacher questions," etc., and the pupils' opportunity to make choices for themselves is limited.[17]

Important health problems are usually made known with the help of the teacher. He or she often leads the way in discovering such items as community health hazards, causes of accidents and illnesses in school, causes of school absences, difficulties in eating, and personal unhappiness.

Problems are solved when children recognize the problems, gather pertinent data, verify and interpret the data, and present conclusions. Data may be gathered by reading, looking at pictures, viewing a film, taking a trip, experimenting, listening to a transcription, asking someone who is an authority, making a survey, and discussing the way we feel about a situation. Conclusions should be made in a general way so that they represent at least one solution to the problem.

Experiment. In many ways the experimental method of teaching health is related to problem solving. It is more formal, but it is founded on the same kind of pupil interest and is successful when there is a burning curiosity to *find out* why we act as we do.

This method is especially stimulating to upper grade schoolchildren who are entering the adventuresome period where they rise quickly to almost any challenge to discover and explore. This is the period that Charles Kettering spoke of when he expressed his views on his own aspirations at an early age. He was always intrigued with the "why." He wanted to know "why" the black cow could eat green grass and give pure white milk. It drove him to experiment in chemistry and biology and became a moving force in initiating his famous career.

---

[17]Russell, William. "A Method for Accommodating the Will—a New View," *Journal of Education*, 154:15–20, December 1971.

True conviction comes from testing and trying things out by oneself. Sometimes simple classroom or laboratory experiments involving the principles of food decay, moisture, or cleanliness, carry more conviction than many of the elaborately printed materials and expensive films one may obtain on the topic. The really effective experimental method requires a thorough organization. This is just as true with second graders as it is with secondary school pupils. Some of the points to keep in mind when setting up a health experiment are as follows:

1. Keep the experiment simple. Simple homemade equipment is often more satisfactory than the more elaborate kind.

2. Perform experiments or have them performed in such a manner as to cause children to think. Do not tell the answers or have the pupils read them. Permit them to experiment and find out.

3. Plan experiments carefully and let the pupils do much of the planning. If the plan fails, the pupils have some basis for deciding why it did not work since they were the ones who made the plan.

4. Warn pupils not to make sweeping generalizations from one small experiment. Most pupil experiments do not *prove* anything. They merely help pupils answer a question or understand an idea.

5. Permit pupils to perform the experiment themselves. They should work in groups if sufficient materials are available;

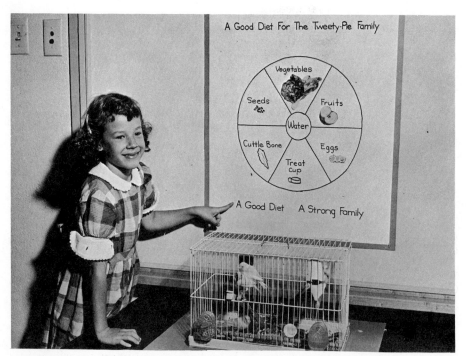

Figure 9–7. Bird feeding experiment. (Courtesy *Health Education Journal,* Los Angeles City Schools.)

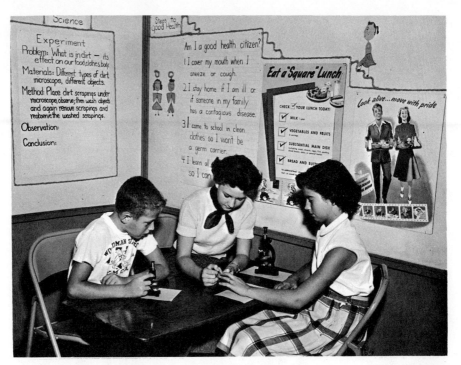

Figure 9–8. Examining fingernail dirt under the microscope. (Courtesy *Health Education Journal,* Los Angeles City Schools.)

otherwise the experiment should be carried out where all can see it.

6. Encourage children to originate experiments in order to solve a problem. If one pupil asks the teacher what would happen if the body did not get enough calcium, with a little encouragement another pupil might suggest an animal feeding experiment (Figures 9–7 and 9–8).

7. The basic purpose for performing an experiment is something much broader than just to answer the question raised. An experiment, to be worthwhile, should answer questions about things children see in the world about them. Too often this application to real-life situations is overlooked.

8. It is not necessary to have records of all experiments performed in the elementary school. The teacher may be guided by the idea, "Is there any reason for writing anything about this experiment?"

Children can experiment at every age. Even second graders can study moisture as it related to colds and sore throats by holding a damp cloth over a heater and observing what happens. Third graders can watch mold appear on a crust of bread and draw valid conclusions without going into any further experimentation. Some of the health experiments that have proven especially valuable over the years include:

Animal feeding experiments to measure the effect of certain foods on growth.

Individual height-weight measurements.

Decay of foods under different situations.

Analysis of the action of useful molds and bacteria in the making of vinegar and cheese.

The making of a satisfactory tooth powder.

Measuring air and water pollution.

Canning of foods.

Oxygen-consuming experiments involving the lighted candle in a glass jar over water, or done with a mouse instead of a candle.

Testing for starch and sugar in various foods.

Assessing sound levels.

Experiment—Starch

Directions for the Pupil

Problem

    a. How can we test for starch in foods?

    b. Do milk and the other foods listed have starch in them?

Materials

cornstarch	test tubes
baking soda	iodine
milk (dry)	dropper
sugar	test tube holders
potato	(optional)
hard-cooked egg	test tube rack
knife	(optional)

What to do

    a. Place about one half teaspoon of cornstarch in a test tube. Fill the test tube one half full of water. Add a drop of iodine. What happens? Make the same test with baking soda. Does the same thing happen?

    b. Try each of the other foods suggested under "Materials." In all cases soften the food thoroughly with water as is suggested for the cornstarch. In the case of potato and other solid foods, it is best to use scrapings. Look for any change in color in the water or on the bits of food.

What did you observe?

What do you think this experiment shows?

Supplementary Aids for the Teacher's Use

The test

    When a blue color is formed with iodine, starch is present. Cornstarch, which children know as a form of starch, gives the blue color as does potato. Soda, sugar, egg whites, and milk do not.

Testing additional foods

    Other foods may be brought from home to test, such as bread, oatmeal, cornmeal, ripe banana, apple, meat. The test shows best on solid foods. Omit dark-colored foods since the test is a color test. Of the above foods, only bread and cereals give the test for starch.

Equipment

    Cups might be used in place of test tubes. However, children like to use test tubes and this test offers an easy experience in handling chemical equipment. Test tubes, test tube holders, and a test tube rack might be borrowed from children's chemistry sets.

Use a tincture of about 1 per cent iodine. The test does not show well with strong iodine. It may be made weaker with alcohol or water.

Related questions and activities

Plants make starch. Where do they store their starch? Read to find out.

Do we use many foods that contain starch in our daily meals? If so, why?

What happens if you eat more food than your body uses for energy? If you are fat, name some foods of which you might eat less.

Babies, at first, use only milk in their diets. How, then, do they get what starch supplies in your food?

If a microscope is available, observe starch grains under the microscope. Drop a solution of iodine on the slide and observe again through the microscope. (Each grain of starch takes on a shiny bluish-purple appearance.)

The following animal experiment illustrates better than almost anything else the powerful motivational force inherent in a properly conceived and implemented experimental method. Throughout the experiment there is demonstrated a sustained interest of high degree. This is the report of a sixth grade experiment conducted, written up, and presented to the author by Annette Marco Penan of Jacksonville, Florida.

A Rat Experiment in the Sixth Grade

We received two white, albino, laboratory raised mice, 28 days old, from the National Dairy Council. Both were males; one weighed approximately 48 grams, the other 50 grams. They were brought to us on a Thursday morning complete with instructions regarding their care, a pair of white workman's gloves, and a gram scale.

Thursday and Friday we discussed the habits of rats, types, and differences, diseases, control, etc. We used the encyclopedias, science books, nature books, read the Pied Piper of Hamlin and played games. We compared rat ages with human ages, and made charts. Some of the boys made age comparison charts on many different types of animals—dogs, horses, elephants, etc.

The first thing I did was to go up and down the aisles and let every child touch the rats while I held them. I did not insist on everyone touching. I then explained how to pick them up so as not to frighten or bruise them, made them all promise to wear at least one glove to protect both the rat and themselves, and opened the rats mouths and showed the little sharp teeth. The entire time I caressed and petted the little things so that all the children could see how very gentle I was with them.

For fear of injury we all decided that possibly they had been handled too much already. After each and every child came by me and touched them again, we put them back in their box and they were not handled any more that day.

As soon as they settled down (both rats and children), we began to plan. I would have liked cages but the children made different arrangements—a bird cage and the case from a record player brought from home. (I still wonder what happened to the record player, but you never in your life saw such a fancy rat cage: the top with wire, the sides painted glass, fancy food dishes, little decorated boxes for them to sleep in, etc.) We kept the rats together until Monday when we began our experiment.

We discussed what we might be able to prove, and we decided to use good and poor breakfasts. We made rules for the care and feeding as well as the handling of the rats, agreed that the children would have to bring a note from home if they wanted to take one home to care for over the weekend, and that they would give the rats only the diets we planned. We would schedule the weekend home visits after the notes arrived. I took them the first weekend to avoid confusion.

Friday, while their cage was being cleaned, the children were permitted to handle the rats themselves, and those poor little things visited on every one of 36 desks that day.

Both rats had the same diet until Monday at which time they were both weighed and measured; there was still approximately 2 grams difference in their weight. The children put the heavier one on the good diet; the other on the poor.

After being weighed, each rat was put in a separate labeled cage. The class suggested names which we voted upon, and the rats' charts read like this:

Name of rat—Mr. Kingsize
Weight of rat at beginning_____
Weight of rat at completion_____
Age of rat at beginning_____
Age of rat at completion _____
Date demontration starts _____
Diet of rat: Whole grain bread or cereal, plus milk, plus fruit, plus bread and butter, plus egg

Name of rat—Mr. Regular
Weight of rat at beginning_____
Weight of rat at completion_____
Age of rat at beginning_____
Age of rat at completion _____
Date demonstration starts_____
Diet of rat: Sweet roll and coffee

The children brought in the food which we kept in containers. Milk and coffee were fresh every day from the lunch room.

Daily records were kept of their appearance, activity disposition, etc. Every Monday morning they were weighed and their weight charted on a large line graph. The children kept a small graph on graph paper in their note books.

During the weeks that followed we studied about the basic foods, had posters and charts on display, made posters and charts, wrote stories, kept a diary on the daily changes in the rats, made booklets, worked arithmetic problems comparing ages, plotted weights (gains and losses), studied weights and measures, graphs (line and bar), charts, printing. The children took care of the rats—committees to clean, others to feed, others to weigh and chart, etc.

Rat cartoons appeared, booklet covers were made, the mothers came to see the progress, and children started eating good breakfasts. Other children in the school came into the room to see the rats, so we issued a weekly bulletin on the changes appearing, the weights and dispositions.

The rats performed beautifully. Mr. King-size became tremendous, developed full of mischief. Poor little Mr. Regular developed a scaly, spotted tail, feet and ears became dry and rough, hair shaggy and dull, a definite contrast to the beautiful ermine coat of Mr. Kingsize. Mr. Regular became sulky and twice I was afraid we were going to lose him, but I cheated after the children went home and I gave him a little milk and dry oatmeal and he'd perk up a little. After four weeks the contrast was great and the children were beginning to worry. Since one of the purposes had been served, the children were delighted when I suggested not continuing for the full six weeks that we had originally decided upon.

We voted to see if we should reverse the diets or to just put Mr. Regular on the same diet as Mr. Kingsize. It was unanimous that the diets *not* be reversed, so both rats then had the same diet. Within two weeks' time Mr. Regular started catching up to Mr. Kingsize and there was a sharp upsweep on the graphs. By the end of four weeks they weighed almost the same, and Mr. Regular's tail lost its scaly look, his eyes became larger and brighter, and his fur grew in thickness and became shiny. (As one of the little boys pointed out to me though, there was still a difference in their sex organs. I hadn't noticed, but there was.)

All these weeks the children had been making booklets about the experiments. We took pictures each week and then made a booklet to give to the Dairy Council containing selections from the children's booklets and pictures by the children together with the photographs.

The experiment over, and the children much more aware of the need of a balanced diet, they became more conscious of their own growth and development. They were more alert in the mornings; only one or two ever fell asleep in class (TV late show—not lack of breakfast). Some mothers complained that they had to fix breakfast now, others were happy. One child fixed his own breakfast, but became a problem when selecting food; he insisted on buying certain items.

Any child who brought a note from home saying he could have a rat had his name put in a box. At the Christmas party we drew the names, and the rats went home with two little girls. The last week of school Mr. Regular came back to visit with us for the day. The children greeted him with great excitement—their little friend was hale and hearty. They were sorry that Mr. Kingsize had been sent to rat heaven by a neighborhood dog, but they were glad that it hadn't been Mr. Regular, who had been such a good sport and had taught them so much.

The number of health-related learnings that can be brought about through experimentation is great indeed. In one city classroom in Niagara Falls, New York, elementary level children experimented with the incubation of fertile chicken eggs and caring for the chicks through adulthood. They were active students in the process, exhibiting the following behaviors.[18]

> *Observed* the daily development of the embryo by candling the eggs and viewing slides.
>
> *Used* a stethescope to discover that no heartbeat was heard until after the third day of incubation
>
> *Saw* eyes develop from tiny specks within a day's time
>
> *Made* charts recording incubator temperature, stages and rate of growth, and later food consumption
>
> *Explored* mitosis, fertilization and birth
>
> *Preserved* specimens of growth stages from a three-year-old embryo to a nineteen-day-old chick, using formaldehyde
>
> *Discussed* dominant strains after a Columbia Wyandotte rooster fertilized the eggs of Rhode Island Red hens one year
>
> *Tested* chickens' responses to noises
>
> *Gave talks* on hatching chicks to other classes of students
>
> *Explained* to visiting primary grade pupils that the incubator takes the place of the mother hen
>
> *Described* how chicks are able to peck their way out of shells
>
> *Investigated* why chicks must be inoculated by a veterinarian to prevent respiratory ailments
>
> *Investigated* differences between chickens bred for egg laying and for meat
>
> *Compared* the baby chicks' brief period of helplessness at birth with the longer period for the human baby
>
> *Identified* gestation periods for several animals and noted how early they adapt to their environment

---

[18]Adapted from the report of Isobel K. Hobba. "Hatching Chicks and Concepts," *Instructor*, April 1971, p. 42

Shared fresh eggs laid by hens they had grown from incubator to maturity

Primary school children can easily experiment. In the air and water pollution areas they may ask:

1. *What pollutants appear in the air?*

    Procedure: a) First collect pictures showing industrial smoke and smog. Post these.

                b) Put the cap on a large clean mayonnaise jar to represent clean air.

                c) Hold a similar jar upside down and burn 4 to 5 wooden matches in it. Put the cap on right away. It will represent dirty air.

    Note: The dirty air will contain oxides of sulfur and nitrogen, as well as hydrocarbons and carbon monoxide.

    Outcome questions:

                a) Would we like breathing this air?

                b) How does it affect throat, lungs, and breathing?

                c) How can we get rid of air pollutants?

2. *Do oceans become polluted?*

    Procedure: a) Place a large dishpan on the table.

                b) Toss into the pan a few tin cans, a paper tissue, some pieces of glass, some leftover food, some food coloring to represent industrial chemicals, and a cup of hot water to represent nuclear energy plant wastes.

    Outcome questions:

                a) Could fish and other marine life live in this "ocean"?

                b) Is there a way to stop polluting the oceans and other large bodies of water?

Help in setting up a number of experiments for students to carry out may be obtained from several sources. Nelson and Lorbeer have an easy-to-use manual.[19] Fodor and Glass, in their manual, set up numerous sixth grade experiments that tie in directly with preconceived concepts and behavioral objectives.[20] Experiments cover such topics as pulse rate, blood pressure, emphysema, bell jar activity, senses of taste and smell, mini-lung, goldfish, and water demonstrations, and others. Somewhat along the same line, but to a far lesser degree of concentration, is the U.S. Public Health Service booklet, *Smoking and Health Experiments, Demonstrations, and Exhibits* which is available through the U.S. Government Printing Office. Experimentation with foods in the classroom is advanced in the booklet, *The Evaporated Milk Story*. It is available from the U.S. Public Health Service, 910 Seventeenth Street, N.W., Washington, D.C. 20006. The National Dairy Council has done the same with foods but in greater detail in their two booklets, *Let's Take Milk Apart.*

---

[19]Nelson, Leslie W. and Lorbeer, George C. *Science Activities for Elementary Children*, Dubuque: William C. Brown Co., Publishers, 1975.

[20]Fodor, John T. and Glass, Lennia H. *Cigarette Smoking and Health—A Teacher's Guide*. Granada Hills, California: HRA Inc., 1971.

Demonstration.　Children like to be entertained; they like to see things done before their eyes, especially if there is an element of the mysterious which they do not understand. The teacher who describes some phase of the body function through skillful demonstration encourages the class to want to do it themselves.

A sixth grade health class, in studying the principles of respiration, may observe a demonstration of artificial resuscitation or cardiopulmonary resuscitation and follow this by a practice period in which everyone gets an opportunity to "revive" and "be revived." In one primary grade the cleanliness of animals was discussed. In class the children watched a real cat clean itself with its paws. One of the pupils combed and brushed a long-haired dog. Another pupil demonstrated how elephants in South Africa saunter down to the nearest river toward sundown and drink and bathe. This was effective.

Actually, there are three kinds of demonstrations: teacher demonstrations, individual pupil demonstrations, and group demonstrations. All three require pre-planning in order to be effective. Individual and group demonstrations often promote more class interest than those performed by the teacher.

Examples of demonstrations that may be performed by class members for everyone to see follow:

A. *Air Pollution and Smog*
1. The best way to see that the air is clean is to keep as much dirt as possible from getting into it.
2. Controls have included "smog alerts" that have closed down factories and stopped motor traffic when serious pollution threatened.
3. *Produce smog* by the condensation of water vapor on solid particles like smoke.
   a. Insert a lighted match in a gallon jug to make a small amount of smoke.
   b. Blow, with the mouth pressed firmly on the mouth of the jug, and release the compressed air quickly. A smog will form in the jug.
   c. Repeat the activity without the smoke from the match.

B. *Ecology and Clean Water*
1. Most of the earth's surface is covered with water and every type of water area supports living creatures, each interdependent in the life chain.
2. Our limited water supply must be preserved and in some cases purified.
3. *Illustrate the life chain.*
   a. Put together a glass dish view of water, soil, roots, and soil animals. (Details may be obtained from *Water World Heroes Teacher's Guide,* supplied free from Nabisco, Inc., Cambridge, Massachusetts 02139.)

Glass dish allows view of water, soil, roots, and soil animals. Screen confines insect larvae and adults.

This shows the requirements for plant growth, water, nutrients (soil), support (soil), and light. The plants are producers; insect larvae feeding on the leaves are examples of consumers. Dead leaves and insects drop to soil and decay. Soil animals, like the earthworm, help to break down this material.

C. *Water Pollution*
   1. Water flows because of land elevations, from high mountains to streams, and into lakes, rivers, and swamps, and eventually to the sea.
   2. *Illustrate land erosion and water pollution.*

   Water sprinkled on the painted foil will flow down "gullies," collect in "lakes," overflow these into larger streams or "rivers" on the way to collection tray (ocean). Paint will wash off where water flows leaving a chart of a "watershed."

D. *Smoking Machine*
   1. The amount of tar in one or more cigarettes can be shown by a tar separating apparatus.

2. Varying amounts of tar in different brands of cigarettes can be compared by "smoking" filtered and unfiltered cigarettes and collecting the residue.

3. *Assemble a smoking machine.*

Equipment:
Large gallon jar with a two-hole stopper
Cigarettes
Delivery tubes (glass)
Cigarette holder
Vacuum pump

Procedure:
Assemble cigarette tar separating apparatus as shown in diagram.
Fill the gallon jar half full with water.
Place cigarette in intake and light.
Pump vacuum pump so as to draw smoke from cigarette into gallon jar and water.
Pump until cigarette is burned completely. Replace with additional cigarettes until tars can be seen in water.
Examine color of water and smell the liquid.

E. *Breathing and Disease*

1. Respiration depends upon lung elasticity and the power to contract.

2. *Assemble a bell jar* for demonstration.

Equipment:
Bell jar
Forked glass tubing
One-hole rubber stopper
Rubber sheet or membrane
Balloons similar in size and elasticity

Procedure:
Blow up one balloon and allow it to remain inflated for a day or two. When ready for demonstration, deflate the balloon and note that it remains enlarged and stretched.
Insert an unused balloon into the used one and note the space or air pocket surrounding the new balloon.
Attach a new single balloon to one of the ends of the forked glass tube and the double balloon to the end of the other tube. Fasten a rubber sheet or membrane across the bottom of the bell jar to simulate the diaphragm.

Pull down on the center of the rubber membrane and observe the balloons fill with air. Note the effect of the double balloon on amount of expansion which takes place. Push the rubber membrane back up into the jar a short way to simulate exhaling. Note the difference in the deflation of the "lungs."

The action of filling and emptying the balloons may be compared to respiration; if both lungs are functioning properly, they inflate and deflate properly. But if the alveoli of the lungs have been stretched too thin, as in emphysema, air pockets form in the lung tissue. The contractile power of the lungs is destroyed.

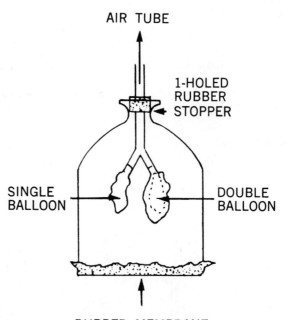

AIR TUBE

1-HOLED RUBBER STOPPER

SINGLE BALLOON

DOUBLE BALLOON

RUBBER MEMBRANE

Small Group Study. Small groups generally work independently on a problem in which all are interested. Three or four pupils may work together or there may be as many as ten or twelve. One health topic may be initiated by the creation of four or five small groups who will consider the several aspects of the topic.

Dramatic Play and Dramatization. To the child, play is real. It is full of meaning. Through this natural expression, a wealth of learning is acquired. Mimetics and action stories are common activities in the play of growing boys and girls. One sees children imitating the athlete, the mother, the physician, the nurse, and many other personalities from everyday life.

Dramatic play is unrestrained and unrehearsed. In the kindergarten and first grade the pupils generally prefer to play alone. Eight year olds will begin to play as a group. The teacher often finds that one has only to suggest a theme and eager, creative children will start to dramatize it as they see fit. Because of the high pupil interest in dramatizations, the method is a good one to use in teaching health.

All seasons of the year lend themselves to dramatizations of health topics. At Thanksgiving time, for example, the story of the nutritious and tasty cranberry can be told. It is a colorful fruit to consider for stories.[21] So highly were cranberries prized by the Indian tribes in southeastern Massachusetts that they made a gift of them to the Pilgrims who cooked them into a sauce to serve with wild turkey and geese. It is believed that cranberries brightened the Pilgrims' first Thanksgiving feast in 1621. Moreover, the health-giving qualities of cranberries were recognized almost immediately and in the early period of America's development, whenever vessels left New England's shores, they carried barrels of cranberries in the hold—not for trade but for the sailors to eat. Just as the English seamen prevented scurvy by eating limes, so American sailors ate cranberries, and in the Middle West, where scurvy was a scourge of the logging camps, cranberries were served regularly.

Health plays, created by the pupils from a classroom experience, are generally the most valuable. In discussing the maintenance of one's personal health through proper physical examinations, the class may decide to dramatize a visit to the school health service or the office of the family physician.

For many years puppets have been successfully used to put across certain concepts in elementary education. Puppets are fascinating to the average boy and girl; they can make statements that will be remembered longer than those made by the teacher. Interest is maintained at an even higher level when the puppets are made by the members of the class (see Figure 9–1).

In using puppets for health teaching, fantasy and imagination must be separated from accurate health information. Timmreck supplies a number of essential details about puppet playhouses, student puppeteers, and the proper use of puppets to teach health concepts.[22]

Sometimes the dramatization takes the form of an organized play. There are a number of practical ways of making the play effective:

1. Try to get as many pupils associated with the play as possible.
2. Use a small stage or platform instead of the crowded classroom if this can be arranged. Do not worry about the absence of backdrops and props; it is part of the fun and, after all, "the play's the thing."
3. Try an arena-style performance. Here the audience surrounds the actors on all four sides, adding to the intimacy of the situation and helping even the most detached pupil to feel that he or she is a part of the performance.
4. Simply assign children to parts and proceed to read the play without attempting to act it out. Although less effective than the acted version, this method does promote discussion.

The Health Project. This has much in common with the problem-solving method. It calls for the study of a problem which is organized by the teacher and pupils in the form of a project or task to be accomplished. It may mean experimenting or carrying on a sur-

---

[21]For a useful teacher's guidebook, *Cranberries, America's Native Fruit,* write to Ocean Spray Cranberries, Inc., Hanson, Mass.

[22]Timmreck, Thomas C. "Creative Health Education Through Puppetry," *Health Education,* 9:40–41, January/February 1978.

vey, interview, or discussion in an effort to ascertain the facts applicable to the particular health question.

The first requirement in a project is to identify and define a health problem which merits study. Goals are established as in the problem-solving method but they appear to be broader in the project method.

Creative Activities. When children express themselves without restraint and without teacher control, they are usually being creative to some degree. Imaginative and creative children may develop and act upon a health topic in several ways—through dramatizations, mimetics, and creative play. These have already been referred to. Another way is through creative writing. Older children who enjoy writing are capable of treating a health problem rationally by writing about it. The outlet for this activity is through the school paper or possibly through the local newspaper.

Creative rhythms is another technique in teaching that is generally overlooked. Creative dance permits the child to express, communicate, and enjoy. In the process of dance-making the pupil plans, experiments, selects, and appraises a number of movements with the help of the teacher. The dance may be interpretive, such as playing the part of a "happy toothbrush," or it may be dramatic and be a part of a story danced by the whole group. Usually it is descriptive—a poem, song, or an idea is conveyed through movement—high like a cloud, low like a caterpillar, fast like a squirrel, or slow like a snowman melting in the sun.

Teachers have to be creative too. Their task is to encourage pupils to see new relationships. They need to ask the question: "Can you imagine" more often. Food, for example, can be discussed unimaginatively in terms of vitamin and mineral content or it can be explored in terms of its color, taste, smell, and general attractiveness where it is served.

Once the imagination is stimulated, it is possible for creativity to emerge. Furthermore, it is fostered when each pupil is allowed to think about a health issue all by himself or herself—with no right or wrong answer required immediately. William Glasser, who wrote *The Identity Society,* would agree; for he sees the problem of school failure in all subject matter areas very much related to pupil feelings and personal identity. This is another reason why value clarification, mentioned earlier in this chapter, is so important in health teaching.

Consider the opportunity for creative activity in a health unit where the teacher gets close enough to children to reach value indicators. This can be accomplished by choosing somewhat innovative learning activities. For example, upper elementary students studying mental health will find the coat of arms activity most rewarding.

Each student is given a mimeographed sheet with the outline of a coat of arms. It is divided into six different sections. In each of the sections, the children use symbols, pictures, and numbers to correspond to: 1) Two things I do well, 2) Three things I would wish for, 3) My proudest moment, 4) A value I wouldn't budge from, 5) The saddest moment of my life, and 6) Two words I would like people to use to describe me and two words I would not like people to use to describe me. Or, there could be variations for third or fourth grade children as follows:

Coat of Arms

Two things you do well	Two things you're working toward
Two beliefs you have that won't change	Two things you love
Two things that represent the world to you	Two things you would change

Although a number of studies have found values clarification to be helpful in reaching health goals, Meeks cautions that using this method just for "fun" serves no real purpose; it must be "integrated with decision-making skills, behavioral objectives, content, and evaluation."[23]

Field Trips.   In one New York school, the second grade planned a trip to the zoo to observe the eating habits of animals. They asked the following questions:

"What do we want to know?"
"How shall we go?"
"How shall we prepare?"
"How shall we behave on the trip?"
"What will we need to do?"

They decided on the following:

Talk with parents, friends, neighbors, and teachers
Obtain further information from books and other aids
Trace the route on a map of the city
Use money
Estimate time and distance
Prepare a report about the trip

Although the trip was a short-term experience, it was beneficial in terms of health instruction and in relating to other subject matter fields such as art, music, mathematics, science, language arts, and social studies.

---

[23]Meeks, Linda. "The Use and Abuse of Values Clarification in the Lifestyle Approach to Health Education," *Health Values: Achieving High-Level Wellness,* 1:82–85, March/April 1977.

The health area is rich in opportunities for impressive field trips. Worthwhile excursions may be taken to the dentist's office, the police department, the cannery, the bakery, the dairy, the food-processing plant, and the water works. Exercise caution because it is easy to abuse this method of instruction. Trips should be made only when there is a real reason for going. The excursion is made as an integral part of the school health lesson that is in progress. Children studying the source of a water supply and how and why it is made pure may have a natural curiosity for wells, streams, types of soil, germs, purification, and the city water works. At this stage in the topic, they are ready to plan a trip to the water works to see how water is purified, what filter beds look like, how chlorine and sodium fluoride are added to the water supply to protect the health of the people, and many other items that are appropriate to consider at the time. A follow-up discussion is engaged in upon returning to the classroom; this tends to anchor the experience in the minds of the pupils. Thus "going to see" can be a most enjoyable and instructive way to learn.

Construction Activities.   Construction activities include everything from using the hammer and saw to build a model playground to using paste, tape, and staples to set up a novel three-sided health exhibit. There can be as much work involved in this method of instruction as there is in the project or problem-solving methods. Research, reading, discussion, and creative expression are background activities for the successful completion of an item under construction.

Pupil interests have much to do with method. In one study of Chicago schoolchildren, it was discovered that about 92 per cent of the first and second graders said that they like to make or construct things. It is possible, therefore, that teachers have underestimated the value of working with the hands.[24]

Health teaching in the primary grades permits the sandbox to be used for building grocery stores, farms, irrigation ditches, and city roads and parks. Several work tables, complete with tools, encourage the construction of models of such items as teeth from clay, toothbrush holders from wood, safety patrol emblems from tin, napkin rings from leather, metal, or wood, shower room slippers from cardboard, attractive handkerchiefs from colored pieces of cloth, and many other health related items. The object, of course, is to make sure that all constructed items are directly related to the health instruction topic.

Some examples of construction activities which may be related to health teaching are:

1. Construct simple wastebaskets.
2. Make simple pencil clips to help impress children with the need for carrying pencils safely.
3. As a workshop project, intermediate grade students can make a baseball equipment rack.

---

[24]Pupils must do things with their own hands. Because the potter works with his hands in shaping the clay, and because he is sensitive to the properties of the mix and its relationship to firing, color, and texture, he becomes changed as a person. He is as much transformed by his art as the clay is.

① CUT THE ABOVE PATTERN FROM A SHEET OF CARDBOARD 26" X 16". (LARGER OR SMALLER BASKETS MAY BE MADE IF DESIRED.)

② BEND ON DOTTED LINES TO SHAPE OF BASKET.

③ GLUE FLAPS TO MAKE SECURE.

Although cleverly constructed items encourage other children to try their skill and do likewise, their greatest value is obtained at the moment the individual or small group works on the particular project. There is genuine meaning to the child in a spot map built with colored pins to show the different types of accidents in the school and on the school grounds. There is value in mounting pictures, building charts and graphs, painting a picture of human anatomy, assembling a collection of foods, diagramming the local fire alarm system, putting together bird feeding trays, constructing a health museum, and dozens of similar purposeful activities.

Educational Games. Almost everyone knows that if something can be made to seem like play, it can be learned quickly. Purposely making a game of something, therefore, is sound methodology.

Slow learners, say researchers, are the chief beneficiaries of games—especially when games supplement other educational programs, making real and vivid material that sometimes seems abstract in a textbook.

Games should be carefully planned and the children should know what the goals are. Games provide many opportunities for an expression of characteristics conducive to optimum social health. Properly conceived, there are many chances for each child to demonstrate cooperation, group loyalty, leadership, and fair play.

Numerous examples can be cited showing how to use a game situation to further the learning of a particular health topic. Some illustrations follow:

1. Use a posture relay in teaching about posture. This is a regular relay race, except that the pupils running must carry a flat object such as a blackboard eraser on their heads. Point out to the class the difficulty in this feat when one does not assume a plumbline posture.

2. Make up riddles. Divide the class into two teams. For example, in discussing the teeth, one pupil says, "I am thinking of something we should do before going to school each morning." Using his or her watch, the teacher notes the time it takes for the other team to guess the correct answer. Riddles are alternated between teams, with the winning team being the one that has the lowest total time.

3. To teach pedestrian safety to primary graders, have pupils draw a floor map of a busy intersection. Assign children as

HEY, LOOK A SMOKING PUZZLE!

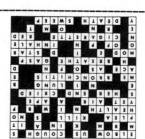

Published by National Tuberculosis and Respiratory Disease Association   12/70

CHRISTMAS SEALS FIGHT
Emphysema...TB...Air Pollution...Smoking
IT'S A MATTER OF LIFE AND BREATH
© NTRDA

Across

1. Arm Joint.
4. We.
*6. Smokers often suffer from annoying, chronic _____.
10. Opposite of "out".
11. In a game of tag, the person who must catch the others is _____.
*12. An appeal. (Begging someone to stop smoking for their own good health.)
*15. To cause death (Cigarettes _____ many smokers.)
16. Opposite of "yes".
*17. Freedom from physical disease or pain. (Everyone wants to have good _____.)
22. Rhymes with "bet".
*23. Cigarette smoke pollutes the _____ we breathe.
25. A large monkey.
27. He and she, or him and _____.
*28. If one must smoke, it is best not to smoke the cigarette to the _____ because the tar and nicotine become more concentrated.
30. Past tense of cry.
*32. A cigarette smoker runs ten times as great a risk of death from _____ cancer as a nonsmoker.
34. Myself.
*36. A serious lung disease characterized by an inflammation in the lining of the bronchial tubes.
38. In playing cards it is higher than a King and lower than a Two.
39. To the same extent. (She swam _____ well as he did.)
*40. Emphysema patients find it hard to _____ .

Down

*41. Many emphysema sufferers actually have to _____ for breath.
45. Contemporary clothing style
48. Solar system twinkler.
*50. From, as a cause or motive. (To die _____ lung cancer.)
*53. Every time you _____ a cigarette you let in a complex mixture of smoke particles and gases, many of which are poisonous.
*54. Leaves a bad taste in your mouth and smells up your clothes.
56. Bright color.
*58. The _____ rate of smokers is about 70% higher than that of nonsmokers.
*59. Cilia act like little brooms to _____ the dirt from the lungs.

Down

*1. A respiratory disease. The lungs lose their elasticity and hold in too much air.
*2. Smoking can cause shortness of _____. (One of the reasons athletes don't smoke!)
3. Abbreviation for "William".
*5. Smoking stains and yellows the _____ on one's fingers.
*6. Efficient little brooms which clean our lungs, but can be paralyzed by cigarette smoke.
7. Opposite of "off".
8. Automobile fuel.
*9. If a cigarette smoker will _____ smoking, his life expectancy will increase.
11. See #10 across.
13. Name of boy or girl.
14. Short for Albert.
*18. Mixture in cigarettes that coats the lungs and slows down their normal action.
19. Short for "hello".
*20. Cigarette manufacturers are required by law to print a _____ on all packages.
21. Small insect which makes honey.
24. Syllable on the musical scale between "do" and "mi".
26. Farm animals from which we get ham.
*29. A poison in cigarettes that makes the heart beat faster and quickens breathing.
*30. If a person is unable to quit smoking, he should at least _____ down.
*31. The preferred entrance for outside air into the respiratory system.
*32. A cigarette smoker can take as many as 8 years off his _____ .
*33. A great many fires are caused by people who smoke in _____, and fall asleep.
35. A repetition of sound, a resounding.
*37. Lung cancer was a _____ disease until smoking became widespread.
*42. Smoking is messy, and often leaves _____ on clothing and furniture.
*43. It is smart not to even _____ smoking.
44. People who are ill often have little color and are _____ .
*45. Cigarettes are costly and a waste of _____ .
46. Nickname for doctor.
*47. Many more smokers than nonsmokers _____ from heart disease and lung cancer.
49. #56 across.
*51. One-fourth of all accidental _____ is caused by careless smokers.
*52. Heavy smokers often puff and _____ as they climb stairs.
55. A type of truck which pulls cars.
57. #34 across.

* Terms which apply to smoking and health.

(May be torn off)

SOLUTION

police officers, pedestrians, and automobile drivers. Cardboard discs may be fashioned as steering wheels. Simulate normal traffic conditions.

4. Use a playhouse situation and emphasize home safety. Children play the parts of different family members.

5. A simple group game of "squat tag" may contribute to mental health, especially if the pupils realize that they are accepting the rules of the game and are having fun playing. The person being chased simply has to squat down to keep from being "It."

6. Play a game of "Health Detectives." Children report on what they have seen and heard each day that pertains to health. One child may have seen the soccer team practicing; a bicycle rider may have seen someone else riding at night without a light; one child may have noticed that children do not run up and down the stairs in the school; someone else may casually point out that Sally Jones has a runny nose—and many more.

7. Use mimetics in primary grades. When discussing pets and home safety, have the class walk like cats, run like dogs, or hop like rabbits. Music may be used and rhythm developed around a theme. For example, sunflowers grow tall in the sun. As a posture activity the children may stretch high with their arms in an effort to grow high like sunflowers.

8. Identify objects by taste, odor, or sound while blindfolded. Divide the class into teams. This will help motivate the class in studying the interrelationship of the senses. Some materials to have on hand for the game might include a piece of chocolate, a spoiled orange, sour milk, or a musical record.

9. Distribute copies of the smoking crossword puzzle available from the National Tuberculosis and Respiratory Disease Association.

10. Play the game where a pupil spins a wheel made out of oaktag or heavy cardboard. The wheel is divided into triangular sections. Each section contains a group of unassoci-

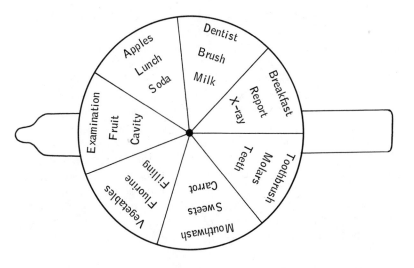

ated words. The pupil writes sentences using one of the words in each section.
Sample sentences:

The dentist filled my tooth.
I brush my teeth after eating.
Milk is good for my teeth.
I will eat candy only at the end of meals.

11. Ask children to bring colorful pictures of food clipped from magazines. Mount these illustrations on lightweight cardboard and cut to make a jig-saw puzzle.
12. Write "mixed-up" words on the chalkboard or duplicate lists and distribute them to children. Let pupils unscramble the letters to make words which are names of foods. Here are examples:

iklm	milk
draeb	bread
gge	egg
epalp	apple

13. Play food charades. Pupils may take turns acting out something to do with food, such as making a cake, peeling an apple, and so on. Whoever guesses the answer has the next turn of being "It."

Programmed Instruction. Programmed health instruction has been employed in a number of communities because it provides the individual pupil with organized health information which can be learned with an immediate knowledge of results.

The Behavioral Research Laboratories programmed a *First Aid* manual which Johnson & Johnson took over for distribution. It has been used with thousands of students throughout the country and is designed for sixth grade use. There is a procedure for using the manual and the first aid film strip which accompanies it. A teacher's instruction manual and a test manual are also available on a complimentary basis. Students work with their own manual and since it is different from most workbooks, the novelty seems to appeal to children.

Other health programs which are a part of the American Health and Safety Series and are distributed by Behavioral Research Laboratories include programmed instruction titles: *Body Structure and Function, Personal Health, Nutrition, Safety,* and *Prevention of Communicable Disease*. These programmed learning experiences provide continuity between the easier and the more difficult health concepts by acquainting the pupil with the organized nature of knowledge. Because the learner can proceed at his or her own speed, he or she is not threatened by the task; the pupil knows he or she is learning and anxiety should be somewhat reduced.

Youth to Youth. As already indicated in Chapter 8, under smoking education, the use of older children to instruct younger children can be a very effective kind of education for healthful living.

In this case the relationship between the "teacher" and the "pupil" is often an exciting experience for both, with the enthusiasm of the one affecting the other. Such a person-to-person contact frequently stimulates student actions that no other teaching ingredient can match.

Role Playing. Health concepts can be explored, feelings expressed, and self-concepts improved when pupils act out a role. There is usually opportunity for spontaneous dramatization, a chance to switch roles, and an evaluation-discussion. The teacher has the responsibility of assisting students in identifying and defining what they are experiencing.[24]

Miscellaneous Techniques. *Storytelling,* an age-old device, has always been a powerful way of impressing youngsters with health facts, especially if the information is accurate and the storyteller skilled in the art. Numerous good health stories are available in textbooks and supplementary readers.

The *guest speaker*—the physician, dentist, police officer or dogcatcher, for example—is often a welcome relief in the average classroom. Such people bring life to the class. They are from the world of reality outside the school and are sometimes able to put across a particular health recommendation when the regular classroom teacher has difficulty.

---

[24]For a number of examples see Teper-Singer, Lynn, "The Many Faces of Role Playing," *Health Education,* 7:34–35, November/December 1975.

Figure 9–9. Enjoying the seriousness of role playing. (Courtesy American Alliance for Health, Physical Education, and Recreation.)

Oral presentations have their place in health teaching. Good reports resulting from research, problem-solving, experimentation, library work, and readings need to be skillfully presented to the class. Individual pupil presentations of this nature, followed by class discussion, represent a useful instruction technique.

The *anecdote* represents an interesting tale, narrative, or description of some person or event in health. It is used, for example, to give an account of the life of a man like Lister or Pasteur, or to depict the conditions present in a disease-ridden land such as Egypt.

Counseling with groups or with individuals has become one of the most successful ways of changing health behavior. In dealing less with health facts and more with individual personalities, it tends to "hit home" and bring about changes in health practices and attitudes. It is not a classroom technique but is one especially suited to the school setting where the teacher has a few moments here and there to talk with and guide the members of the class.

The use of *student leaders* is a first-rate method of teaching. Leaders may assist in the classroom and on the playground. They may help the teacher inspect for cleanliness or form patrols for safety. New leaders should be chosen as often as possible.

Independent study may be employed when certain individuals show a keen interest in a health topic. It may be a short-term topic but some phase of it is of such concern to some pupil or pupils that permission is granted to pursue the topic further to satisfy personal curiosity. This may be done with or without infringing on class time and it permits the teacher to provide challenging work and study for the especially gifted child.

A *Health Education Fair* has been carried on with much general interest in a number of schools. Its purpose is not only to motivate students in health education but also to enlist the support of community groups in assisting the schools. Students prepare health projects which are exhibited and judged by representatives of the community health agencies. In Norfolk, Virginia, the fair has gone on for several years and health projects have been judged on the basis of their originality, scientific accuracy, and overall quality. Several thousand students prepare fair exhibits each year. For young people a fair is both fun and informative and provides the motivation that many children need to become involved in a health activity.[25]

The *analysis of current events,* both in the community and the world at large, is one method that has been used for years to make geography and science stimulating. Not a day goes by that there is not some occurrence, phenomenon, or discovery taking place which has either direct or indirect health consequences. Radio, television, and local newspapers invariably refer to such news items as an improved sewer system for a nearby town, a child rushed to the hospital because he swallowed poison, a search for a rabid dog, an automobile and bicycle accident, news of a new method of aiding some disease, or another city setting up plans to fluoridate the water supply. Using current events so that they tie in with the health topic of

---

[25]For greater detail see Pratt, Le Etta, "A Health Fair for Elementary Children," *Health Education,* 8:25–26, July/August 1976.

the moment requires little extra planning and represents an easy technique to employ. From news articles may come group discussions relative to misbehavior in social situations, such as stealing, lying, fighting, or drunkenness. This is an opportunity for intermediate graders to better understand human relationships, thus leading to a better comprehension of mental health.

School-Community Activities. The day has long since passed when the school was considered a self-sufficient agency occupying a building in the center of town. Today, community life is the life of the school and much of school life is the life of the community. Education is a two-way street. Community personnel and their accompanying ideas come into the school and classroom health facts and figures arrive in the home to indirectly educate the parents.

The services of the community resources will vary in the degree to which they make a health contribution. Finding and using these resources is the teacher's job. A good place to begin is *people;* this is followed by *places* and *materials.*

People in the community who are usually willing to give assistance to health teachers include:

Health officer	Satistician
School physician	Laboratory technician
School nurse	Health educator
Public health nurse	Safety director
Dentist	Welfare director
Sanitary engineer	Hospital superintendent
Practicing physician	Social worker
Water plant operator	Farmer
Home demonstration agent	Dairy plant operator
Sewage disposal plant operator	

Places in the community that are especially helpful in health instruction include:[26]

Health department	Farm
Dairy	Recreation facility
Milk pasteurization plant	Water purification plant
Industrial plant	Sewage disposal plant
Food Freezer plant	Housing project
Experimental station	Fire department
Dental clinic	Police department
Laundry	Restaurant
Bakery	City playground
Home garden	Home water supply
Utility company	Meat packing plant

Parents, perhaps more than any other group in the community, are equipped to work closely with the schools in the health program. If there is any one modern method of teaching health, it is to get

---

[26]For a useful list of voluntary, professional, and commercial organizations see Chapter 10.

pupils to carry out at home what they have learned in the classroom. Teachers, therefore, assign homework in health that involves action about the home and encourages classroom-home cooperation.

CORRELATION AND INTEGRATION OF HEALTH INSTRUCTION

There is an interrelationship between direct teaching, correlation, and integration. It is difficult to say that one is better than the other, for all three methods of instruction may be used in health instruction.

There is a distinct difference between correlation and integration. *Correlation involves the use of other areas within the curriculum by which health material is taught.* Health, therefore, is correlated with physical education, science, and social studies. It may also be correlated with additional areas such as art, arithmetic, and English. In the elementary classroom, in which there is less formality and the teachers have their own pupils most of the day, it is not difficult to relate the materials in one subject matter discussion to that of another. True correlation means that the teacher, when thinking of English, must plan for some health teaching in the English lesson. The same is true for other lessons. In discussing ventilation and heating in the sixth grade science period, some definite reference to the personal and community health aspects of the topic would be provided. In social studies the teacher purposely plans to talk about health conditions and the practice of bloodletting during the colonization days at Plymouth and Jamestown. Likewise, health is correlated with physical education games, stunts, and dances by definitely organizing the time available so that specific reference may be made to items such as playground safety, exercise, food, rest, and personal cleanliness. There are many opportunities for correlating health teaching with art through the preparation of posters and charts relating to health problems under study and in the making of puppets to dramatize an idea.

It may be seen that almost any school activity can be correlated with health.

Social Studies
    History of foods
    Eating habits over the world
    Food preparation for the party
Art
    Discussing and arranging flowers for table
    Making place mats
    Poster drawing
    Foods modeled from clay
Arithmetic
    Counting: "How many will eat with me?"
    Building number vocabulary: quart of milk, one-half slice of toast, pound of butter
    Concept of time: time needed to eat breakfast
Science
    How foods grow

The effect of climate and weather on foods
Animal experiments with foods

Physical Education
Food and energy for play
Rest and recreation
Overeating and undereating

Reading
Health textbooks
Charts and posters about good foods
Captions under food ads in magazines and newspapers

Good health instruction helps make correlation a two-way process. Not only is health taught through English but also through proper speech, writing, and spelling. An example of this kind of cooperation is illustrated by the story of what happened in one elementary school. The teacher of a third grade class felt that the parents were not always aware of what meals were served in the school cafeteria. So the class copied the cafeteria menu for the next day as part of their writing lesson. This was taken home to the family. The children were encouraged to use their best handwriting so that their parents would really know what they were going to have to eat.

Integration involves an oranization of learning experiences around a central objective. It differs from correlation by relating parts to the whole. The "whole" can be anything. A well-integrated bicycle, for instance, is one in which all parts—wheels, chain, nuts, bolts, seat, handlebars, fenders—fit perfectly together to afford the rider a safe and pleasant journey. By the same token, a well-integated child is one who has been exposed to the hundreds of educational stimuli and has emerged to take his or her place in society as a "whole" person. The well-integrated person is like a giant mosaic—all the unique parts make a compete being. This may be accomplished by the well-integrated curriculum, one which is balanced, refined, and embraces many areas of instruction.

Instruction in the lower grades is very often based on centering the attention of pupils on broad topics rather than dividing the school time into periods for different subject matter areas. Here, arithmetic, art, spelling, social studies, science, and health are interrelated as part of a broad learning experience. As an example, third grade children in Baltimore studied housing problems. A dilapidated old house being rejuvenated according to the Baltimore Plan was dramatized by the children. They acted the parts of germs, trash, garbage, and mice, and declared that this was no longer a home for them. In the same school there were other examples of integration. One second grade study was built around the quality of Baltimore's water supply. Health aspects were considered with social study aspects. Moreover, the choice of words and ease in speaking gave proof to the observer that these elementary grade children understood the importance of good water.

No subject in the elementary curriculum can long remain divorced from the total program. An overlapping of topics is necessary in order to give appropriate meaning to the various pieces of information. As it is, too many children know a great many health facts but fail to see their usefulness in the world they live in. This may be due to the fact that we live in an integrated society but we often continue to formally study the parts without in any way relating them to the whole. This is somewhat true at all educational levels. It has only been in recent years that physiology, sociology, and psychology have been examined together with the resulting emphasis today on human ecology.

MATERIAL AIDS IN HEALTH TEACHING

Thinking directly in terms of color, tones, images, is a different operation technically from thinking in words. . . . If all meanings could be adequately expressed by words, the arts of painting and music would not exist. There are values and meanings that can be expressed only by immediately visible and audible qualities and to ask what they mean in the sense of something that can be put into words is to deny their distinctive existence.

—John Dewey
Art as Expression

Education is more than just exposing a learner to information. Somehow he or she must be involved in the process by taking part in it. One has to *do* something *with* something. And because it is purposeful activity, one has to feel, listen, smell, and acquire health concepts *through the use of material things.* Homer once said, "Greater glory hath no man than that which he wins with his own feet and hands." Therefore, we may say that children learn some from what they hear, more from what they see and hear, and most from what they do. If something appeals to children because they have heard or read about it, they usually want to "try it out," "feel it," and "work it." One seeks a rich, full-bodied experience that is the bedrock of all education. It is the unabridged version of life itself—commonly referred to as "something you can sink your teeth into." This alone is reason enough for the existence of good instructional materials and the continuous search for better ones.

THE NATURE OF INSTRUCTIONAL MATERIALS

Instructional materials, by definition, exist to aid in the instructional program. They are not a substitute for good teaching—they are only a supplementary item. They are *aids,* and their effectiveness is well supported by research. When properly used in the teaching situation they accomplish the following:

They supply a concrete basis for conceptual thinking and hence reduce meaningless word-responses of students.

They have a high degree of interest for students.

They make learning more permanent.

They offer a reality of experience which stimulates self-activity on the part of pupils.

They develop a continuity of thought; this is especially true of motion pictures.

They contribute to growth of meaning and hence to vocabulary development.

They provide experiences not easily obtained through other materials and contribute to the efficiency, depth, and variety of learning.

THE PROPER USE OF HEALTH TEACHING MATERIALS

The numerous audio-visual materials and other teaching aids cannot take the place of the teacher. It is the teacher who determines the opportune time for each type of instructional material. Whether teaching aids are successful or not depends upon preplanning and effective usage. In one grade five class, for example, a filmstrip was shown to start pupils thinking about drug use and drug abuse. Following this a display of pertinent materials was set up consisting of empty containers or various medicines from aspirin to prescription drugs.

It is interesting to note when considering the proper use of instructional materials that Comenius, in his *Orbis Pictus* (a book of "sense objects" numbered to tie in with English and Latin words), warned his students about making pictures and other materials the main part of education. Materials were to be used chiefly to avoid verbalistic teaching. They were not to be an end in themselves.

Edgar Dale stresses eight ways of evaluating these materials.[27] They may be readily applied to the general use of all health teaching materials:

"Do the materials give a true picture of the ideas they present?" Is there some distortion of truth in order to make a point? Is there a built-in bias of some kind? Several existing films on alcohol present this weakness.

"Do they contribute meaningful content to the topic under study?" The only way to really answer this question in a health class is to evaluate the results of teaching. Do the pupils know any more about the topic? Are practices improved and attitudes changed because of the materials used? We say that "a picture is worth ten thousand words," but is just any picture that effective? One may have an elaborate and highly authentic display of alcohol and tobacco pictures, pamphlets, and other supplementary materials but it may not alter behavior any more than a movie or a talk by the school nurse. Probably the chief reason more television is not used in schools is not because sets and programs are difficult to obtain; it is because, in the minds of some people, there is a question whether television is a highly effective educational aid.

"Is the material appropriate for the age, intelligence, and experience of the learners?" One of the common mistakes of inexperienced teachers is to use materials with the wrong age group. A cancer film that appears interesting to the teacher may leave her primary grade

---

[27]Dale, Edgar. *Audio-Visual Methods in Teaching.* New York: Dryden Press, revised 1964.

class "cold." A lesson on the making of tooth powder may insult the intelligence of an upper grader yet be most appropriate for the second grade boy and girl. Certain health textbooks are difficult when used alone but when supplemented with other materials they become usable.

The appropriateness of materials is best determined by ascertaining the common custom and practice in their use. Many school systems today employ personnel to manage materials through an educational media center and to be of service to teachers. These people have the evidence and the educational listings; they make it their business to know which teaching aids are satisfactory for a certain grade level. Beyond this, some experimentation by the teacher is necessary.

"Is the physical condition of the materials satisfactory?" Few things can detract more from a teaching aid than untidiness and uncleanliness. A broken working model of the eye, a dirty graph, a grimy poster, or a film with a noisy sound track can hurt the teaching lesson measurably. Health teaching exhibits, drawings, and models should be fresh and almost sparkling in appearance.

"Is there a teacher's guide available to provide help in effective use of the materials?" Ideally, every teacher should preview materials before they are used. A good guide can provide a detailed understanding of the items being used and offer numerous practical suggestions.

One of the finest sources of teaching aids may be found in the teacher's guides distributed with the health reading books of several of the larger book publishers.[28] These guides are often as well prepared as the texts they are made to accompany.

"Do they make students better thinkers, critical-minded?" Because children usually enjoy moving pictures, it is not difficult for them to be lulled into accepting and believing something that they might otherwise challenge if they had examined it critically. On the other hand, experience demonstrates that children become quite critical of smoking when they experiment with a simple smoking machine such as the Mini-lung (see Figure 9–10).

"Do they tend to improve human relations?" Children learn to live together harmoniously not only by studying about it but also by practicing it as they live together in the school. Human relations is a continuous process. The use of a wide variety of materials in teaching health tends to pave the way for cooperative effort, sharing of ideas and objects, and understanding the skills and feelings of the other person.

"Is the material worth the time, expense, and effort involved?" This, of course, is the culminating question. In every educational endeavor it becomes necessary sooner or later to appraise fully the expended efforts of teachers. It is at such a time as this that the criterion of economy is applied. Just how costly, in terms of time and money, is the project? In a third grade class studying cleanliness, is it

---

[28]Notably Scott, Foresman, & Co., Laidlaw Brothers, Bobbs-Merrill Co., and J. B. Lippincott Co.

Figure 9–10. The mini-lung teaching aid fosters critical thinking. (Courtesy Spenco Corporation, Waco, Texas.)

better to draw posters for a poster contest than to view a ten-minute film on some phase of community sanitation? In a fifth grade class studying the relationship of food to personal vigor, is a rat-feeding experiment worth all the time it takes to feed the animals, clean the cages, keep the records, and secure the food?

VARIETIES OF TEACHING AIDS IN HEALTH EDUCATION

There are few fields of educational endeavor that are as fertile for the use of teaching aids as health education. Health has a biological, sociological, and psychological basis that cuts across traditional subject boundaries. It is concerned with total human welfare: mind, body, and spirit. Because of this, practically every known teaching aid can in some way be used in the health instruction program. But school time is at a premium; one must be scientific in the use of methods and supplementary aids.

Variety in the use of material aids is as important as varying the method of teaching from time to time. Children welcome a change and since some pupils prefer one aid to another, it is only fair to everyone to be flexible in the use of the various materials. By the same token, some material aids are better than others at a particular grade level. To children who cannot read, a typical poster may be less effective than a flat photograph. A colored slide, for instance, may do a better job of depicting the relationship of food colors to one's appetite than almost any other available means.

Numerous errors are committed in the name of variety. Care must be taken not to forget eye and ear appeal nor to lose sight of the fact that materials should be pertinent to the health lesson. Also, materials should be free from objectionable commercial advertisements.

MATERIALS AVAILABLE TO THE CLASSROOM TEACHER

The following materials are not easily made in class and should be available to the teacher:

Essential in Health Teaching

Catalogs of films
Catalogs of equipment
Card file of films
Model boards
Bulletin boards
Chalkboard
Picture file
Filmstrip projector and filmstrips
Motion picture projector
Portable screen
Overhead projector
Record player

Desirable in Health Teaching

Daylight projection screen
Camera (bl. & wh. and 35 mm color)
Movie camera
Opaque projector
Tape recorder
Public address system
Slide projector and 35 mm slides

In the larger elementary schools in which there are satisfactory media centers, the average classroom teacher will have little trouble securing the necessary aids. In fact, by selecting from the "Desirable" list, it will be possible to experiment somewhat with other items. The teacher may try out a tape recorder in class or borrow a 35 mm camera and take his or her own pictures of the pupils in action to be shown on the slide projector at a later date.

SOURCES OF INSTRUCTIONAL MATERIALS

It is no small task to find new techniques and clever materials for putting across a particular health lesson. Magazines such as *Instruc-*

tor and *the Grade Teacher* are rich in ideas for new teaching materials every month. (Creative ways of developing inexpensive materials appear in several back issues of *Instructor* in full detail.)

The teacher with an open mind who is searching for new ideas and sources of information on the selection, preparation, and use of audio-visual materials will find most of the following sources helpful:

Printed Materials

Aids to Learning, grades one to eight, a project of Creative Playthings, Inc., Princeton, N.J.

Educator's Grade Guide to Free Curriculum Materials, edited by Patricia H. Suttles and published annually by Educator's Progress Service, Randolph, Wisconsin.

Educational Media Index, a project of the Educational Media Council, New York, McGraw-Hill Book Co. Contains a vast range of materials; volumes 1 and 2 refer to health and safety materials for kindergarten through sixth grade.

Free and Inexpensive Learning Materials, published annually by George Peabody College for Teachers, Nashville, Tennessee.

Guide Book Describing Pamphlets, Posters, and Films on Health and Disease, published periodically by the Maryland State Department of Health, Baltimore, Maryland.

Lacey, Richard A. *Seeing With Feeling: Film in the Classroom,* Philadelphia: W. B. Saunders Co., 1972.

Lowndes, Douglas. *Film Making in Schools,* New York: Watson-Guptill Publications, 1968.

Mallery, David. *The School and the Art of Motion Pictures.* Revised ed. Boston: National Association of Independent Schools.

Sources of Free Pictures, edited by Merton B. Osborn and Bruce Miller, published periodically by Bruce Miller Publications, Riverside, California.

Sources of Information on Educational Media, edited by John R. Molstad of Education Media Council in cooperation with U.S. Office of Health, Education, and Welfare, Washington, D.C. (available from U.S. Government Printing Office).

Vertical File Index, published monthly with an annual cumulative volume by R. R. Bowker Co., New York, New York. Lists free and inexpensive materials from private and public sources.

Periodicals

Audio-Visual Instruction. Washington, D.C.: National Education Association Department of Audio-Visual Instruction, 1201 16th Street, N.W. Nine issues.

Children's Record Reviews. Box 192, Woodmere, New York 11598.

Educational Screen and Audio-Visual Guide. Chicago: 2000 Lincoln Park West. Ten issues.

EFLA Film Review Digest. New York: Educational Film Library Association, 345 E. 46th Street. Eight issues.

Journal of Physical Education and Recreation. Washington, D.C.: American Alliance for Health, Physical Education, and Recreation, 1201 16th Street, N.W. Nine issues. Each issue contains an audio-visual section.

Journal of School Health. Kent, Ohio: The American School Health Association, 515 E. Main Street. Ten issues. Most issues contain specific references to new teaching aids.

Junior Scholastic. New York: Scholastic Magazines, 33 West 42nd Street. A weekly for grades six to eight. Features material on plays, short stories, science, health, radio, TV, records, personal guidance and hobbies.

Health Education. Washington, D.C.: American Association for Health, Physical Education, and Recreation, 1201 16th Street, N.W. Nine issues. Each issue contains a section on resources for school health programs.

Current Health. Curriculum Innovations, Inc., Highwood, Ill. 60040.

Audio-Visual Materials in Health Instruction

W. Eugene Smith, a man *Camera* magazine refers to as the most important photographer the 20th century has produced, points out that photography is a small voice at best but sometimes one photograph or a group of them can lure our senses into awareness. When the photograph summons enough emotion, it can be a catalyst to thought.

Of the dozens of techniques and aids being used in the elementary schools, some are more common than others. A brief discussion of each follows this paragraph. It begins with the more spectacular projected materials involving motion, sound, electricity, and electronics and moves to the older and more elemental forms of nonprojected materials. One cannot accurately say that a certain photograph or similar aid is superior to another without qualifying the statement in terms of the objectives. To say that one material aid is better than the other depends upon a number of variables such as the teacher's ability and the make-up of the class. Each classroom teacher will have to determine to what extent the following material aids can be successfully used in classes of health instruction.

1. Motion Pictures. In one breath we can say that the use of motion pictures to convey health messages is almost as badly abused as the use of pamphlets; they cannot stand alone in putting messages across. In the next breath, however, we can state with certainty that motion pictures may well be one of the finest media for presenting health ideas in readily acceptable terms. Why the extreme difference in these two statements? One answer lies in the meaning of the film. Lacey asks, "Meaning for whom?"[29] Aren't children different? Don't

---

[29]Lacey, Richard A. *Seeing With Feeling: Film in the Classroom,* Philadelphia: W. B. Saunders Co., 1972, p. 18.

they find a variety of meanings in a film? They should react with feelings ("Fantastic movie") as well as thoughts and they shouldn't be *compelled* to intellectualize the movie, says Lacey, or they will miss the experience.

Another answer lies in planning. *When good planning takes place, health interest and health understanding increase.* Specifically, health education instructional films are planned to reach certain goals. They may be used:

As an introduction to a unit to stimulate interest or give an overview.

In the direct teaching of a health lesson, i.e., to help develop an idea or attitude, to convey certain facts, or to help solve or correct certain problems.

As a review or summary of previous learnings.

a. The *preliminary steps* are:

Familiarize yourself with the film before showing it.

Make a list of the important points in the film that you want the audience to understand and remember.

Prepare some thought-provoking questions which will stimulate discussions.

Introduce the film to the class, bringing out the points you want them to look for.

b. The *presentation* is a challenge:

The viewing distance of the farthest seat from the screen is approximately six times the width of the picture for pupils in the front row.

c. The *follow-up* "sets" the experience:

Review with the class the main points of the film.

Clear up any existing questions concerning the film.

Ask the class questions (oral or written) for the purpose of evaluating the film and its effectiveness.

Repeat film showing if time permits and some points appear to need reemphasis.

Engage in follow-up activities, i.e., tests, papers, drawings, demonstrations, experiments, as necessary to insure a practical understanding of the topic.

d. The *evaluation* is as important as any of the above points. Standard evaluation forms may be obtained from the Educational Film Library Association, Inc. Teacher-made forms for elementary classroom appraisal should include answers to a number of questions.

It takes time to become familiar with the large number and variety of health films appropriate for the primary and intermediate grade levels. Such a list would more than fill this book. A good start may be made by reviewing Chapter 10 which deals with the sources of materials. Also the lists of producers and distributors are continually being revised. For a wide coverage of current sources, consult the following:

The Blue Book of Audio-Visual Materials. Chicago: Educational Screen, 64 East Lake Street. Included here are films, filmstrips, slides, and recordings.
Educator's Guide to Free Films, Educator's Guide to Free Film Strips, Educator's

Guide to Free Transcriptions, Tapes and Scripts. Randolph, Wisconsin: Educator's Progress Service. An annually revised guide with title index, subject classification, brief descriptions, and cross references.

Public Health Service Film Catalog. Washington, D.C.: U.S. Public Health Service, U.S. Government Printing Office, annual.

Visual Materials in Safety Education, Supplement II. Washington, D.C.: National Commission on Safety Education, 1201 16th Street, N.W. A bibliography. (Revised periodically.)

U.S. Government Films for Public Educational Use, compiled for the U.S. Dept of Health, Education, and Welfare and published by the Government Printing Office, Washington, D.C., annual.

It sometimes makes a good project to produce a health film at school. The teacher who can operate a movie camera and knows something about the composition of pictures can often make an 8 mm or 16 mm colored film that may be used from year to year. A good homemade film does not outgrow its usefulness very soon. Future classes enjoy seeing their older friends in the moving picture and the class that makes the film has a wonderful opportunity to integrate the health message with other subject matter areas. In writing the script, the various scenes are tied in closely with the narration. This, like the use of all instructional aids, takes conscientious planning but it can be quite worthwhile, for there is a tremendous range of health problems that can be approached by this teaching technique. Some examples of films produced by classes include first aid to the injured child, boating safety, swimming safety, garbage disposal, and shopping for safe vegetables and fruits. Even a simple on-the-spot movie of a field trip to the dairy or of a group of happy youngsters surrounding an animal feeding demonstration can be a motivating device for children in succeeding years. Also, a good

Figure 9–11. Following the showing of a safety film the teacher reviews key points. (Courtesy National Safety Council.)

amount of fun may be had in filming the bicycle skills of several children riding about the school playground. Ideas for a local film could come from viewing the excellent Eastman Kodak Company booklet, *Movies With a Purpose* (free), which is a teacher's guide to planning and producing 8 mm movies for classroom use.

A very fine teaching aid is the silent cartridge *loop film*. This is a short (several minutes) presentation to drive home a point. Shown on the single-concept film projector, it can be used with other media.

2. Filmstrips. Much that has already been said about the selection, presentation, and evaluation of movie films can be applied to the utilization of filmstrips.

Filmstrips are a very convenient technique of showing a series of still pictures. They are mounted on a continuous strip of 35 mm film and vary in length from 18 frames to several times that number.

The advantages of filmstrips for elementary health teaching are:

They are lightweight and easy to handle in the classroom. The projector is simple enough for a primary grade pupil to operate.

They are relatively inexpensive—one of the cheapest projected visual aids.

They are available in vivid colors.

They may be obtained for use with a sound recording.

There is a wide variety to choose from in health.

Body functions and specific health implications can be effectively broken down and presented through a sequence of filmstrip projections.

The teacher can pause as long as he or she likes on any one picture.

Many filmstrips are designed to accompany textbooks.

Recent BFA Educational Media produced a series of four color and sound filmstrips to integrate language art with health for upper elementary age students. Included are filmstrips *Fighting Disease– Past and Present, Formula for a Healthy Body,* and *Mind and Body Working Together.* Skill development exercises are included in the kit of cassettes. (BFA, 2211 Michigan Ave., P.O. Box 1795, Santa Monica, California 90406.)

3. Slides. Slides, like filmstrips, are easy to use and relatively inexpensive. One can make a slide or filmstrip from anything that is drawn, written, typewritten, printed, or photographed—and it can be done in full color. Drawings may be made with pencil on etched glass or with special slide ink. It would not be difficult in an intermediate grade class, for example, to sketch the skeleton of the body on glass and project it life-size on a screen. So many slides are readily available today that it often proves more economical in terms of teacher time to purchase ready-made slides.

Most slides are 2 inches × 2 inches; however, the 3½ inch × 4 inch variety is sometimes employed. The latter are more readily used in adapting charts, pictures, tables, and the like from magazines and books since more detail can be shown. Also they can be made by hand more easily. Most slides of a health and biological nature are photographically produced. They may be shown on any one of a number of easy-to-operate projectors. One type of tape recorder is available which will automatically change the slides in a slide projector. This can be a very effective means of putting over a health topic at an exhibit or as part of a display in the main corridor of the school.

4. Opaque Projector. The light from any flat picture may be reflected directly on the screen by means of mirrors and lenses. The opaque projector is flexible enough to handle anything up to six inches square; anything larger can be inserted into it and moved around until the desired part of the picture is on the screen. Its use in the lower grades for showing almost any flat object is great. Although it is heavy to move about, it is inexpensive to use. Small clippings from a newspaper or magazine can be greatly enlarged on a screen. The same is true for poison labels and medical prescription instructions. It is a good health motivating device, for children love to see their own health pictures, drawings, charts, and graphs projected on a big screen before the whole class.

5. Overhead Projector. For the teacher of health it is a simple matter to sketch, write, or draw on a strip of cellophane with a ceramic or wax pencil, and in color if desired. The chief advantage of this projector is that the teacher can readily project all the details of a lecture while facing the class.

6. Transparencies. With the use of the overhead projector has come an increasing amount of good transparencies.

Some of the finest prepared health education transparencies, ready to use and in sharp colors, are distributed by such companies as the Minnesota Mining and Manufacturing Company (3M), National Dairy Council, American Dental Association, Popular Science, Milton Bradley in Springfield, Massachusetts, American Cancer Society, Western Publishing Company, Hubbard Scientific Company, and Dennoyer-Geppert Company. Other full-color transparencies especially good in depicting physiological functions are distributed by Medi Visuals, Inc., 342 Madison Avenue, New York, N.Y. 10017.

Overlay transparencies are useful in showing the structure of items such as body organs, cells, muscle tissue, human skin as it would appear under the microscope, sense organs, and major areas of the brain.

7. Radio. One teacher has said, "Our boys and girls like to listen to others their own age. It seems to me they learn more from them."

The radio in the classroom is an inexpensive device that is realistic, is authentic, and has emotional impact. It may be used directly by scheduling classes to coincide with some radio programs in order to hear health lectures, interviews, or panel discussions. It may also be used within the classroom as a simulated broadcast with class members taking part in the production.

From the point of view of health actions, pupils need to be taught how to use the radio and be selective and critical of radio programs. Just as children are taught not to accept everything that appears in print, so they must learn to appraise that which is presented over the radio and television channels.

8. Portable Conference Telephone. A whole class can talk on the telephone with the help of one set. While all listen, a public health official can explain the need for precautions against the flu germ or a senator can be engaged in conversation a thousand miles away. This device weighs less than 20 pounds and can plug into any standard telephone jack. There are dozens of ways it can enliven health teaching.

9. Television. A number of schools have access to educational television. Health programs are staged for school audiences. Both professional personnel and schoolchildren may be employed as performers. This can be a fine medium for motivation providing, as in the case of moving picture films, there is some pertinent discussion prior to and following television presentation. Here sight and sound are combined to teach an entire community. Several intermediate grade school classes, for example, could watch the actual pulling of a bad tooth in a dentist's chair, followed by a special message from the dentist.

If programs are carefully related to classroom activity, especially following the presentation, it seems logical to expect television to become an effective tool in the promotion of health. However, it must always be evaluated against alternate tools that are available.

Cassettes are now available from several educational film makers for classroom use. Columbia Broadcasting System has a selection (EVR cassettes) at 51 W. 52nd Street, New York, N.Y. 10019. Videotaping is also becoming popular in the schools. All kinds of student activities, trips, and experiments are recorded on videotape and replayed later.

The Agency for Instructional Television, a non-profit American-Canadian organization, employs television and other technologies to advance health education. Main offices are in Bloomington, Indiana 47401 (Box A). Their "Inside/Out" program provides young people with a "feeling" approach to health education. This is an interdisciplinary series of 15-minute programs to help 8 to 10 year olds cope with their emotions. Another popular program for 11 to 13 year olds personally involves youngsters in the health problem-solving process. Throughout this television program, there is a reliance on student listening, valuing, and decision-making rather than on "rules for healthy living."

Home television may be used for pupil assignments somewhat the same way as radio has been used for years, i.e., to appraise "health" commercials and advertising and to listen to special health talks, demonstrations, news, and plays.

10. Records. Records are easy to play, are relatively inexpensive, and are available in many schools today. Disc recordings are owned by children who often enjoy sharing their records with the rest of the group. They give meaning to numerous events, bring authentic sounds into the classroom, and improve the listening habits of boys and girls. They constitute two-way communication and can be stopped and discussed with the class.

In the teaching of health, commercial records may be used for health songs and action stories. The Stanley Bowmar Company, Valhalla, N.Y. 10595, has a wide selection of these.

11. Tape Recordings. The tape recorder opens a great many areas to the teacher of health. Tape recorders are not difficult to operate and the tape is easy to edit and repair. In many respects the tape recorder has more uses in the classroom than the radio or television set. Tape recordings may be purchased. (The periodical *Tape Recording* lists most of the tapes available from commercial companies. See also *Educator's Guide to Free Transcriptions, Tapes, and Scripts,* Educator's Progress Service, Randolph, Wis.)

From a health instruction viewpoint, tape recordings make learning more complete by:

a. Bringing health authorities into the classroom. A committee of two or three pupils can visit a busy physician, bakery manager, or water department superintendent and record the answer to prearranged classroom questions. Distance is no problem. The world is brought to the classroom.

b. Recording home radio and television commercials, plays, and talks to be used for class discussion and appraisal.

c. Providing a variety of approaches to the same subject. A recording of a health lesson may be reviewed two weeks later with profit. Gives both pupils and teacher an opportunity for self-evaluation.

d. Bringing to the classroom some of the health problems of the community. The teacher's ability to verbalize about a health problem—alcoholism and drug abuse, for example—is at best limited. The tape recorder brings to the students the actual voices of community members who know the problem at first hand. The teacher can use this information, emphasize it, and elaborate upon it; but the raw material of life is here, not lost in abstract verbiage.

Figure 9–12. Headset listening assures student attention. (Courtesy Anedex, Incorporated.)

Moreover, it can be identified in a social peer group setting where it is especially revealing.

One of the most valuable uses of a tape recorder is to play it back to the pupils so that they hear how their own voices sound. Several statements pertaining to a health lesson may actually be read into the machine and played back the next day for class use. A "traveling recorder team" may survey the pupils and teachers for their opinions relative to some current health idea or they may venture into the business area of town to interview the "passing citizen." A sixth grade class in one New York State community questioned quite a number of leading citizens on their opinions relative to fluoridating the city water supply. Another idea often used is to put together a simple story and have it taped exactly as desired for future presentation. A single topic combining humor with good advice is "How to Burn Down Your House."

12. Textbooks. Earlier, textbooks were reviewed as a method of teaching. If they are up-to-date and are more than just another reading book, they have value. If not, then they are very much the way historian Oscar Handlin described them—"dogmatic and dull, an obstacle rather than an aid to learning." Shopping for the most useful textbook is not an easy task. However, Scheer has developed a criteria sheet and scoring system so that textbooks may be evaluated.[30] Overlooked by many teachers is the reading level. Many times, reading level will vary considerably within a grade, yet learning materials are at one grade level only. Above and below-the-grade level texts should be on hand.

When the book is accurate in the presentation of facts and illustrations and orderly in the arrangement of materials, it can be used as an effective guide to the health program at a certain grade level. This is particularly true if the pupils are asked to discover things for themselves, answer questions, engage in learning activities, and respond to diagrams and situations. Listed below are the publishers of textbooks primarily concerned with health in the elementary school:

Benziger, Inc., *Becoming a Person Grades 1–8*. (1972) 866 Third Ave., New York, New York 10022.

The Bobbs-Merrill Co., Inc., Indianapolis, Indiana, *Health for Young America Series,* grades 1–8 (Revised).

Harcourt, Brace, Jovanovich, *Health Decisions for Growth,* Level 1–6 (1977).

Houghton Mifflin, Boston, Massachusetts, *Investigating Your Health.* (Grade 6) (1977).

Laidlaw Brothers, River Forest, Illinois, *The Healthful Living Program,* grades 1–8 (1977).

J. B. Lippincott Co., Philadelphia, Pennsylvania, *Basic Health Science Series,* (Grades 1–6) (1972).

Prentice-Hall, Inc. *Systems of the Body Series*—Ages 8–12, Englewood Cliffs, New Jersey 07632 (1972).

Scott Foresman & Company, Glenview, Illinois. *You and Your Health* K–8 (1978).

13. Pamphlets. Pamphlets need to be simple and have a definite message. They should be in bold print with lots of color and illustrations and contain some white space so that what is written will stand out. These criteria should also be followed when health leaflets or "handouts" are made in class for home distribution.

---

[30]Scheer, Judith K. "Shopping for the Best Text," *Health Education, 8*:26–27, November/December 1977.

Pamphlets for school use may be obtained from numerous official and nonofficial health agencies. Most of the large insurance companies, the American Medical Association, the Florida Citrus Commission, The Cereal Institute, National Society for Prevention of Blindness, and the National Dairy Council represent organizations which distribute particularly well-fashioned leaflets and bookets suitable for elementary school classroom use. In recent years there has been a reduction in the number of free materials available for teachers. However, the quality of the inexpensive materials has improved measurably. For years the National Dairy Council has made its wide variety of health leaflets available to teachers in sufficient quanity so that each pupil may have one. *The Story of the Cow* has been written for 12 different grade levels. Third graders are able to use the little 3 inch × 4 inch colored leaflet on the four basic food areas, both in the classroom and at home. This is printed in Spanish as well as English. Attractive "handouts" such as these may be used in a number of effective ways; however, a pamphlet cannot be expected to influence attitudes and behavior without being used in conjunction with other methods of health education.

Finally, a word about the use of magazines. The Research Division of the National Education Association has discovered that some of the most imaginative classroom projects are sparked by materials appearing in magazines. Their most common usage is to develop bulletin board displays. They are also employed for useful reference information, for independent reading, and for stimulation of student writing.

14. Encyclopedias. Sets of encyclopedias form a wealth of background materials for the classroom. By following the library method of teaching, real use may be made of this two-way reference material. Many a statement in an encyclopedia has triggered ideas for pupil activities. Even more important, perhaps, is the fact that encyclopedias can be used directly by pupils in their search for facts and comments relative to the health unit being studied.

15. Clippings. One of the finest uses of the health clipping is to tack it to a designated space on a bulletin board where everyone can see it. Clippings from magazines and newspapers include pictures, stories, reports, research, and advertising. Every health topic, particularly in grades four to six, can be bolstered with appropriate clippings. Hardly a week passes by without some of the magazines having an item suited for a health lesson. Pictures of foods, drawings of body parts, and facial expressions may all be posted on a bulletin board or projected on a large screen.

16. Study Guides and Workbooks. There is some use in health teaching for these aids providing they encourage students to be active—to try something out, to experiment, to listen, to observe, or to discuss.

17. Pictures and Photographs. Pictures crystallize ideas and form much of the basis for thinking. Industry and business spend a fortune each year on pictures to put their story across. Pictures are everywhere today in magazines, folders, and booklets. Good photographs are also available or may be made through a school project.

Once used, the outstanding pictures and photographs should be filed in an accessible folder for future use.

Suitable health instruction pictures should include items such as groups of healthy children with smiling faces; pictures of pets and other animals eating the same foods as children (pigs drinking milk, rabbits eating green vegetables, chickens picking up grain in the barnyard); the fire engine en route to a fire, and the police officer directing traffic.

A multitude of heterogeneous pictures will only confuse a student. To obtain the best results with pictures, use only a few well-chosen ones for a pertinent illustration. Pictorial materials may be mounted and passed around for individual inspection or exhibited on a board. They may also be projected by the opaque projector.

18. Posters. The thousands of billboards spread across the land have only one purpose: to convey an idea in one fleeting glance. Posters accomplish the same purpose.

Posters have become an expressive form of American art. Their chief purpose is stimulation. Thus, they may be used to introduce a unit or call attention to some facts in a phase of instruction. A good poster should be simple, large (28 inches × 22 inches), have bold and colored lettering that is easily read and understood. If it can be interesting enough to cause a chuckle, adroit enough to promote discussion, and clever enough to haunt the memory, it has just about everything that is needed to make it a useful teaching aid. If, however, it functions only as another implement, requiring the support of more basic teaching aids, then it is of limited value. Too often posters have been used solely as a wall decoration, having been left on display far beyond the point of attractive notice. They are effective only when they are *frequently changed*.

Numerous manufacturers of foods, toothpastes, school furniture, and dairy products are excellent sources of poster materials. Practically all of the large insurance companies distribute, free of charge, colorful wall posters relating to health and safety practices. Some examples of the more effective free posters for primary and intermediate grade use may be obtained from:*

American Cancer Society
American Dental Association
American Heart Association
American Medical Association
Bicycle Institute of America
Educators Mutual Life Insurance Co.
Equitable Life Assurance Society
Florida Citrus Commission
Instructor (Every month in this magazine)
The National Dairy Council
National Institute of Mental Health
National Livestock and Meat Board
Personal Products Corporation
National Commission on Safety Education
Sunkist Growers
The National Safety Council
Travelers Insurance Co.

---

*Addresses may be found in Chapter 10.

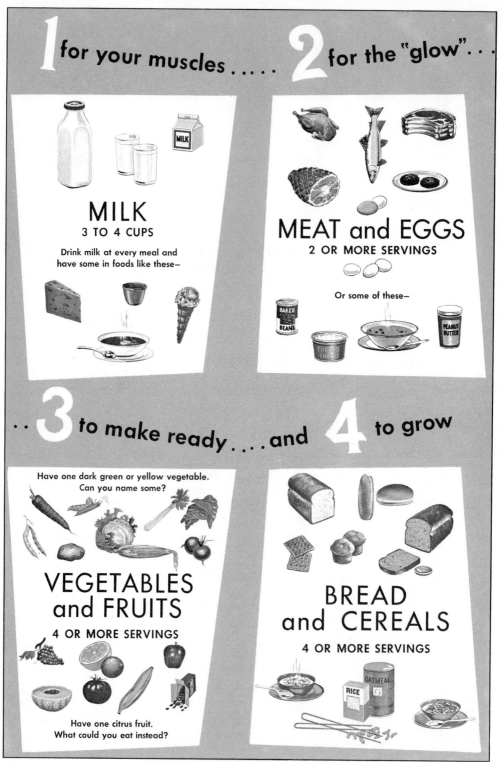

Figure 9–13. (Courtesy National Dairy Council.)

In working with posters the best learning probably takes place when children make their own. This is especially true when the poster making is directly related to the particular health topic, is clear and forceful, is well designed, is colorful, and has easily understood titles with brief captions. An example of a poster that meets these qualifications and would be attractive on a fourth grade bulletin board is Figure 9–13.

Artistic posters may be fashioned from wrapping paper, scrap tin, tinfoil, box tops, magazine pictures, wallpaper, and the usual art supplies. Even comic book clippings and newspaper cartoons may be used in making the poster. These sometimes serve to make the poster more attractive and humorous.

Once health posters are discussed in class they may be hung about the room for a short period. The better ones may be selected for a main corridor bulletin board, the lunchroom, or the physical education locker room.

More and more posters are employing cut-out figures and superimposed materials over the foundation surface. Items are readily tacked, stapled, or glued to the surface and provide another dimension for observation. Simple line expressions can tell more sometimes than fancy drawings. Mental health is well depicted this way:

SIMPLE LINE EXPRESSIONS

YELL   LAUGH   SHY   SMILE

19. The Health Mobile. Under the direction of the clever teacher an eye-catching health "mobile" may be constructed. This may consist of wooden signs, printed on both sides, a wire frame, and string. To learn about food values a fourth grade class might build and hang a mobile such as the following. This mobile is different enough from the usual display that the pupils can learn the four basic food groups more easily. Here they also see the values inherent in each group. The wooden signs may be made in class or in the elementary industrial arts laboratory. These are superior to cardboard signs. Also, as an alternative to using signs for vitamin and mineral values, the class might cut out and hang pictures of the various human organs affected such as the eyeball for vitamin A or the skeleton for calcium.

20. Cartoons. The perfect cartoon needs no caption. The symbolism conveys the message, for the best cartoons make their point immediately.

MAN

WOODEN SIGNS
PRINTED ON BOTH SIDES

FOOD

| 1 | 2 | 3 | 4 | — 4 BASIC FOOD AREAS |

— VITAMIN AND MINERAL VALUES

If the teacher will watch carefully for cartoons having to do with health, he or she will find a number of excellent ones appearing each week in popular magazines and newspapers.

In some respects, cartoons work better with intermediate grade children, probably because a first-rate cartoon has emotional impact. This is arranged by the clever cartoonist who is able to play with humor, mockery, or satire—qualities that are generally appreciated more by older children.

In using such a medium in health teaching, one must be careful that pupils do not accept the message of the cartoon uncritically.

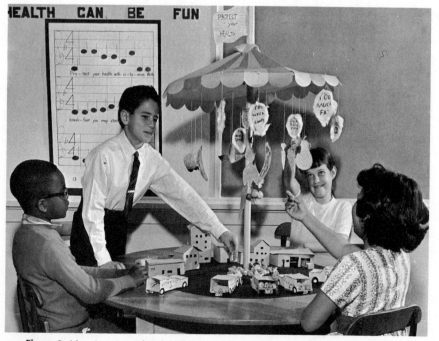

Figure 9–14. A variety of mobile. (Courtesy *Health Education Journal*, Los Angeles City Schools.)

Figure 9–15. "Why should I wash—I'm inoculated against everything, ain't I?" Reproduced through courtesy of Irwin Caplan, McNaught Syndicate, Inc., and the *American Legion Magazine.*

Cartoons are very often all "black" or "white," or they oversimplify without qualification. Moreover, they cannot be used repeatedly as can pictures and photographs. They become outdated rapidly. They must be considered because surveys indicate that they are among the most popular aids used by teachers. And where they are not obtained from other sources they may be made in the classroom. In fact, original health cartoons frequently help students think for themselves and apply what they know about health to the cartoon.

21. Sketches and Drawings. A pencil sketch or drawing made with a pen, pencil, or special crayon may make health facts more vivid. A class studying posture, for example, may see what is involved in a straight line type of posture when a simple sketch is drawn of building blocks.

Drawings and diagrams are valuable at all age levels. Primary grade children seem to appreciate the line drawing that outlines a process. In a study of foods, an outline of how the grain passes from the farmer's field to the bakery and ultimately to the bread on the table is of real interest. The diagram of a water supply from the original source to the clean glass or the story of milk from the cow to the table are other examples that may be nicely diagrammed. Some of these items may be put on transparencies by pupils themselves.

Drawings, sketches, and diagrams may also be put together by the teacher or the class using magazine prints, newsprint, wrapping paper, window shades, or anything else that can be brought to class to work with. These materials may be large sheets of paper, chart cloth, old bedsheets, large paper panels, or classroom chalkboards.

22. Strip Drawings ("Comics"). Here a story is told through a series of drawings, frequently called "comics."

A number of free health comic books are available from the Food and Drug Administration, U.S. Public Health Service. So are the several "Sparky" fire stories distributed by the National Fire Protection Association: *Early Man and Fire, Man Learns More about Fire, and Hello, I Am Fire, Is This Your Home?*

23. Writing Pads. These pads of paper may be as big as or bigger than 2 feet × 3 feet. They are usually supported on an easel and used very much the same as a chalkboard. They have a distinct advantage over the chalkboard in that sketches, diagrams, and notes may be prepared well in advance of the class period. This is especially helpful in the crowded school with inadequate blackboard space. To many children it is simply a different medium—a fact to keep in mind when new sources of motivation are sought.

24. Charts and Tables. Information is arranged in lists. Facts, figures, and even pictures are organized in some way so that the visible parts are related to the whole. The ramifications of a whole concept or idea are presented at once. The danger here is that the table or chart may include too much detail or too many words.

A proper chart should have a title large enough to be seen across an ordinary classroom. Lettering should be clear with strong colors on a neutral or light background. It may be several square feet in size and hung from the ceiling or small enough to be duplicated and distributed to each pupil. It may be mounted on heavy paper, a bulletin board, or ordinary flannel. In any case, it should not remain on display beyond its period of usefulness.

Health charts with the most instructional value are those which the pupils make themselves and are based on data which they have assembled. In one Southern school the primary grade boys and girls put together a chart which they called *A Trip Through Healthland*.[31] It was constructed with felt mounted on heavy paper. The medium of light colors was also applied to make it attractive.

At each "stop" on the "trip through healthland" the importance of that area was discussed and personal problems were talked about.

Every elementary teacher should have a chance to look over the *Good Health Record* charts distributed by the Kellogg Company, Battle Creek, Michigan. The students keep these current on a day-to-day basis, recording habits of cleanliness, eating, sleeping, and helping at home and at school. Most children enjoy charting their progress and keeping their own records. This becomes a kind of self-testing activity—a means of comparing oneself today with what one did yesterday or with someone else in the class.

Another attractive chart used especially in health teaching is one for measuring pupil height in the ordinary classroom. The *How Tall Chart* of the Travelers Insurance Company, Hartford, Connecticut, fits inconspicuously on a closet door or wall. It hangs so that the bottom of the chart is 2½ feet above the floor. Height may be measured to the nearest quarter inch.

25. Graphs and Maps. A graph diagrams quantity, development, function, or relationship of factors. There are graphs that are

---

[31] Originated and reported by Mary Charles Garrett of Gainesville, Fla.

A TRIP THROUGH HEALTHLAND

SUNSHINE VALLEY

SWEET MILK FALLS

PLAY MEADOW

LONG SLEEP MOUNTAIN

BROWN BREAD HILL

SAFETY LAKE

DOCTOR CROSSING

HOT SOUP SPRINGS

BREAKFAST NOOK

BATHTUB VILLE

TOOTHBRUSH RIDGE

horizontal or bar, line, pictorial, and circular or pie. All may be effectively used in health teaching. Excellent multi-colored bar graphs for health teaching may be obtained from the Evaporated Milk Association and the National Dairy Council.

A map is something more than a diagram or line drawing. It generally starts somewhere and goes somewhere. A map may be made on any health subject. It is different from the physical, economic, and political maps made available by a supplier and used in geography and social studies; it is generally made by the students. Primary graders, for example, may derive considerable benefit from mapping the route from home to school. In one school, as a part of a lesson on safety, all pupils drew a picture map showing the route from home to school. They are encouraged to make them complete, even to including such hazards as water holes, angry dogs, inviting junkyards, houses under construction, a pile of dirt, and the like. When the maps were completed they were studied by the class so that the hazardous places could be discussed. Some new routes were created to avoid the hazards. The routes were further appraised from the point of view of the bicycle rider. The maps were so revealing that the pupils carried the discussion beyond walking and bicycling to automobile and bus safety.

Another map particularly suited to health teaching in the elementary school is the spot map. It may be a map of the community or an ordinary road map. It could be stuck with a small colored-head pin to show the exact spot where an automobile accident occurred during the preceding month. In one school, the pupils marked the spots on the map of the school grounds where accidents occurred. They counted everything from cut elbows, scraped knees, and blisters, to serious falls and minor emergencies. Once the map was well covered with pins, the class stopped to analyze the situation in an attempt to do something about it.

26. Flash Cards and Flip Charts. Flash cards have titles printed on each side for use in flashing certain information before the pupils. An idea is brought home on a small card. These cards may be in the form of charts, such as the food value charts of the National Dairy Council, and they may be mounted on hinged display panels and flipped one at a time by the teacher.

Flash cards and flip charts may be used to develop quick reaction and correct responses. To many pupils they are a novelty and as such command attention. A series of questions and answers on school safety may be displayed before the class on 13 inch × 22 inch panels, or the logical progress of a certain food may be followed through the processes of assimilation, digestion, and elimination.

A series of 36 large flip charts, expressly created for kindergarten or grade one pupils, are the *How About You?* health charts published by Ginn and Company. These 17 × 20 inch full color charts were described on page 165, Chapter 7.

Teaching with flash cards permits the teacher to put over a concept that is brief and to the point. The word *Stop* or *Go* or *Caution* has a message all by itself. A series of words arranged to cover health instruction in one class period might read (1) Health, (2) Food, (3) Music, (4) Rest, and (5) Happiness. As the essential ingredients of a healthy person are mentioned, the particular key word on the chart or card is flipped for the class to see. Finally, if the flip chart is helpful in keeping the pupils' minds on the speaker's track, it is equally helpful in keeping the speaker's mind on it.

27. The Bulletin Board. Practically every classroom or corridor has some kind of bulletin board which is used from time to time to display health materials. The materials displayed should have a unifying theme. They should be authentic and easy to read. Simplicity should be the rule in organizing material for elementary schoolchildren. One should ask these questions:

Is there a center of interest?
Is there beauty of line and form?
Do the materials go well together?
Is the total arrangement well-balanced?
Is there repetition of color?
Is a feeling of unity created?
Does the arrangement tell a story?

Captions for bulletin boards have great value. A challenging question or statement accompanying the material may have much to do with the value derived from the display. Captions which tell little, such as *Foods for Health,* or *This Is Posture Week,* can be improved by making them read *Eat Your Way to Good Health* and *How Do You Look to Your Friends?* Other captions which relate to health clippings or the health topic being studied might read: *Have You Seen These? Do You Know? Stop–Look–Read.*

Notice that in arranging the pictures or other materials the teacher places the largest number of pictures in the bottom row to give strength to the arrangement. The same procedure is followed when color is used—the darkest colors are concentrated near the bottom of the display.

The bulletin board, when used in health teaching, can arouse interest in many things such as special health week (safety, heart), seasonal wearing apparel, current discussion topics, or local health

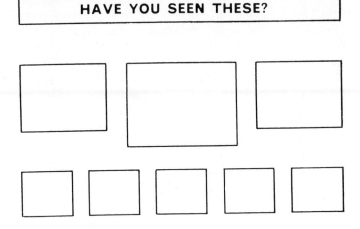

HAVE YOU SEEN THESE?

events. If bulletin boards are especially colorful and make a good first impression early in September, there is a fairly good chance they will be purposely seen by pupils whenever they pass by them. Needless to say, the materials must be changed frequently.

Three-dimensional display can enhance the appearance of the bulletin board. Real objects brought from home may be hung or tacked to the board with particular attention given to space, color, and shape. In fact, when children help plan and organize the bulletin board display, it is more apt to be read than otherwise. The pupils

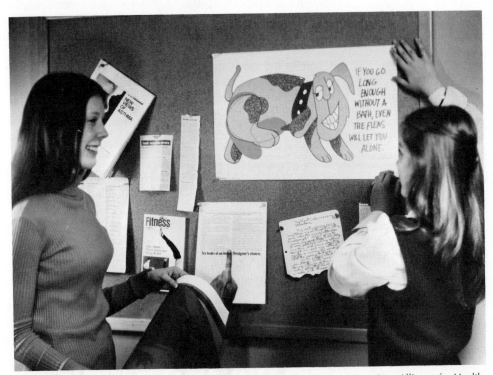

Figure 9–16. Experimenting with a bulletin board display. (Courtesy American Alliance for Health, Physical Education, and Recreation.)

may print their own captions, mount their materials, and take care to label each item with the name of the child who made it or brought it to school. An odorless and stainless bulletin board wax may be used in place of thumbtacks to hold three-dimensional as well as flat objects.

28. Flannel Boards and Felt Boards.   Flannel or felt is unique in that once the background is constructed it may be developed into any type of diagram, graph, chart, or bulletin board. Moreover, this may be done while the class watches, and, like a blackboard or chalk talk, the teacher can add portions of the chart or diagram as the lesson unfolds until the story is complete.

The flannel or felt is stretched over a 2 foot ×3 foot stiff board, usually on an easel. Velvet, velveteen, suede cloth, or flocking may also be used. Material which will cling to this includes coarse sandpaper, flannel, felt, terry cloth, or Floktite. All titles, captions, letters, and models are pasted to one of these adhering substances. It is a simple matter after this to arrange and rearrange the board materials. In one school a pie graph of the four basic food groups was put together piece by piece in four operations while the teacher told the class about each category of food. By the time she added piece Number 4 the class was well on the way to visualizing how the parts make up the whole—the balanced diet. Here, the pie graph and the felt board techniques were effectively employed to give meaning to a health lesson which would be difficult to duplicate through some other medium.

In a second grade class in Garden City, New York, the children made up pictures of a large number of food items which were attached to the board. They were then asked to select from the board those foods that would make a good breakfast, lunch, and dinner. With practice the pupils were able to do a reasonably good job in planning a full day's diet. Such a technique in learning is another worthy way to help boys and girls of varying abilities engage in a stimulating learning experience.

29. Magnetic Boards. Closely associated with the flannel board is the magnetic board. This is essentially a metal sheet upon which magnets may be attached for a number of purposes of representation. The board may be covered with a thin layer of cardboard or oilcloth or some other material which will not hinder the action of the magnet. One form of this board is truly flexible in all situations. Not only is it permanently magnetized but it has a chalk writing surface and is available with brighty colored plastic symbols and indicators enabling the teacher to plan and illustrate almost anything. In terms of health instruction, this aid may be used to teach things such as fire routes for fire drills, moving foods from one plate to another, showing the spread of cold germs, illustrating the hands of the clock at bedtime, showing children and equipment on the school playground, and as many others as the teacher's imagination will permit.

30. Collections and Specimens. Newspaper clippings, magazine articles, and cartoons may be collected for bulletin board display. Other items such as eight or ten animal teeth for a dental health lesson present a challenge to the average nine or ten year old if he or she is asked to locate them. In one fourth grade class, the boys and girls made a collection of empty cereal boxes. Every known cooked and dry cereal was represented and displayed. This was done to initiate a unit on breakfasts. It promoted much interest, especially after the boxes were examined to see what food values the cereals contained. In a fourth grade class that was talking about food spoilage, several persons were asked to bring a good item and a spoiled one to class, for example, a good grapefruit and a bad one, a sound potato and an unsound one, a fresh stalk of celery and a withered one. There was as much interest created by the bad specimen as by almost anything else brought to class that school year.

Other ideas for collections of health-centered articles include:

Canned food labels
Foods that clean teeth
   (apples, celery)
Household cleaning
   agents
Animals and human teeth
   (also bones and hair)
Potentially dangerous
   implements (knives, axes,
   sharp pencils, chisels)

Candy bar wrappers
Samples of good and poor
   sneakers
Varieties of apples
Drinking utensils used over
   the years
Pressed leaves and stalks
   of edible plants (wild)

31. Models. The true value of a model lies in its degree of accuracy. It helps also if it has several characteristics to attract the eye. An excellent sample of an attractive, natural size model is *Resusci Anne,* used for over 18 years for resuscitation training. It is a mannequin so real that using it to teach artificial lung ventilation and external cardiac compression (cardiopulmonary resuscitation or

CPR) is like working on a real person. (Available from Laerdal Medical Corporation, 1 Labriola Court, Arnack, N.Y. 10504.)

A number of biological supply houses sell excellent models of the various body parts. Merely demonstrating or exhibiting these, however, does not necessarily promote understandings and appreciations. Associating a model of the digestive system with a machine that processes foods or a model of the heart with a mechanical instrument is not enough. The teacher must project the idea that the digestive tract or heart or anything else is merely a part of the whole person, that humans are not machines—for no machine repairs itself or reproduces itself. In other words, a model is, at best, only a poor copy of the real thing but it may be quite helpful in creating favorable concepts. A model of the human ear, for instance, may help teach the fact that careless blowing of the nose can be dangerous. This is more important to understand than learning all of the names of the parts of the inner ear. An exploratory examination of the mechanics of the inner ear, however, may be the item that impresses the children the most. The way the model is used is probably more important than the model itself. If somehow the student can get the idea that the human body is the greatest of wonders, a real appreciation will be born.

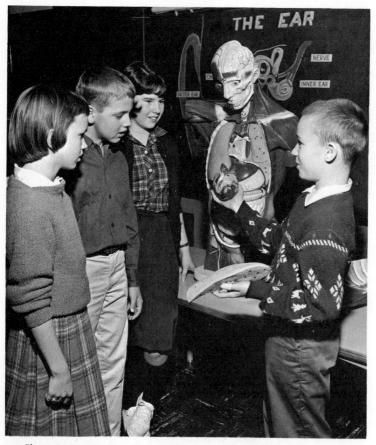

Figure 9–17. Studying the special senses via the model. (Courtesy Cincinnati Public Schools.)

Humanity wonders over many things, said St. Augustine, but "man himself is the most wonderful."

32. Mirrors. A large share of health teaching is concerned with personal appearance. The use of a single full length mirror can do much to impress growing boys and girls. Children may look at themselves in terms of cleanliness and neatness. They may view their own eyes, teeth and tongue at close range. Many children have never seen themselves in a full length mirror. Also, when it comes to posture improvement, there is no finer medium than the mirror. Full length mirrors hinged together are the most desirable for they allow several viewing angles.

33. Exhibits and Museums. The educational exhibit, whether a simple affair in the corner of a classroom or an elaborate museum layout, has considerable value in the health instruction area. It tends to have its greatest value when it is a product of the pupils who help to design and develop it.

A good health exhibit takes careful planning and time to prepare. Here are some useful standards to follow for making school exhibits:

Use only one central idea in the exhibit.

Place the exhibit where it is certain to be seen.

The exhibit is something to look at, not to read.

Make all labels short and simple, uniform and legible.

Motion attracts attention.

See that the exhibit is well lighted.

Use color to add interest and attractiveness.

Employ sound and various mechanisms to add charm to the exhibit.

The construction method of teaching is applicable to the building of displays for exhibits and museums. Children have excellent ideas when it comes to presenting these materials. The exhibits that stand out in almost any room are those which employ color and motion. Colored posters, colored paper, paint, or cloth add spice to the display. A simple battery-driven device or a turntable from a discarded phonograph puts motion into the exhibit. Music and other sounds may be supplied by automatic record players. Questions may be asked and answers given over a simple telephone circuit. Most local telephone companies are happy to cooperate in such a project by lending the necessary equipment to the teacher. In fact, there are many people in every community who willingly go out of their way to help the classroom teacher. An orthodontist, for example, will lend plaster casts of teeth, which may be displayed along with the teeth of horses and cows and the jawbones of other animals. A taxidermist in Florida will lend alligator teeth, while his or her colleague in Wyoming will lend one of the elk.

At almost any time of the year displays may be obtained for exhibit purposes from official and non-official health agencies. Many state health departments have such displays. In New York State two of the most popular have dealt with tuberculosis and fluoridation. Other displays may be obtained from the local heart or mental health association, the county health association, the National Foundation,

Figure 9–18. "Juno," world-famous transparent talking woman. (Courtesy Cleveland Health Museum.)

the American Red Cross, the American Dental Association, the National Safety Council, and many other health organizations. Safety displays are often prepared by traffic safety personnel in industry and business. And, of course, one should not overlook the local police department and its safety efforts.

The way an exhibit is used is the key to whether or not pupil behavior is changed in any appreciable way. Generally, there is an intrinsic interest in pupil-built exhibits—an interest that may accompany a particular display *if the teacher requires the pupils to use the materials.* Children should be permitted to touch, feel, and otherwise examine much of the exhibit. There should be answers to their questions. Even a formal listing of questions on a sheet of paper may help to guide some students in securing answers from the exhibit. More than one teacher has employed a simple version of the true-false questionnaire for the pupil to complete as he or she studies the exhibit.

Additional activity may be involved when electric buttons are pressed or little doors are opened. In the Cleveland Health Museum there is a food facts and fallacies exhibit which employs the "lift-up door" technique.[32] Here, a question is asked, such as "Are celery and fish special brain foods?" After the pupil ponders the answer for a few seconds, he or she simply lifts the hinged door and finds the answer. "No. There are no such things as brain foods." Other examples from this excellent display which support this method of teaching include the following:

Q. "Are raw eggs more digestible than cooked eggs?"
A. "No. Soft or hard cooked eggs are more digestible."
Q. "Is Vitamin A margarine as good as butter?"
A. "Yes. Vitamin A margarine contains the same amount of vitamin A as butter."
Q. "Is it safe to leave food standing in open tin cans?"
A. "Yes, if food is properly refrigerated."

True-false questions may be also used with this "lift-up door" technique. Following are two examples used for sixth graders in the Cleveland Health Museum:

Q. "Potatoes have more minerals and vitamins than a head of lettuce. True or false."
A. "True. Lettuce has few minerals and vitamins while potatoes contain iron, vitamins B and C."
Q. "Calcium pills are a good substitute for milk. True or False."
A. "False. Milk contains valuable minerals, vitamins, and proteins in addition to calcium."

The elementary school health museum may be built in a spare room or in the corner of a large classroom, but this is not easy to accomplish. A museum differs from the usual exhibit in that it is permanent. For this reason very few schools have a museum. Space is at a premium in most buildings and unless the whole school has easy access to the museum, it will soon lose its usefulness. The short-term exhibit, therefore, will be more practical for elementary school use and the museum will be more practical if set up as a resource area in the community.

Permanent museums have been gaining in popularity since the Century of Progress World's Fair in Chicago (1933–1934). One of the first to be established was the Mayo Foundation Museum of Hygiene and Medicine in Rochester, Minnesota, opened in 1935. A year later the Cleveland Health Museum was incorporated. The Dallas (Texas) Health Museum was organized in 1946 and in 1952 the now famous Lankenau Hospital Health Museum opened in a suburb of Philadelphia. This was followed by the establishment of the Hinsdale Health Museum in a Chicago suburb in 1959 and by 1963 the Reading (Pennsylvania) Hospital had its health museum in operation. In 1972

---

[32]The Cleveland Health Museum, Cleveland, Ohio, has a long history of experimenting with the more effective ways of visualizing health concepts. Among its most successful attempts has been the production of a series of suitcase exhibits created for classroom use.

the Hall of Health at the California Museum of Science and Industry opened in Los Angeles. It features the "Circulatory Man," the "Neuroman," and the "Transparent Woman." People of all ages are discovering that the value of a permanent health museum is great indeed; it is an educational institution, alive and vital—not a static, smelly mausoleum.

There is little doubt that the community health museum is a real force in the area of public health and school health education. The constantly replaced and modernized exhibits of the Dallas Health and Science Museum make it one of the outstanding educational forces in that section of the United States. The Cleveland Health Museum is without doubt the finest example of a museum set up to educate in matters of health. For almost three decades thousands of schoolchildren and adults have visited this institution to see superb exhibits such as: Human Genetics; the Hall of Health, which shows how the body is put together and how it works; the plastic engravings, "From Egg to Embryo"; the transparent talking woman; the transparent tooth; the famous Dickinson sculptured models showing human birth and growth; the sound of the beating heart; truths and misconceptions relative to food and nutrition; and many more. The educational department of this one museum supplies hundreds of schools annually with materials for use in various phases of health and human biology.

One of the most successful projects originated by the Cleveland Health Museum is that of the portable exhibits for health teaching in the classroom. These suitcase exhibits have traveled widely and teachers and nurses have been instructed in teaching from the materials presented. To facilitate this, a seven-minute magnetic tape recording was made for each exhibit, describing in detail and giving teachers pointers on what to stress at different grade levels as well as suggestions for class projects. A mimeographed teacher's manual was also developed.

Finally, and perhaps more important than anything else, the modern health museum is a place where one goes to look at something that is available without obvious propaganda and where one is saved from any kind of commercialism.

THE MEDIA CENTER

One of the problems confronting teachers is the storage of materials and equipment. For the teacher of several decades ago who was concerned primarily with one textbook for each subject, the problem of selection, handling, and storage of these materials was relatively simple. However, with the increase in variety and quantity of instructional aids came the problem of their management. This has been resolved in some of the larger elementary schools by the organization of a resource or materials center—more recently called a media center.

Such a center is a vital force in the health instruction program, especially if one person is given the responsibility for its direction.

Figure 9–19. Class of schoolchildren hear a museum staff instructor talk on "Wonder of Life" display. (Courtesy Cleveland Health Museum.)

Figure 9–20. Materials galore. Making ice cream in Grade One.

Regardless of size, a few of the services which the center can offer classroom teachers and pupils are:

Make available a central source for all types of teaching materials.

Assist in locating and obtaining needed teaching aids.

Assist with the production of classroom materials.

Organize and keep current a file of all health instructional materials and equipment in the school building and a file of community resources.

Maintain equipment and materials in a good state of repair.

Inform teachers of new materials.

Organize in-service training in the use of equipment for pupils and teachers.

In an open plan school, whose hub is the mediacenter, teaching is quite different. Groups of pupils choose the medium which helps them learn best. Such flexibility in a center encourages exploration, problem-solving projects, and independent study.

QUESTIONS FOR DISCUSSION

1. To what extent are teaching aids being used?

2. Does there appear to be any one teaching method that works more effectively than others in the teaching of health at the elementary school level? Explain.

3. What are your impressions about the use of values clarification methods in schools? Is it realistic to expect to reach the decision-making stage through value awareness activities? (See Dalis and Strasser; also Read, Simon, and Goodman in *Selected References.*)

4. In your opinion, what is the difference between seeing a good film dealing with the work of the heart or some other organ and hearing an interesting broadcast on this function?

5. Do you see the health museum as influential in helping students form concepts of healthful living? Does it have more or less to offer than a well-run classroom program in school?

6. As a classroom teacher interested in health instruction, what value would there seem to be in coordinating the activities and materials of the community health agencies with those of the school?

SUGGESTED ACTIVITIES

1. Go to a curriculum library and look over several brands of health textbooks suitable for primary or intermediate grade pupils. Generally, the level of word difficulty and the pictures will approximate the age level of the pupils for which the text is intended. However, the content may vary considerably between brand books for a particular grade level. What are some of your specific observations?

2. Review an article or two about innovation in teaching. Are there ways of teaching that literally "turn kids on"? List the essential points set forth in the article you review; follow this up with your comments.

3. Review several books listed under *Selected References* and compare their view on effective teaching. Which methods seem to be stressed today? Which methods appear to be the least popular? Are there research data given in support of a particular teaching method?

4. Visit a media center that has been established to serve the varied needs of teachers in a school system. Find out how it functions and how regularly it is used by the elementary classroom teachers.

5. Observe the teaching method being practiced in an elementary school classroom. After the class is dismissed, ask the teacher *why* the particular method was chosen. Ask also if the method has replaced another method or has been changed at any time during the last year or two. In short, are teachers flexible in the use of methods?

6. Design an experiment to appraise the effects of three different methods of teaching on health behavior. The health topic and methods selected may be of your own choosing.

SELECTED REFERENCES

Bedworth, David A. and Bedworth, Albert E. *Health Education: A Process for Human Effectiveness,* New York: Harper & Row, 1978, Chapters 8 and 12.

Brown, George I. *The Live Curriculum.* New York: The Viking Press, 1975.

Bruess, Clint E. and Gay, John E. *Implementing Comprehensive School Health,* New York: Macmillan Publishing Co., 1978.

Dacey, John S. *New Ways to Learn: The Psychology of Education.* Stamford, Connecticut: Greylock Publishers, 1976, Part 1.

Dalis, Gus T. and Strasser, Ben B. *Teaching Strategies for Value Awareness and Decision Making in Health Education.* Thorofare, N.J.: Charles B. Slack, Inc., 1977.

_____ "A Concept of Value for the Classroom." *Health Education, 7*:12–13, March/April 1976.

Ensor, Phyllis G. and Means, Richard K. *Instructor's Resource and Methods Handbook for Health Education,* 2nd ed., Boston: Allyn and Bacon, Inc., 1977.

Erickson, Carlton W. and Curl, D. C. *Fundamentals of Teaching Audio-Visual Technology.* New York: Macmillan Publishing Co., 1972.

Funk, Hal D. and Olberg, Robert T. *Learning to Teach in the Elementary School.* New York: Dodd, Mead & Co., 1971.

Galli, Nicholas. *Foundations and Principles of Health Education.* New York: John Wiley and Sons, Inc., 1977, Chapter 6.

Good, Thomas L., et al. *Teachers Make a Difference,* New York: Holt, Rinehart & Winston, 1975.

Gray, William A. and Gerrard, Brian A. *Learning By Doing: Developing Teaching Skills.* Boston: Addison-Wesley Publishing Co., Inc., 1977.

Greenberg, Jerrold S. *Student-Centered Health Instruction: A Humanistic Approach.* Boston: Addison-Wesley Publishing Co., 1978.

Hash, Virginia. *Values: Awareness, Significance and Action.* Dubuque: Kendall/Hunt Publishing Co., 1975.

Hubbard, Nancy E. "Motivation for Health Learning: Taped 'Live Experience'," *Journal of School Health, 42*:548–550, November, 1972.

Kime, Robert E., Schlaadt, Richard H. and Tritsch, Leonard E. *Health Instruction: An Action Approach.* Englewood Cliffs: Prentice-Hall, Inc., 1977, Chapter 7.

Kniker, Charles R. *You and Value Education.* Columbus, Ohio: Charles E. Merrill Publishing Co., 1977.

Lacey, Richard A. *Seeing With Feeling: Film in the Classroom.* Philadelphia: W. B. Saunders Co., 1972.

Miller, John P. *Humanizing the Classroom: Models of Teaching in Affective Education.* New York: Praeger Publishers, 1976.

Nelson, L. W. and Lorbeer, G. C. *Science Activities for Elementary Children.* 5th ed., Dubuque: William C. Brown Co., Publishers, 1975.

Nakamura, Raymond. "Health 4 Fun: A Game of Knowledge," *Health Education,* 9:35, September/October 1977.

Read, Donald A. *Looking In: Exploring One's Personal Health Values.* Englewood Cliffs, N.J: Prentice-Hall, Inc., 1977.

—————————, Simon, Sidney B., and Goodman, J. B. *Health Education: The Search for Values.* Englewood Cliffs, N.J.: Prentice-Hall, Inc., 1977.

————————— and Greene, Walter H. *Creative Teaching in Health.* 2nd ed., New York: Macmillan Publishing Co., 1975.

Shart, Philip A. "Sixth Grade Film Making," *Instructor, 81*:43, June/July 1972.

Simon, Sidney B. "Promoting the Search for Values," *School Health Review, 2*:21–25, February 1971.

Snow, David L. "Behavior Modification Techniques in School Setting," *Journal of School Health, 44*:198–204, April 1974.

Sorochan, Walter D. and Bender, Stephen J. *Teaching Elementary Health Science,* Boston: Addison-Wesley Publishing Co., 1975.

Stone, Donald B., O'Reilly, Lawrence B. and Brown, James D. *Elementary School Health Education.* Dubuque: William C. Brown Co., Publishers, 1976.

Torrance, E. P. and Myers, R. E. *Creative Learning and Teaching.* New York: Dodd, Mead and Co., 1971.

Wiist, William A. "Television Production for A Community Health Project," *Health Education, 6*:39–40, November/December 1975.

Willgoose, Carl E. *Health Teaching In Secondary Schools,* 2nd ed., Philadelphia: W. B. Saunders Co., 1977, Chapter 9.

Sources of Free
and Inexpensive
Teaching Aids

10

The health curriculum, having lost its old-fashioned rigidity, now employs a variety of health materials to supplement books and teacher lectures; this is a practical means of recording and reporting the current scene. But it requires considerable work on the part of the teacher to locate and select these materials for classroom use. A vast amount of material is available because many organizations are interested in child health.

A number of organizations and agencies have educational consultants who are of real help to teachers. Others simply make materials available on request; they are usually free or relatively inexpensive. When ordering materials, it is well to mention the age group to be served and the special area of interest. Some companies or agencies will then go out of their way to supply useful aids to learning.

The Reliability of Health Information

Health information must be evaluated before it is used in the classroom. How reliable is this material? Is it loaded with advertising in order to sell a product? Ordinarily there is little reason to question the materials and aids of a well-known organization such as the American Red Cross or the American Medical Association. And there are numerous commercial organizations that conscientiously promote health as their primary purpose, followed by the promotion of their own product. This is well demonstrated by the fact that it is sometimes difficult to find the name of the commercial organization or its product on the school health literature.

The evaluation of health information, whether it is read, heard, or seen, may be determined in part by appraising the publisher, association, or agency. One might ask the following questions:

Is the agency recognized as having a good reputation in the field of health?

Why has the health information been presented?

Is the purpose of the communication to give facts on which to base personal opinion and beliefs? To improve living?

Is the purpose to sell specific products or ideas without reference to the scientific value of the product?

433

Is the purpose simply to entertain?

What are the qualifications of the specific author?

Is the material up to date?

What is the opinion of others, such as medical experts, public or private agencies and reliable friends, familiar with the topic?

OFFICIAL HEALTH AGENCIES

Organizations that have been established by law to accomplish specific health maintenance, promotion, and control are generally designated as official health agencies. These include city, county, state, and federal government organizations. Very often a wealth of free teaching aids is available from these groups:

City and County Health Departments—Child health material in the form of pamphlets for teacher use. Films and certain poster material may also be on hand.

State Health Departments—In almost every state there are many child and teacher health pamphlets, monthly magazines or bulletins, films, special health exhibits, and speakers available for school use. In addition to this, several states publish catalogs dealing specifically with sources of health education materials and selected audio-visual aids.

State Universities—In many states the unit of the state university having to do with public health or school health provides pamphlets, bulletins, and special charts for school use within the state. Other institutions, such as Indiana University, Syracuse University, or Boston University, have an extensive division which supplies a wide variety of audio-visual aids. See table on opposite page.

NON-OFFICIAL HEALTH AGENCIES

In almost every American community there are groups of citizens banded together for the express purpose of promoting health. Generally their interest is centered on some special disease or abnormality such as malnutrition, mental illness, heart disease, or handicapped children. This groups are, without a doubt, in a position to be of immense service to the schoolteacher if the teacher will call upon them.

Non-official agencies generally include *voluntary health agencies, commercial organizations,* and *professional associations.* Their scope of influence is great and includes health education services for the entire community, its industries, and its schools. If the agency is a state or national one, its sphere of influence is almost unlimited.

With the tremendous growth in the number of charitable institutions and foundations in this country over the last quarter century, it is becoming increasingly difficult to differentiate between a purely voluntary health organization and a professional association. Many voluntary health organizations began at the local level with a handful of volunteers and blossomed through the years into full-fledged national groups with considerable professional zeal. In any case, both categories of organization exist to help in any way they can.

Federal Government

Department of Health, Education, and Welfare, Office of Education, Washington, D.C. 20025	Special booklets, primarily for teacher use, on food, alcohol, drugs, environmental pollution, consumer health, prevention and control of illness. Lists of materials are available with no charge for single copies.

General Services Administration

National Archives and Records Service, National Audiovisual Center, Washington, D.C. 20409	Extensive list of films on all major health problems. For rent or sale.
National Interagency on Smoking and Health, P.O. Box 3650, Arlington, Virginia 22203	Extensive material on smoking research and smoking education programs.
National Coordinating Council on Drug Abuse, P.O. Box 19400, Washington, D.C. 20036	Program materials on drug abuse; for school and community use.
National Institute of Mental Health, Chevy Chase, Maryland 20015	Teaching aids pertaining to mental health and related areas.
U.S. Environmental Protection Agency, Office of Public Affairs, Washingington, D.C. 20460	Environmental, ecological, and conservation literature.
Superintendent of Documents, U.S. Government Printing Office, Washington, D.C. 20025	Considerable health information for teacher use which may be adapted to healthful school living and health teaching. A catalog should be secured before materials are ordered.
U.S. Public Health Service, Washington, D.C. 20201	This organization has many health interests including the National Institutes of Health, health research, statistics, and promotion.
U.S. Children's Bureau, Division of Reports, Washington, D.C. 20025	Numerous catalogs, child health pamphlets, and lists.
The United Nations World Health Organization, Geneva, Switzerland (or New York, N.Y. 20006)	A large number of picture booklets dealing with world health conditions. Useful in studying community health and social studies.

The staff and members of these citizen and professional worker groups help the schools enrich curricula, add resources, carry on research, and improve the school health programs. The schools in turn offer to these agencies an excellent channel for working towards personal and community health. Certainly there are common goals: "child health is everybody's business." Moreover, there are common activities involving the home and the school. Some of the agency activities include:

Making available to school personnel the latest health information.

Providing teaching aids.

Helping in the preparation of resource units.

Helping with special short-term projects.

Helping with in-service education of teachers.

Providing the means for demonstrations and studies.

Enriching the curriculum.

Interpreting the school health program and needs of the community to parents and others.

Voluntary and Professional Health Agencies

A selected number of the more productive voluntary and professional health agencies that have proved to be of immeasurable service to elementary teachers are as follows:

Alcoholics Anonymous, P.O. Box 429, Grand Central Annex, New York, N.Y. 10017.

American Academy of Pediatrics, 1801 Hinmon Avenue, Box 1034, Evanston, Ill. 60204.

American Alliance for Health, Physical Education, and Recreation, Department of the National Education Association, 1201 16th Street, N.W., Washington, D.C. 20036.

American Association of Poison Control Centers, c/o Academy of Medicine of Cleveland, 10525 Carnegie Ave., Cleveland, Ohio 44106.

American Cancer Society, 219 E. 42nd Street, New York, N.Y. 10017.

American Dental Association, 211 E. Chicago Avenue, Chicago, Ill. 60611.

American Foundation for the Blind, 15 W. 16th Street, New York, N.Y. 10011.

American Hearing Society, 919 18th Street, N.W., Washington, D.C. 20006.

American Heart Association, 44 E. 23rd Street, New York, N.Y. 10010.

American Hospital Association, 840 N. Lake Shore Drive, Chicago, Ill. 60611.

American Institute of Family Relations, 5287 Sunset Boulevard, Los Angeles, Calif. 90027.

American Lung Association, 51 Sleeper St., Boston, Mass. 02210.

American Medical Association, 535 N. Dearborn Street, Chicago, Ill. 60610.

American National Red Cross, 17th and D Streets, N.W., Washington, D.C. 20006.

American Optometric Association, Department of Public Affairs, 700 Chippewa Street, St. Louis, Mo. 63119.

American Public Health Association, 1790 Broadway, New York, N.Y. 10019.

American School Health Association, 515 E. Main Street, Kent, Ohio 44241.

American Social Health Association, 1740 Broadway, New York, N.Y. 10019.

Arthritis Foundation, 23 West 45th Street, New York, N.Y. 10019.

Better Vision Institute, 630 Fifth Avenue, New York, N.Y. 10020.

Child Study Association of America, 9 East 89th Street, New York, N.Y. 10028.

Cleveland Health Museum, 8911 Euclid Avenue, Cleveland, Ohio 44106.

Hogg Foundation for Mental Health, University of Texas, Austin, Tex. 78712.

Muscular Dystrophy Associations of America, 1790 Broadway, New York, N.Y. 10019.

National Association of Hearing and Speech Agencies, 919 18th Street, N.W., Washington, D.C. 20006.

National Congress of Parents and Teachers, 700 N. Rush St., Chicago, Ill. 60637.

National Coordinating Council on Drug Abuse, P.O. Box 19400, Washington, D.C. 20036.

National Council on Alcoholism, 2 Park Avenue, New York, N.Y. 10016.

National Education Association, Division of Elementary Education, 1201 16th Street, N.W., Washington, D.C. 20036.

National Foundation, 800 Second Avenue, New York, N.Y. 10017.

National Multiple Sclerosis Society, 257 Park Avenue South, New York, N.Y. 10010.

National Nutrition Education Clearing House, P.O. Box 931, Berkeley, Calif. 94701.

National Safety Council, 425 N. Michigan Avenue, Chicago, Ill. 60611.

National Society for Crippled Children and Adults, Inc., 2023 W. Ogden Avenue, Chicago, Ill. 60603.

National Society for the Prevention of Blindness, Inc., 79 Madison Avenue, New York, N.Y. 10016.

Nutrition Foundation, Inc., 99 Park Avenue, New York, N.Y. 10016.

Planned Parenthood Federation of America, Inc., 515 Madison Avenue, New York, N.Y. 10022.

Public Affairs Committee, 381 Park Avenue South, New York, N.Y. 10016.

Rutgers Center for Alcohol Studies, The State University, Rutgers, New Brunswick, N.J. 08901.

Sex Education and Information Council of U.S. (SEICUS), 1855 Broadway, New York, N.Y. 10023.

United Cerebral Palsy Associations, Inc., 321 W. 44th Street, New York, N.Y. 10017.

Commercial Organizations and Associations of Industry

There are many business and commercial agencies which publish materials especially fitted for elementary school use. The list of individual industries that offer printed matter is a long one. It is customary today for practically every commercial organization to promote its product through bulletins, brochures, posters, and other advertising media. Many of these companies have suitable products that are legitimate in terms of health promotion. In the area of foods there are a number of firms that sell a healthful product and employ sound health teaching techniques to promote it. There is also a large number of companies which promote a valid health concept as a public service item. For instance, a company promoting dental health through charts, leaflets, and films puts over a basic idea. This in turn is good business, for it sells more dental products. When people buy more dental products, this is an indication that their health behavior has been favorably changed. In view of this, a number of commercial firms in several areas have formed their own association. These associations of industry make available, often in unlimited quantity, a number of health items for the classroom teacher to use with the pupils.

There follows a partial list of national sources of especially reliable and generous companies and associations of industry. No attempt is made here to list specific materials offered by these sources but in many cases catalogs are available and in most cases the name of the agency will indicate to some extent the subject matter and scope of its material.

Aetna Life Affiliated Companies, Education Department, 151 Farmington Avenue, Hartford, Conn. 06115. Leaflets and motion pictures on safety for teachers and pupils, special tests.

American Automobile Association, Traffic Safety Department, 1712 G Street, N.W., Washington, D.C. 20036. Pamphlets and films on traffic safety; also safety project materials.

American Institute of Baking, Consumer Service Department, 400 E. Ontario Street, Chicago, Ill. 60611. Pamphlets, posters, self-testing charts, colorful guides to eating, record forms.

American Insurance Association, Safety Department, 85 John Street, New York, N.Y. 10038.

Armour and Company, Public Relations Department, 401 N. Wabash Street, Chicago, Ill. 60690. Maps, charts on foods.

Association of American Soap and Glycerine Products, Inc., Cleanliness Bureau, 295 Madison Avenue, New York, N.Y. 10016. Pamphlets, posters, radio and TV scripts.

Athletic Institute, 805 Merchandise Mart, Chicago, Ill. 60650.

Behavioral Research Laboratories, Box 577, Palo Alto, Calif. 94300.

Bicycle Institute of America, 122 E. 42nd Street, New York, N.Y. 10017.

Blue Cross Association, 840 N. Lake Shore Drive, Chicago, Ill. 60611.

The Borden Company, The Borden Building, 350 Madison Avenue, New York, N.Y. 10017. Pamphlets on milk values and uses.

Cereal Institute, Inc., Educational Director, 1111 Plaza Drive, Schaumburg, Ill. 60195. Classroom teaching units, food charts, and graphs.

Colgate Palmolive Company, 300 Park Avenue, New York, N.Y. 10022. Toothbrushing kits and dental health teaching materials.

Consumer Union of U.S., Inc., Mount Vernon, N.Y. 10550. Consumer health pamphlets and booklets.

Cream of Wheat Corporation, Box M, Minneapolis, Minn. 55413.

Educational Activities Inc., Box 392, Freeport, N.Y. 11520. Action records for physical fitness and rhythmics.

Eli Lilly and Company, 740 South Alabama Street, Indianapolis, Indiana 46206. Materials on safety and control of infectious diseases.

Employers Mutuals of Wausau, 407 Grant Street, Wausau, Wisc. 55402.

Encyclopaedia Britannica Educational Corporation, Britannica Building, 425 N. Michigan Avenue, Wilmette, Ill. 60611. Filmstrips, slide films, movies, cartoons, and records. (Rentals only.)

Evaporated Milk Association, 228 North LaSalle Street, Chicago, Ill. 60601. Flash cards, graphs, and leaflets on milk equivalent values.

Florida Citrus Commission, P.O. Box 148, Lakeland, Fla. 33802. Posters, pamphlets, movies on citrus fruits.

Ford Motor Company, Information Department, Dearborn, Mich. 48127. Traffic safety materials.

General Mills, Inc., Education Section, 9200 Wayzata Boulevard, Minneapolis, Minn. 55426. Nutrition education teaching aids.

H. J. Heinz Company, P.O. Box 57, Pittsburgh, Pa. 15230. Food charts and stories of origin of various foods.

Johnson & Johnson, Educational Division, New Brunswick, N.J. 08903. Charts, pamphlets, films on first aid and safety and programmed first aid instruction for grade six.

Kansas Wheat Commission, 1021 N. Main Street, Hutchinson, Kan. 67501.

Kellogg Company, Department of Home Economics Services, Battle Creek, Mich. 49016. Breakfast food pamphlets and charts.

Kimberly-Clark Corporation, Educational Department, Neenah, Wis. 54947. Menstrual physiology chart and films; pamphlets, guides on common cold.

Kraft Cheese Company, 500 Peshtigo Court, Chicago, Ill. 60690. Nutrition items.

Lederle Laboratories Division, American Cyanamid Co., Pearl River, N.Y. 10965. Child health and nutrition information.

Licensed Beverage Industries, Inc., 155 E. 44th Street, New York, N.Y. 10017.

Metropolitan Life Insurance Company, Health and Welfare Division, 1 Madison Avenue, New York, N.Y. 10010. Catalogs, exhibits, films, filmstrips, booklets for teachers on all diseases and the school health instruction program; health bulletin for teachers.

Money Management Institute, Prudential Plaza, Chicago, Ill. 60601. Consumer health materials.

National Board of Fire Underwriters, 85 John Street, New York, N.Y. 10038.

National Dairy Council, Program Service Department, 111 N. Canal Street, Chicago, Ill. 60606. Health education materials, exhibits, films, filmstrips, displays, animals for feeding experiments. Local chapters are rich in materials especially suited for primary and intermediate grades; health bulletins for teachers.

National Fire Protection Association, Public Relations Department, 60 Batterymarch Street, Boston, Mass. 02110. Posters, pamphlets, safety lists, comics, fire inspection blanks, charts, quizzes.

National Livestock and Meat Board, 36 S. Wabash Avenue, Chicago, Ill. 60603. Self-testing charts, food graphs, colored posters of the various cuts of meat, pamphlets on food values of meat.

North Dakota State Wheat Commission, 316 N. Fifth Street, Bismarck, North Dakota 58501.

Ocean Spray Cranberries, Inc., Executive Offices, Hanson, Mass. 02341. Pamphlets, films, food recipes, and food record charts.

Personal Products Company, Milltown, N.J. 08850. Charts, posters, leaflets regarding menstruation.

Pet Milk Co., 1406 Arcade Building, St. Louis, Mo. 63101. Nutrition pamphlets and charts.

Pharmaceutical Manufacturers Association, 1155 15th Street, N.W., Washington, D.C. 20005. Films and booklets on general health topics.

The Procter and Gamble Company, P.O. Box 171, Cincinnati, Ohio 45201. Booklets and materials for dental health. Several excellent posters in color.

Schering Laboratories, Kenilworth, N.J. 07033.

Scholastic Book Services, 904 Sylvan Avenue, Englewood Cliffs, N.J. 07632.

Scott Paper Company, Home Service Center, Philadelphia, Pa. 19913. Menstrual health pamphlets.

Sealtest Foods Consumer Service, 605 3rd Avenue, New York, N.Y. 10016. Food charts and graphs.

Social Studies School Service, 10,000 Culver Blvd., Culver City, Col. 90230.

South Dakota Wheat Commission, P.O. Box 549, Pierre, South Dakota 57501.

Spenco Medical Corporation, Box 8113, Waco, Tex. 76710.

Stanley Bowmar Company, Inc., Valhalla, N.Y. 10595. Records for creative activities and rhythmics.

Sunkist Growers, Box 7888, Valley Annex, Van Nuys, Calif. 91409. Teaching units on nutrition, posters, pamphlets.

Swift and Co., Union Stockyards, Chicago, Ill. 60609.

Tampax, Incorporated, Educational Director, 5 Dakota Drive, Lake Success, New York 11045. Anatomical charts, student pamphlets, and special instruction materials for teachers on the subject of menstruation.

The Travelers Insurance Company, Hartford, Conn. 06115. Charts on growth, height-weight, and posture, and several colorful posters.

United Fresh Fruit and Vegetable Association, 777 14th Street, N.W., Washington, D.C. 20005. Leaflets on foods for elementary level.

United States Beet Sugar Association, Tower Building, Washington, D.C. 20005. Teaching kits and charts.

Washington Wheat Commission, 409 Great Western Building, Spokane, Wash. 99201.

Wheat Flour Institute, Supervisor of Distribution, 14 E. Jackson Boulevard, Chicago, Ill. 60604. Posters, filmstrips, pamphlets, and catalogs pertaining to nutritious breakfast foods.

SOURCES OF AIDS FOR HEALTH TEACHING UNITS

A list of sources of health teaching materials for a major area of study cannot contain every known aid, nor would one want it to, because some sources are better than others for teaching a certain health topic. The teacher's time is at a premium and following up several leads to sources takes time. It is the purpose of the author, therefore, to limit the following list to those sources of *teaching aids which have proved to be especially valuable in the health instruction program in the elementary schools.*[1] All sources listed are for the students to read or see themselves. They have been carefully selected with this in mind.

In previous editions of this book, there were long lists of pamphlets and leaflets for each major health area. These have now been eliminated because their titles and content change from year to year. It is recommended that teachers contact organizations and companies for a current list of their written materials.

The sources are set up by health topics which are in keeping with the major activity areas referred to in Chapter 8. The type of teaching aid (e.g., film, filmstrip, poster), the specific name of the aid, and the name of the agency supplying it are listed.

---

[1]For additional sources see *Educator's Guide to Free Films, Filmstrips, Transcriptions, Tapes and Scripts,* Educators Progress Services, Randolph, Wis. 53956 (annual).

1. Personal Cleanliness and Appearance*

a. Films**

Alexander Has A Good Day, Coronet Instructional Films.
Body Care and Grooming, McGraw-Hill Book Company.
Care of the Hair and Nails, Encyclopaedia Britannica.
Care of the Skin, Encyclopaedia Britannica.
Choosing Clothes for Health, Coronet Instructional Films.
Cleanliness and Health, Coronet Instructional Films.
Hear Better: Healthy Ears, Coronet Instructional Films.
Health: The Dirt Witch Cleans Up, Encyclopaedia Britannica.
How Billy Keeps Clean, Coronet Instructional Films.
How the Ear Functions, Knowledge Builders.
Joan Avoids a Cold, Coronet Instructional Films.
Johnny's New World, National Society for the Prevention of Blindness.
Kitty Keeps Clean, Young America Films.
Let's Be Clean and Neat, Coronet Instructional Films.
Platform Posture, Young America Films.
Running for Sheriff, Charles Cahill and Associates.
See Better: Healthy Eyes, Coronet Instructional Films.
Ways to Good Habits, Coronet Instructional Films.
Your Cleanliness, Young America Films.
Your Ears, Young America Films.
Your Eyes, Young America Films.
Your Friend the Doctor, Coronet Instructional Films.
Your Health at School, Coronet Instructional Films.
Your Teeth, Young America Films.

b. Filmstrips

Care of the Hair and Nails (Health story), Encyclopaedia Britannica.
Care of the Skin (Health story), Encyclopaedia Britannica.
Healthy, Happy, and Wise, Popular Science.
How Your Ears Work, Popular Science.
Keep Yourself Clean, Scholastic Book Services.
Keeping Clean, McGraw-Hill Book Company.
Keeping Well, McGraw-Hill Book Company.
Let's Stand Tall, Society for Visual Education.
Protecting Our Eyes and Ears, McGraw-Hill Book Company.
The Ears, Young America Films.
The Eyes, Young America Films.
The Neat Bird, Walt Disney Education Media Company.
The Science of Personal Appearance, McGraw-Hill Book Company.
The Wizard of Good Appearance, Walt Disney Educational Media Company.
This Is You, Encyclopaedia Britannica.
You and Your Clothes, Young America Films.
You and Your Ears, Encyclopaedia Britannica.
Your Eyes at Work, Popular Science.
Your Skin and Its Care, Popular Science.

c. Posters

A Bath Can Be Man's Best Friend, Spenco Medical Corporation.
Clean Is a Neat Word, Spenco Medical Corporation.
Be Fair—Cover Your Coughs and Sneezes, National Tuberculosis Association.
How to Catch a Cold, Kimberly-Clark Corporation.
Physical Fitness Posters, National Dairy Council.
Reading Takes Seeing, American Optometric Association.
School Time, Vision Exam Time, American Optometric Association.
To Fight Germs—Wash Your Hands, National Tuberculosis Association.
Wash Thoroughly, National Safety Council.

d. Charts

Cross Section of the Eye, National Society for the Prevention of Blindness.
One Out of Four Children Needs Eye Care, National Society for the Prevention of Blindness.

---

*Includes the care of the special senses.
**The addresses of film and filmstrip sources may be found on page 465.

Snellen, Symbol E Charts, National Society for the Prevention of Blindness.
The Ivory Inspection Patrol, Procter and Gamble.

e. Radio Scripts

(From University of Texas, Bureau of Research in Education by Radio)
Care of the Skin
Cleanliness
Importance of Good Vision
We Wash Our Hands Before We Eat

f. Tape Recordings

Health Is Wealth (HC15), New York State University College of Agriculture, Cornell
University, Ithaca, N.Y.
Are We Responsible for Our Own Good Health? Audio-Visual Aids Service, University
of Illinois.

g. Selected Stories for Children

(P) Primary Level, (I) Intermediate Level

About Glasses for Gladys (I), Mary K. Erickson (Melmont).
All Ready for Winter (P), Leone Adelson (McKay).
Big and Little (P), J. P. Miller (Random).
Health Can Be Fun (P), Munro Leaf (Lippincott).
Lesson in Loveliness (I), J. W. Scott (Macrae, Smith).
Look at Your Eyes (I), Paul Showers (Crowell).
Manners Can Be Fun (P), Munro Leaf (Lippincott).
Much Bigger Than Martin (I), Stephen Kellogg (Dial).
Nothing to Wear but Clothes (I), F. K. Jupo (Aladdin).
Our Senses and How They Work (I), H. Zimm (Morrow).
Our Wonderful Eyes (P), J. Perry (McGraw-Hill).
Somebody Called Boo (P), L. Gardner (Watts).
Story of Your Coat (P,I), Clara Hollos (International Publishing Co.)
The Clean Pig (P), Leonard Weisgard (Scribner).
Tim and His Hearing Aid (I), E. C. Ronnei and Joan and Max Porter (Dodd).
Time Out for Living (P), D. E. Patridge and C. Mooney (American Book).
True Book of Health (P), O. U. Haynes (Children's Press).
You and Your Senses (I), L. Schneider (Harcourt).
Your Ears (I), Irving and Ruth Adler (John Day).
Your Eyes, (I), Irving and Ruth Adler (John Day).
Your Manners Are Showing (I), B. Betz (Grossett).

2. Activity, Sleep, Rest, and Relaxation

a. Films

America Goes Camping, Bicycle Institute of America.
American Square Dance, Coronet Instructional Films.
Day at the Fair, Coronet Instructional Films.
Exercise and Health, Coronet Instructional Films.
Fun That Builds Good Health, Coronet Instructional Films.
How the Body Uses Energy, McGraw-Hill Book Company.
Improving Your Posture, Coronet Instructional Films.
Play in the Snow, Encyclopaedia Britannica.
Playtown U.S.A., The Athletic Institute.
Safety: Playground Spirits, Encyclopaedia Britannica.
Ski the Outer Limits, Bicycle Institute of America.
Sleep for Health, Encyclopaedia Britannica.
Water Safety, Young America Films.
You and Your Helpers, Coronet Instructional Films.
Your Child's Health and Fitness, American Alliance for Health, Physical Education,
and Recreation AAHPER, Washington, D.C. 20036.
Your Exercise and Posture, Coronet Instructional Films.

b. Filmstrips

At Home in the Evening, Popular Science.
Checking Your Health, Encyclopaedia Britannica.

Exercise and Health, American Alliance for Health, Physical Education, and Recreation.
Exercise for Happy Living, Encyclopaedia Britannica.
Feeling Fit, Scholastic Book Services.
Getting Ready for Bed, Popular Science.
Learning About Growth and Exercise, Encyclopaedia Britannica.
Learning About Sleep and Rest, Encyclopaedia Britannica.
Physical Fitness and Health, Walt Disney Educational Media Company.
Rest and Sleep, McGraw-Hill Book Company.
Rest and Sleep, Young America Films.
Sleep and Rest, Popular Science.
Sleep for Health, Encyclopaedia Britannica.
The Muscular System, Encyclopaedia Britannica.
The Skeletal System, Encyclopaedia Britannica.
Working and Playing Together, McGraw-Hill Book Company.

c. Posters

Activity Strengthens; Inactivity Weakens—Hippocrates, Spenco Medical Corporation.
A Day with the Wide Awakes, General Mills, Inc.
Health Is Not Just Luck, General Mills, Inc.
Keep Physically Fit, Florida Citrus Commission.
Lift with Your Legs, Not Your Back, American Medical Association.
Physical Fitness (4), Educational Activities, Inc.
Physical Fitness (9), National Dairy Council.
Physical Fitness Posters (4), Stanley Bowmar Co.
We Help You Keep Fit, Florida Citrus Commission.

d. Charts

Ball Handling Skills, Athletic Institute.
Day to Day Good Health Records, Kellogg Company.
Your Heart and How It Works, American Heart Association.

e. Radio Scripts

Batter Up, National Safety Council.
Fresh Air and Sunshine, Bureau of Research in Education by Radio, University of Texas.
Sleep and Rest, Bureau of Research in Education by Radio, University of Texas.
Swimming Is Fun, National Safety Council.
Vacation Daze, National Safety Council.

f. Comics

The Adventures of Eva, Pora, and Ted, Evaporated Milk Association.

g. Records

Another Rainy Days Record, Educational Activities.
Around the World in Dance, Educational Activities.
Classroom Rhythms, Stanley Bowmar Co.
Exercise Every Day, Educational Activities, Inc.
Honor Your Partner Records, Educational Activities, Inc.
Let's Do Some Posture Exercises, Educational Activities, Inc.
Lullabies for Sleepy Heads, Dorothy Olsen, RCA Victor.
Modern Square Dancing, Stanley Bowmar Co.
Music for Relaxation, Melochrino Strings, RCA Victor.
Play Party-Singing Games, Stanley Bowmar Co.
Physical Fitness Activities, Album 14, Primary Grades (Durlacher), Stanley Bowmar Co.
Rhythms and Game Songs, Stanley Bowmar Co.
Rhythmic Play Series (K–3), Educational Record Sales.
Toy Shop Album (A4—Grades 1–6), Activity Records.

h. Selected Stories for Children

(P) Primary Level, (I) Intermediate Level

Bedtime for Frances (P), H. Hoban (Harper and Bros.)
Boo, Who Used to Be Scared of the Dark (P), Munro Leaf (Random House).
Child's Good Night Book (P), Margaret Wise Brown (W. R. Scott).
Child's Treasury of Things to Do (P), Caroline Horowitz (Hart).
Do You Move As I Do? (P), Helen Borten (Abelard).

Forty Rainy Day Games and Play Alone Fun (P), Caroline Horowitz (Hart).
Going to Camp (P,I), Helen Beck (Daye).
Health Can Be Fun (P), Munro Leaf (Lippincott).
Hustle and Bustle (P), Louis Slobodkin (Macmillan).
Jimmy's Own Basketball (I), M. B. Renick (Scribner).
Joey Gets the Golf Bug (I), J. Sherman (Little, Brown).
Lifeline (I), L. Schneider (Harcourt).
Mr. Tall and Mr. Small (I), Barbara Brenner (W. R. Scott).
Sleepy ABC (P), Margaret Wise Brown (Lothrop).
Switch on the Night (P), R. Bradbury (Pantheon).
The Dream Book (P), Margaret Wise Brown (Random House).
Time for Sleep (I), Millicent Selsam (W. R. Scott).
Touchdown for Tommy (I), M. Christopher (Little, Brown).
While Susie Sleeps (P), Nina Scheider (W. R. Scott).
Who's Afraid of Thunder? (I), H. E. Sandman (Sterling).

3. Nutrition and Growth

a. Films

Better Breakfasts, U.S.A., Cereal Institutes, Inc.
Big Dinner Table, National Dairy Council.
Changing Foods in Changing Times, Cereal Institute.
Digestion of Foods, Encyclopaedia Britannica.
Eat for Health, Encyclopaedia Britannica.
Food, Energy and You, National Dairy Council.
Food and Growth, Encyclopaedia Britannica.
Food, the Color of Life, National Dairy Council.
Foods That Build Good Health, Coronet Instructional Films.
Foundation Foods, Avis Films, Inc.
Fundamentals of Diet, Encyclopaedia Britannica.
Good Eating Habits, Coronet Instructional Films.
Good Table Manners, Coronet Instructional Films.
Growing Up Day by Day, Encyclopaedia Britannica.
Judy Learns About Milk, Young America Films.
Health—You and Your Helpers, Charles Cahill and Associates.
Learning About Foods We Eat, Coronet Films.
Milk, Encyclopaedia Britannica.
Nutrition and Weight Control, Metropolitan Life Insurance Company.
Something You Didn't Eat, Association Films.
The Best Way to Eat, Florida Citrus Commission.
The King Who Came to Breakfast, Association Films.
The Wheat Farmer, Encyclopaedia Britannica.
Two Little Rats, National Dairy Council.
Uncle Jim's Dairy Farm, National Dairy Council.
Understanding Vitamins, Encyclopaedia Britannica.
Vegetables for All Seasons, Arthur Barr Productions, Inc.
Visit to Dairyland U.S.A., National Dairy Council.
Vitamins from Food, National Dairy Council.
Water We Drink, Coronet Instructional Films.
Whenever You Eat, Association Films.
You and Your Food, National Dairy Council.
Your Food, McGraw-Hill Book Company.
Your Food, Young America Films.

b. Filmstrips

A Right Breakfast, Society for Visual Education.
Alexander's Breakfast Secret, Cereal Institute.
Beef—From Store to Table, National Livestock and Meat Board.
Bill's Better Breakfast Puppet Show, Cereal Institute, Inc.
Diet and Health, American Alliance for Health, Physical Education, and Recreation.
Digestive System, Young America Films.
Eat Well: Live Well, McGraw-Hill Book Company.
Food Around the World, National Dairy Council.
Foods for Health, Young America Films.
Food We Eat, American Bakers Association.
Grain from Farm to Table, Cereal Institute, Inc.
Guide to Breakfast, Kraft Foods.

How Food Becomes Part of You, Guidance Associates.
How Food Becomes You, National Dairy Council.
How Food Is Digested, McGraw-Hill Book Company.
How We Get Our Foods, Society for Visual Education.
How Your Body Uses Food, National Dairy Council.
Learning About Food, Encyclopaedia Britannica.
Mix and Match for Good Meals, Evaporated Milk Association.
Nutrition for You, Educational Activities.
On the Grow, Scholastic Book Services.
Project AM, Cereal Institute, Inc.
Proper Food, Encyclopaedia Britannica.
Skimpy and a Good Breakfast, Cereal Institute, Inc.
Story of Wheat, Wheat Flour Institute.
The Digestive System, Encyclopedia Britannica.
The Essentials of Diet, McGraw-Hill Book Company.
The Foods We Eat, Singer Society for Visual Education.
The Power of Food, National Livestock and Meat Board.
Vitamin C Makes the Difference, Sunkist Growers.
We Grow, National Dairy Council.
What Is Food? Guidance Associates.
What Foods People Need, Guidance Associates.
What's in Our Food, American Bakers Association.
Why Does Food Spoil?, McGraw-Hill Book Company.
Why Eat a Good Breakfast?, Cereal Institute, Inc.
You and Your Food, Young America Films.

c. Posters

A Basic Breakfast Pattern, Cereal Institute, Inc.
A Day with the Wide Awakes, General Mills, Inc.
A Guide to Good Eating, National Dairy Council.
Child Feeding Posters (3 posters), National Dairy Council.
Citrus Guards Your Health, Florida Citrus Commission.
Eat to Live, Not Live to Eat, Spenco Medical Corporation.
Food Nutrient Posters (6), National Livestock and Meat Board.
Foods, United Fresh Fruit and Vegetable Association.
Foods You Need Every Day, National Livestock and Meat Board.
Foodway to Follow, American Institute of Baking.
Good Breakfast Is Fun, Florida Citrus Commission.
Grains—Origin of Breakfast Cereals, Cereal Institute.
If You Wish to Grow Thinner, Diminish Your Dinner, Spenco Medical Corporation.
Let's Make Butter, National Dairy Council.
Make Lunch Count, National Dairy Council.
Milk from Farm to Family (6 posters), National Dairy Council.
More Milk Please, National Dairy Council.
My Growth Record, National Dairy Council.
Nutrition Ladder to Better Health, Florida Citrus Commission.
Ready for Breakfast, National Dairy Council.
School Lunch, National Dairy Council.
Series of Posters about Citrus Fruits (8), Florida Citrus Commission.
Start a Better Day with a Better Breakfast, National Livestock and Meat Board.
Surprise for Mother Pictures, National Dairy Council.
The Four Food Groups, Florida Citrus Commission.
The Wheel of Good Eating, American Institute of Baking.
What Did You Eat for Breakfast This Morning? National Dairy Council.
Which Are You? General Mills, Inc.

d. Charts

A Basic Breakfast Pattern, Cereal Institute, Inc.
A Guide to Good Eating, National Dairy Council.
Availability Guide for Fruits and Vegetables, United Fresh Fruit and Vegetable Association.
Better Breakfast for Primary Children, Florida Citrus Commission.
Colored Food Value Charts, National Livestock and Meat Board.
Conserving Minerals and Vitamins, General Mills, Inc.
Day to Day Good Health Record, Kellogg Company.
Facts About Foods, H. J. Heinz Company.
Food Chart, General Foods Corporation.
Food Mobile, American Institute of Baking.

Foods for Growing Boys and Girls, Kellogg Company.
For the Calcium You Need, Evaporated Milk Association.
Grains—Origin of Cereal Breakfasts, Cereal Institute, Inc.
It's Always Breakfast Time Somewhere, National Dairy Council.
Kernel of Wheat, Kansas Wheat Commission.
Milk from Farm to Family, National Dairy Council.
Mother Hubbard's Cupboard, General Mills, Inc.
My Daily Food Record, National Livestock and Meat Board.
My Growth Record, National Dairy Council.
Nutritive Values of Fruits and Vegetables, United Fresh Fruit and Vegetable Association.
Potato Calorie Bar Charts, United Fresh Fruit and Vegetable Association.
Safari Breakfast Game, General Mills, Inc.
School Lunch Evaluation Charts, General Mills, Inc.
School Lunch Record, National Dairy Council.
School Teaching Charts on Beet Sugar, United States Beet Sugar Association.
Shield of Good Health, Wheat Flour Institute.
Teaching About Meat, National Livestock and Meat Board.
Vitamin Food Chart, The "Cream of Wheat" Corporation.
Wall Meat Charts, National Livestock and Meat Board.
We Work Together, Wheat Flour Institute.

e. Maps

Armour Food Source Map, Armour and Company.

f. Models

Better Breakfast Cut-outs, Florida Citrus Commission.
Dairy Farm, National Dairy Council.
Food Mobile, Pennsylvania Bakers Association.
Food Model, National Dairy Council.
It's Always Breakfast Time Somewhere, National Dairy Council.
Model Cow, National Dairy Council.
Story Display Banners, United Fresh Fruit and Vegetable Association.
Urban Panorama, National Dairy Council.

g. Comics

How Meat Moves to Market, Swift and Company.

h. Selected Stories for Children

(P) Primary Level, (I) Intermediate Level

About Food and Where It Comes From, (I), T. Shannon (Melmont).
Around the World in Eighty Dishes, (I), L. Blanche (Harper).
At the Bakery (P), L. Colonius and G. Schroeder (Melmont).
Baker Bill (P), Jean Barr (Whitman).
Basketful, the Story of Our Foods, (I), J. Eberle (Crowell).
Brazil, Giant to the South (I), Alice Hagar (Macmillan).
Chickens and How to Raise Them (I), L. Darling (Morrow).
Chocolate Touch (P, I), P. S. Cathing (Morrow).
Cook-A-Meal Cookbook (I), G. Clark (W. R. Scott).
Diet and Dental Health (I), (American Dental Association).
Don't Forget the Bacon (P,I), Pat Hutchins (Greenwillow).
Everybody Eats (P), M. M. Green (W. R. Scott).
Farmer and His Cows (P), L. Floethe (Scribner).
Fish (I), R. Fawcett (Gawthorne).
Fun with Cooking (I), Mae Freeman (Random House).
Great Nutrition Puzzles (I), D. Callahan (Scribner).
It's Always Breakfast Time Somewhere (I), M. C. Letton (National Dairy Council).
Jimmy, the Groceryman (P), Jane Miller (Houghton).
Krista and the Frosty Foods (P,I), H. Olds (Messner).
Let's Take a Trip to a Fishery (P), S. Riedman (Abelard).
Little Pig in the Cupboard (P), Helen Buckley (Lothrop).
Milk for You (P), W. G. Schloat (Scribner).
Miss B's First Cook Book (I), Percy Hoffman (Bobbs).
Nothing to Eat but Food (I), Frank Jupo (Aladdin).
Plants That Feed Us (I), C. Fenton (Day).
Story Book of Foods (P,I), M. Petersham (Winston).
Story Book of Wheat (P), M. Petersham (Winston).
Stories from the Americas (I), F. Henius (Scribner).

Sugar (I), R. Fawcett (Gawthorne).
The Apple That Jack Ate (P), William R. Scott (W. R. Scott).
The Lunchbox Story (P), M. Goldberg (Holiday House).
The Milk That Jack Drank (P), W. R. Scott (Cadmus).
The Wonderful Egg (I), W. G. Schloat (Scribner).
This Is the Bread That Betsy Ate (P), Irma Black (W. R. Scott).
To Market We Go (P), Jane Miller (Houghton).
Walkabout Down Under (I), K. S. Foote (Scribner).
What the World Eats (I), H. H. Webster (Houghton).
Where's the Bunny? (P), Ruth Carroll (Oxford University Press).
Who Dreams of Cheese? (P), Leonard Weisgard (Scribner).
Wonderful Baker (I), M. L. Hunt (Lippincott).
Your Food and You (I), H. S. Zim (Morrow).

4. Dental Health

a. Films

Case of the Missing Tooth, American Dental Association.
D is for Dentist, American Dental Association.
Gateway to Health, National Apple Institute.
Healthy Teeth: Happy Smile, American Dental Association.
How Teeth Grow, Encyclopaedia Britannica.
It Doesn't Hurt, Coronet Instructional Films.
Merlin's Magical Message, American Dental Association.
Project Teeth, American Dental Association.
Save Those Teeth, Encyclopaedia Britannica.
Is Fluoridation the Answer? American Dental Association.
Sights and Sounds Around the Dental Chair, American Dental Association.
Teeth Are for Keeping, American Dental Association.
Teeth, Films Incorporated.
Teeth Are to Keep, Encyclopaedia Britannica.
The Teeth, Encyclopaedia Britannica.
Tommy's Day, Young America Films.
Tommy's Healthy Teeth, Coronet Instructional Films.
Tooth Truth with Mary and Marv, Alfred Higgins Productions, Inc.
What Do You Know about Teeth? American Dental Association.
Your Teeth, Young America Films.

b. Filmstrips

A Tale of Two Teeth, Walt Disney Educational Media Company.
Billy Meets Tommy Tooth, American Dental Association.
Brush Up on Your Teeth, Canadian National Film Board.
Dental Health Stories, Educational Activities.
Enjoy Your Teeth for Life, American Dental Association.
Johnny's Magic Toothbrush, American Dental Association.
Learning About Our Teeth, Encyclopaedia Britannica.
Let's Visit the Dentist, National Dairy Council.
Meet Your Teeth, Walt Disney Educational Media Company.
Primary Grade Health Series, National Dairy Council.
Save Those Teeth, Encyclopaedia Britannica.
Strong Teeth, McGraw-Hill Book Company.
Tale of a Toothache, Society for Visual Education.
Teeth Care, Scholastic Book Service.
Ten Little People and Their Teeth, Canadian National Film Board.
The Magic Potion, Walt Disney Educational Media Company.
The Mouth I Live In, Colgate-Palmolive.
Tooth Wisdom, Harcourt Brace Jovanovich.
The Teeth, Encyclopaedia Britannica.
The Teeth, Young America Films.
Tips on Tooth Care, American Dental Association.
You and Your Dentist, American Dental Association.
Your Body and How to Care for It: Teeth, Guidance Associates.
Your Teeth and Their Care, Popular Science.

c. Posters

Armed to the Teeth, Florida Citrus Commission.
Begin Early, National Dairy Council.
Big Pains, Travelers Insurance Company.
Brush Your Teeth, Eat Good Foods, Visit Your Dentist, National Dairy Council.
Combat Captain Plaque! American Dental Association.
Do You? National Dairy Council.
Do's for Dental Health, Florida Citrus Commission.
Frayed Toothbrush, American Dental Association.
How Teeth Grow, Procter and Gamble.
Healthy Tooth, Procter and Gamble.
How We Take Care of the Teeth, National Dairy Council.
Make Your Teeth the Best, National Dairy Council.
Swish and Swallow, American Dental Association.
Teeth, American Dental Association.
They're Your Teeth, National Dairy Council.

d. Charts

Class Toothbrushing Record, Procter and Gamble.
Flossing Chart, American Dental Association.
Four Food Groups, National Dairy Council.
Honor Roll–Clean Teeth Club, Pepsodent.
How to Brush the Teeth (21" × 25½"), American Dental Association.
Ivory Inspection Patrol Chart, Procter and Gamble Company.
We Can Be Replaced, American Dental Association.

e. Records

Friendly Doctor Drillum Fillum, J-209 Columbia Records.
Recorded Radio Presentations, American Dental Association.
Willie and a Little Tooth, J-184 Columbia Records.

f. Toothbrushing Kits

American Dental Association (M 10 kit), Procter and Gamble Company. (Third grade.)
Colgate-Palmolive Company.

g. Models

Look at Your Teeth–Everyone Else Does, American Dental Association.
Toothbrushing Model (M 13), American Dental Association.

h. Exhibits

Behind the Smile of Health (6½' × 7½'), American Dental Association.
Break the Chain of Tooth Decay (7½' × 5½'), American Dental Association.
Fluoridation (6½' × 7½'), American Dental Association.

i. Comics

The Friendly Ghost, Casper, And The Friendly Dentist, American Dental Association.

j. Loop Films

Cleaning Your Teeth, Encyclopaedia Britannica.
The Nature of Decay, Encyclopaedia Britannica.
What Is a Tooth, Encyclopaedia Britannica.

k. Selected Stories for Children

(P) Primary Level, (I) Intermediate Level

Child's Book of Teeth (I), H. W. Ferguson (World Book).
Diet and Dental Health (I), (American Dental Association).
Let's Be Healthy (P), W. W. Charters (Macmillan).
Let's Go to a Dentist (P), N. Buckheimer (Putnam).
Milk for You (P), W. G. Schloat (Scribner).
Milkman Freddy (I), Elizabeth Hoffman (Messner).
One Morning in Maine (P), R. McClusky (Viking).
The Serpent's Teeth (I), Penelope Farmer (Harcourt).
Your Wonderful Teeth (P,I), W. G. Schloat (Scribner).

5. Body Structure and Operation

a. Films

Breath of Life, American Heart Association.
Breathing, Encyclopaedia Britannica.
Circulation, United World Films.
Cells of Plants and Animals, Coronet Films.
Digestion in Our Bodies, Coronet Instructional Films.
Digestive System, Films Incorporated.
Endocrine Glands, Encyclopaedia Britannica.
Functions of the Nervous System, Knowledge Builders.
Health: Eye-Care Fantasy, Encyclopaedia Britannica.
Healthy Lungs, Coronet Instructional Films.
Heart and Circulatory System, Films Incorporated.
Heart, Lungs, and Circulation, Coronet Instructional Films.
Mechanisms of Breathing, Encyclopaedia Britannica.
Muscles and Bones of the Body, Coronet Instructional Films.
Nature of Life: Respiration in Animals, Coronet Films.
Obesity, National Dairy Council.
Our Wonderful Body: How It Grows, Coronet Instructional Materials.
Rest That Builds Good Health, Coronet Instructional Films.
Sitting Right, Association Films.
Sleep for Health, Encyclopaedia Britannica.
The Huffless, Puffless Dragon, American Cancer Society.
The Human Body, National Dairy Council.
To Live and Breathe, Aetna Life and Casualty Company.
Wonder Engine of the Body, American Heart Association.
Wonder of Our Body, Moody Institute of Science.
You and Your Five Senses, Walt Disney Productions.
Your Nervous System, Coronet Instructional Films.
You–The Human Animal, Walt Disney Educational Media Company.

b. Filmstrips

Every Body's Skin Makes Everybody Kin, American Association for Health, Physical Education, and Recreation.
Eye, Nose and All of Those, Harcourt Brace Jovanovich.
Harvey and Blood Circulation, International Film Bureau.
How the Heart Works, Popular Science.
How to Grow Well and Strong, McGraw-Hill Book Company.
How to Grow Well and Strong, Popular Science.
Human Respiration, Popular Science.
Learning About Our Ears, Encyclopaedia Britannica.
Learning About Our Eyes, Encyclopaedia Britannica.
Learning About Our Skin, Encyclopaedia Britannica.
Nervous System, Young America Films.
Respiratory System, Young America Films.
Sense Organs, BFA Educational Media.
Skin, Hair, and Nails, McGraw-Hill Book Company.
Straight and Tall, Young America Films.
Systems of the Body, Educational Activities, Inc.
Taste, Smell and Touch, Encyclopaedia Britannica.
The Circulatory System, Encyclopaedia Britannica.
The Digestive System, Encyclopaedia Britannica.
The Heart–How It Works, McGraw-Hill Book Company.
The Human Cell, American Cancer Society.
The Story of Human Life, Educational Activities, Inc.
Use of Artificial Respiration, McGraw-Hill Book Company.
We Grow, National Dairy Council.
You and the Living Machine, Encyclopaedia Britannica.
You and Your Ears, Walt Disney Educational Media Company.
You and Your Eyes, Walt Disney Educational Media Company.
Your Blood System, Curriculum Films.
Your Body: Fitness, Growth, Appearance, Guidance Associates.
Your Bones and Muscles, Popular Science.
Your Heart and Lungs, Popular Science.
Your Posture–Good or Bad, Young America Films.

c. Posters

ACS Bulletin Board Posters (7 each), American Cancer Society.
Blood As a Medicine, American National Red Cross.
Give Blood to Give Life, American Medical Association.
Posture on Parade (for girls), National Dairy Council.
Protect Your Eyes, National Safety Council.
The Breath of Life, Aetna Life Insurance Company.

d. Charts

Bone Structure, National Livestock and Meat Board.
Cancer Wall Chart (3' × 4'), Eli Lilly and Company.
Heart Charts (12), American Heart Association.
How Tall, The Travelers Insurance Company.
Human Body (kit), Owen Publishing Company, Danville, N.Y.
My Growth Record, National Dairy Council.
Physical Growth Record for Boys, American Medical Association.
Physical Growth Record for Girls, American Medical Association.
Your Heart and How It Works, American Heart Association.

e. Transparencies

Physiology of the Heart, Media Visuals, Inc.
Physiology of the Nervous System, Media Visuals, Inc.

f. Records

Childhood Rhythms for Intermediate Grades (Evan CHR-3), Stanley Bowmar Company.
Chidhood Rhythms for Lower Grades (Evans CHR-1), Stanley Bowmar Company, Valhalla, N.Y.
Creative Rhythm Album (Burns-Wheeler), Stanley Bowmar Company.
My Heart and I, American Heart Association.

g. Models

Anatomical Models in Health and Disease, Spenco Medical Corporation.
Plastic Anatomical Reproductions, Medical Plastics Laboratory, Gatesville, Texas
The Heart and Circulation, American Heart Association.

h. Selected Stories for Children

(P) Primary Level, (I) Intermediate Level

A Baby Is Born (P), L. I. Mitton and J. N. Seligmann (Simon & Schuster).
A Baby Starts to Grow (P), Paul Showers (Crowell).
A Button in Her Ear (I), A. B. Litchfield (Whitman).
A Drop of Blood (P), Ellen Raskin (Atheneum-Aladdin).
All About the Human Body (I), B. Glemser (Random).
All About Us (I), Eva Evans (Capital).
All Kinds of Babies and How They Grow (P), Selsan Millicent (W. R. Scott).
Brave Gives Blood (I), Philip and Mirina Eisenburg (Messner).
Do You Know What I Know? (P), Helen Borten (Abelard).
Freddie Found a Frog (P), James Napjas (Van Nostrand).
Growing Story (P), Ruth Krauss (Harper).
Growing Up (P), Karl DeSchweintz (Macmillan).
How We Grow (I), P. O'Keefe and C. H. Maxwell (Winston).
How Your Body Works (I), H. Schneider (W. R. Scott).
Linda Goes to the Hospital (I), Nancy Dudley (Coward-McCann).
My Five Senses (I), Aliki (Crowell).
Oxygen Keeps You Alive (P), F. M. Branley (Crowell).
Patrick Will Grow (P), Gladys Baker Bond (Whitman).
The Amazing Bone (P), W. Steig (Farrar, Straus & Giroux).
The Ear Book (I), Al Perkins (Random).
The Smallest Boy in the Class (I), J. Beim (William Morrow).
What's Inside of Me? (I), Herbert S. Zim (Morrow).
What's Inside of Me? (P), Herbert S. Zim (Morrow).
When I Am Big (P), R. P. Smith (Harper).
Wonders Inside You (P), L. Cosgrove (Dodd).
Wonders of the Human Body (I), A. Ranelli (Viking).
Your Body and How It Works (I), P. Lauber (Random House).
Your Bones Are Alive (P), S. Kalina (Lothrop).
Your Heart and How It Works (I), H. Zim (Morrow).

6. Prevention and Control of Disease

a. Films

Avoiding Infections, Encyclopaedia Britannica.
Child With a Cold, Pharmaceutical Manufacturers Association.
Cleanliness and Health, Coronet Instructional Films.
Common Cold, Encyclopaedia Britannica.
Germs and What They Do, Coronet Films.
Goodbye, Mr. Germ, National Tuberculosis Association.
Health: Germs and the Space Visitors, Encyclopaedia Britannica.
Health Heroes: the Battle Against Disease, Metropolitan Life Insurance Co.
House Fly, Encyclopaedia Britannica.
How to Catch a Cold, Walt Disney Educational Media.
I Never Catch a Cold, Coronet Instructional Films.
Immunization, Encyclopaedia Britannica.
Immunization Now, American Educational Films.
Joan Avoids a Cold, Coronet Instructional Films.
Let's Have Fewer Colds, Coronet Instructional Films.
Mr. Galen Comes To Town, Pharmaceutical Manufacturers Association.
Spot Prevention, U.S. Public Health Service.
Story of Dr. Jenner, Teaching Film Custodians.
Story of Louis Pasteur, Teaching Film Custodians.
The Body Fights Bacteria, McGraw-Hill Book Company.
The Fight Against Microbes, International Film Bureau.
The Inside Story, National Tuberculosis Association.
Time for Living, Pharmaceutical Manufacturers Association.
Tiny Water Animals, Encyclopaedia Britannica.
Unmasking the Germ Assassins, International Film Bureau.
Water We Drink, Coronet Instructional Films.
Your Health, Disease and Its Control, Coronet Instructional Films.

b. Filmstrips

Avoiding Infections (Treating a Cold), Encyclopaedia Britannica.
Cancer, the Challenge to Youth, American Cancer Society.
Checking Your Health, Encyclopaedia Britannica.
Common Cold, Encyclopaedia Britannica.
Communicable Diseases, Young America Films.
Controlling Germs, Curriculum Films.
Dear Little Mumps Child, BFA Educational Media.
Fighting Disease, Stanley Bowmar Co.
Florence Nightingale, Metropolitan Life Insurance Company.
Germ Invaders, McGraw-Hill Book Company.
Health Heroes, Metropolitan Life Insurance Company.
Helping the Body Defenses Against Disease, McGraw-Hill Book Company.
Karen Gets a Fever, BFA Educational Media.
Keeping Ourselves Healthy, Curriculum Films.
Keeping Sickness Away, McGraw-Hill Book Company.
Keeping Well, Young America Films.
Learning About Germs, Encyclopaedia Britannica.
Louis Pasteur and the Germ Theory of Disease, Metropolitan Life Insurance Co.
Madame Curie, Metropolitan Life Insurance Company.
Making Water Safe to Drink, McGraw-Hill Book Company.
Shots for Your Health, National Education Association.
The Little Pink Bottle, National Foundation.
The Water We Drink, Young America Films.
Walter Reed and the Conquest of Yellow Fever (with transcription), Metropolitan Life
    Insurance Company.
We Have You Covered, Society for Visual Education.
Witchcraft to Modern Medicine, International Education and Training, Inc.

c. Posters

Germs Can Hatch in a Scratch, National Safety Council.
Help Us Fight Infection, National Safety Council.
How to Catch a Cold, Kimberly-Clark Corporation.
How to Cure a Cold, Kimberly-Clark Corporation.
How to Spread a Cold, Kimberly-Clark Corporation.
We Had Polio Vaccine, National Foundation.

d. Records

Cover Your Mouth, Educational Activities.
Doctors Make History, American Medical Association.
Health Heroes, American Medical Association.
Keep the Germs Away, Educational Activities.
Rainy Days, National Safety Council.
Shots For Your Health, National Education Association.

e. Charts

Cancer Wall Chart (3′ × 4′), Eli Lilly and Company.
Diseases of the Digestive System, Spenco Medical Corporation.
Hazards of Drug Abuse, Spenco Medical Corporation.
I Promise Common Sense, Kimberly-Clark Corporation.
The Good Seed, Eli Lilly and Company.
200 Years of Health and Medicine in the United States, Metropolitan Life Insurance Company.

f. Radio Scripts

(From Bureau of Research in Education by Radio, University of Texas)
Fly Control
Health Living Radio Broadcast (kit of 30 scripts)
Keep Your Cold at Home
Mosquito Control
Safe Water Supply
We Wash Our Hands Before We Eat

g. Selected Stories for Children

(P) Primary Level, (I) Intermediate Level

A Sick Book (I), Marie Winns (Four Winds).
Arnold Roth's Crazy Book of Science (I), A. Roth (Grossett & Dunlap).
Conquest of Disease (I), L. Martin (Coward).
Doctors and Nurses: What They Do (I), C. Greene (Harper & Row).
Doctors and What They Do (I), H. Coy (G. P. Putnam's Sons).
Dr. Trotter and His Big Gold Watch (P), H. Gilbert (Abingdon).
Have a Happy Measle, a Merry Mumps and a Cheery Chickenpox (I), J. Bendick (Whittlesey House).
Health Can Be Fun (P), Munro Leaf (Lippincott).
Johnny Goes to the Hospital (P), J. Sener (Houghton).
Linda Goes to the Hospital (P), N. Dudley (Coward).
Modern Medical Discoveries (I), E. Bigland (Criterion).
Moptop (P), D. Freeman (Viking).
Our Insect Friends and Foes (I), W. A. DuPuy (Winston).
The Clean Pig (P), Leonard Weisgard (Scribner).
The First Book of Microbes (I), L. Lewis (Watts).
The Water That Jack Drank (P), William R. Scott (W. R. Scott).
True Book of Health (P), Mary Brockman (Scribner).
What's Inside of Me? (P), Herbert S. Zim (Morrow).

7. Safety and First Aid

a. Films

A Monkey Tale (Bicycle Safety), Encyclopaedia Britannica.
Bicycle Rules of the Road, Aims Instructional Media Services.
Bicycle Safety Skills, Coronet Instructional Films.
Bike Safety Quiz, American Educational Films.
Bike-Wise, to Be Sure, Centron Films.
Children at Play with Poison, U.S. Public Health Service (Food and Drug Administration).
Drugs, Drinking and Driving, Aims Instructional Media Services.
Emergency 77, Metropolitan Life Insurance Company.
Fifty Thousand Lives, Johnson & Johnson.
Fire Exit Drill at Our School, Coronet Instructional Films.
Fireman, Encyclopaedia Britannica.
First Aid Now, Johnson and Johnson.
First Aid Quiz: Saving a Life, American Education Films.
First Aid Quiz: Treating an Injury, American Education Films.

Halloween Safety, Centron Films.
Health: Eye-Care Fantasy, Encyclopaedia Britannica.
Help Prevent Fires, National Fire Protection Association.
Help Wanted, Johnson & Johnson.
Home Safety: It's Up to You, Centron Films.
If Bicycles Could Talk, Aetna Life and Casualty Company.
I'm No Fool as a Pedestrian, American Automobile Association.
I'm No Fool with a Bicycle, American Automobile Association.
Mouth-to-Mouth Resuscitation, American Heart Association.
Primary Safety: In the School Building, Coronet Instructional Films.
Primary School Bus Safety, Centron Films.
Read the Label and Live, National Fire Protection Association.
Safe Living at Home, Coronet Instructional Films.
Safe Living at School, Coronet Instructional Films.
Safe Living in Your Community, Coronet Instructional Films.
Safe Skateboarding, American Educational Films.
Safe Through Seat Belts, International Film Bureau, Inc.
Safe Use of Tools, Coronet Instructional Films.
Safest Way, American Automobile Association.
Safety: The Helpful Burglars, Encyclopaedia Britannica.
Safety Begins at Home, Young America Films.
Safety Belts for Susie, Charles Cahill and Associates.
Safety in Winter, Coronet Instructional Films.
Safety on the Playground, Encyclopaedia Britannica.
Safety on the Streets, Encyclopaedia Britannica.
Safety on the Way, Coronet Instructional Films.
Safety with Fire, Coronet Instructional Films.
School Bus and You, Progressive Films.
School Rules—How They Help Us, Coronet Instructional Films.
Singing Wheels, Bicycle Institute of America.
Sniffy Escapes Poisoning, Henk Wewenhouse Films.
Stop, Look, and Think, Charles Cahill and Associates.
Water Safety, Young America Films.
You and Your Bicycle, Progressive Films and Employers Mutuals of Wausau.

b. Filmstrips

Artificial Respiration, Sunburst Communication.
Be a Better Pedal Pusher, Society for Visual Education.
Bicycle Safety, Curriculum Films.
Controlling Fire, McGraw-Hill Book Company.
Electrical Hazard, Stanley Bowmar Company.
Elementary Safety, Centron Films.
Goofy over Automobiles, Walt Disney Educational Media.
Happy Hollow Makes the Honor Roll, Society for Visual Education.
Home Safety, Encyclopaedia Britannica.
I'm No Fool Having Fun, McGraw-Hill Book Company.
I'm No Fool with a Bicycle, McGraw-Hill Book Company.
I'm No Fool with Fire, McGraw-Hill Book Company.
Keeping Food Safe to Eat, McGraw-Hill Book Company.
Little Children and Big Poisons, American Association of Poison Control Centers.
Motor Mania, Walt Disney Educational Media.
Play Safety, Encyclopaedia Britannica.
Playing in City Streets, Curriculum Films.
Safe and Sure with Electricity, McGraw-Hill Book Company.
Safety Choice, Scholastic Book Services.
Safety at Play, Scholastic Book Services.
Safety at School, Curriculum Films.
Safety Helpers, Encyclopaedia Britannica.
Safety in the Mouth, Walt Disney Educational Media Company.
Safety in the Summer, Curriculum Films.
School Safety, Encyclopaedia Britannica.
Street Safety, Encyclopaedia Britannica.
Until Help Arrives, Scholastic Book Services.
The Great Race (Bicycle Safety), American Alliance for Health, Physical Education and
    Recreation.
The Happy Bus, American Alliance for Health, Physical Education, and Recreation.
Vacation Safety, Encyclopaedia Britannica.
Wintertime Safety, McGraw-Hill Book Company.

c. Posters

Accidents Occur When Least Expected, National Safety Council.
A Clean House Seldom Burns, National Fire Protection Association.
Always Use Bike Hand Signals, Bicycle Institute of America.
ARC Safety Posters, 1446 and 1447, American National Red Cross.
Be Extra Careful, National Safety Council.
Be Sure Your Bike Is Ready to Go, Bicycle Institute of America.
Bicyclists Use Your Hand Signals, Bicycle Institute of America.
Bike Route, Bicycle Institute of America.
Bike Safety Aids, Bicycle Institute of America.
Exit: Plan Your Way Out, National Fire Protection Association.
Get First Aid Promptly, National Safety Council.
Little People Don't Read Labels, American Association of Poison Control Center.
Poison-Ivy-Oak, National Safety Council.
Prevent Fire, National Fire Protection Association.
Protect Your Eyes, National Safety Council.
Safety Is a Year Round Job, National Safety Council.
Safety Is Always in Season, National Safety Council.
Seat Belts, American Medical Association.
See, Be Seen, Bicycle Institute of America.
Show-offs Get Hurt, National Safety Council.
Sizing Up Strangers, Walt Disney Educational Media Company.
Sports Accidents, American Medical Association.
Stop Fires, Save Lives, American Insurance Association.
Take It Easy on Your Vacation, National Safety Council.
Wait on the Curb for Your Go Signal, American Automobile Association.

d. Charts

First Aid, Metropolitan Life Insurance Company.
First Aid Wall Chart, Johnson and Johnson.
Home Fire Safety Check List, National Fire Protection Association.
Six Month Inspection, Bicycle Institute of America.
Stop-Dial, Aetna Life & Casualty Company.

e. Records

Buckle Your Seatbelt, Educational Activities.
Fire on Thunder Hill, American Forest Products Industries, Inc.
Safety Through Music, Educational Activities.

f. Comics

Dennis the Menace Takes a Poke at Poison, U.S. Public Health Service.
Early Man and Fire, National Fire Protection Association.
Hello, I Am Fire! National Fire Protection Association.
Man Learns More About Fire, National Fire Protection Association.
Sparky, National Fire Protection Association.
Sparky Makes a Home Fire Inspection, National Fire Protection Association.

g. Radio Scripts

Benny, the Matchstick, National Safety Council.
Bobby Grows Up, National Safety Council.
Carl, the Bear Cub, National Safety Council.
Child Safety Stories, National Safety Council.
Danger, Children at Play, National Safety Council.
Fire Prevention, Bureau of Research in Education by Radio, University of Texas.
Fire Safety, National Safety Council.
Happy and Safe Thinking, National Safety Council.
Lady from Safety Land, National Safety Council.
Louis Agazzi Fuertes, National Safety Council.
Make Your City Safer, National Safety Council.
Mary and the Broken Glass, National Safety Council.
Needles and Pins, National Safety Council.
On a Bicycle Not Built for Two, National Safety Council.
Our Animal Show, National Safety Council.
Out of the Night, National Safety Council.
Safe Water Supply, Bureau of Research in Education by Radio, University of Texas.
The Bat Blinky, National Safety Council.
The Safety Elf, National Safety Council.
The Twins Have Safety Trouble, National Safety Council.

To Walk in the Night, National Safety Council.
Worrying Bike, National Safety Council.

h. Loop Films

Preventing Slips and Falls, Encyclopaedia Britannica.
Safety with Pets, Encyclopaedia Britannica.

i. Selected Stories for Children

(P) Primary Level, (I) Intermediate Level

Andy and the School Bus (P), J. Beim (Morrow).
Big Fire (P), E. Olds (Houghton).
Binkey's Fire (P), Sally Scott (Harcourt).
Country Fireman (P), J. Beim (Morrow).
Dr. Squash, the Doll Doctor (P), Margaret Wise Brown (Simon & Schuster).
Fireman for a Day (I), Z. K. McDonald (Messner).
Fireman Fred (P), Jean Barry (Whitman).
First Book of Fireman (I), Mary Elting (Watts).
Forest Fireman (P,I), Bill and Rosalie Brown (Coward).
Going to Blazes (I), R. V. Masters (Sterling).
Hercules, Story of an Old Fashioned Fire Engine (P), Hardie Gramatsky (Putnam).
I Want to Be a Policeman (P), C. Green (Children's Press).
Johnnie Wants to Be a Policeman (I), W. J. Granberg (Aladdin).
Let's Find Out about Safety (I), M. Shapp (Watts).
Mountain Courage (I), D. Hawkins (Doubleday).
Pat and Her Policeman (I), F. Friedman (Morrow).
Rags, the Firehouse Dog (P), E. Morton (Winston).
Red Light, Green Light (P), Margaret Wise Brown (Doubleday).
Safety Can Be Fun (P), Munro Leaf (Lippincott).
The Accident (P), Carol Carrick (Seabury).
The Bike Lesson (P), S. and J. Berenstain (Random House).
The Firefighter (I), H. B. Lent (Macmillan).
The Little Igloo (P), L. Beim (Harcourt Brace Jovanovich).
The New Fire Engine (P), Jay Barnum (Morrow).
Time and the Brass Buttons (P, I), Ruth Tooze (Messner).
Walkabout Down Under (I), K. S. Foote (Scribner).
Watch Out (I), Norah Smaridge (Abington).

8. Mental Health

a. Films

Adventuring Pups, Young America Films.
Are You Popular? Coronet Instructional Films.
Attitudes and Health, Coronet Instructional Films.
But They Might Laugh, National Instructional Television Center.
Curious Alice, National Institute of Mental Health.
Don't Be Afraid, Encyclopaedia Britannica.
Face Yourself, Aetna Life and Casualty Company.
Feeling Left Out, Coronet Instructional Films.
Getting Along With Others, Coronet Instructional Films.
Getting Even, National Instructional Television Center.
Good Sportsmanship, Coronet Instructional Films.
Growing Up, Coronet Instructional Films.
How Do You Do? Young America Films.
How Friendly Are You? Coronet Instructional Films.
How Honest Are You? Coronet Instructional Films.
I Dare You, National Instructional Television Center.
Jimmy Rabbitt, Bailey Films.
Let's Play Fair, Coronet Instructional Films.
Making Life Adjustments, McGraw-Hill Book Company.
Mental Health, Encyclopaedia Britannica.
Mr. Finley's Feelings, Metropolitan Life Insurance Company.
Other Fellow's Feelings, Young America Films.
Out of Orbit, National Council on Alcoholism.
Overcoming Worry, Coronet Instructional Films.
Sky Guy, Coronet Instructional Films.
The Outsider, Young America Films.

The Ugly Duckling, Coronet Instructional Films.
To See Ourselves, Aetna Life and Casualty Company.
To Your Health, World Health Organization.
Understanding Stresses and Strains, Walt Disney Productions.
Ways to Good Habits, Coronet Instructional Films.
What To Do About Upset Feelings, Coronet Films.
What Do Drugs Do?, National Institute of Mental Health.
You and Your Family, Association Films, Inc.
You and Your Friends, Association Films, Inc.
You and Your Time, Association Films, Inc.

b. Filmstrips

Brothers, Sisters, Feelings and You, Guidance Associates.
Getting Acquainted, McGraw-Hill Book Company.
Health Helpers, Encyclopaedia Britannica.
How Do We Know? Harcourt Brace Jovanovich.
How Do You Know What's Fair? Guidance Associates.
Keeping Children Happy, McGraw-Hill Book Company.
Learning To Make Friends, Society For Visual Education.
Let's Have a Party, Society for Visual Education.
Lonely Boy, Stanley Bowmar Co.
Mental Health, Image Publishing Corporation.
Mike Finds out about Friendship, Society for Visual Education.
Orphan Willie, Canadian National Film Board.
Promises Are Made to Keep, Encyclopaedia Britannica.
Reflection, Image Publishing Corporation.
Sense and Nonsense, Popular Science.
Sharing with Neighbors, Encyclopaedia Britannica.
Talk About Good, Talk About Bad, American Cancer Society.
The Little Cloud, Society for Visual Education.
The Nervous System, Encyclopaedia Britannica.
The Raggedy Elf, Society for Visual Education.
The Secret Is You, Harcourt Brace Jovanovich.
Thinking for Yourself, Encyclopaedia Britannica.
Understanding Stresses and Strains, Walt Disney Educational Media Company.
We Play Together, Stanley Bowmar Co.
We Work Together, Stanley Bowmar Co.
Working and Playing Together, McGraw-Hill Book Company.

c. Posters

If at First You Don't Succeed, Spenco Medical Corporation.
Most People Live, Spenco Medical Corporation.

d. Records

Getting To Know Myself, Educational Activities.
Won't You Be My Friend, Educational Activities.

e. Selected Stories for Children

(P) Primary Level, (I) Intermediate Level

A Friend Is Someone Who Likes You (P), J. Walsh (Harcourt Brace Jovanovich).
All It Takes Is Practice (I), Betty Miles (Knopf).
A Name for Obed (P), E. C. Phillips (Houghton).
A Race for Bill (I), M. N. Wallace (Nelson).
Ann and the Sand Dobbies (I), John Colburn (Seabury Press).
"B" Is for Betsy (P), Carolyn Haywood (Harcourt).
Beat the Turtle Drum (I), Constance Greene (Viking).
Ben And Me (I), Robert Lawson (Walt Disney).
Child of the Silent Night (I), Edith Hunter (Houghton Mifflin).
Come Again in the Spring (I), R. Kennedy (Harper & Row).
David's Bad Day (P), Ellen McKean (Vanguard).
Even Steven (P), W. Lipkind (Harcourt).
Fair Play (P), Munro Leaf (Lippincott).
Finders Keepers (P), W. Lipkind (Harcourt).
Goodbye, Grandpa (P), R. Koch (Augsburg).
Grandfather and I (P), Helen Buckley (Lothrop, Lee, Shepherd).
Granite Harbor (I), D. Bud (Macmillan).
Growing Story (P), Ruth Krauss (Harper).
Growing Up (P), Karl DeSchweintz (Macmillan).

Here's a Penny (P), Carolyn Haywood (Harcourt).
How to Behave and Why (I), Munro Leaf (Lippincott).
How To Stand Up for What You Believe (I), H. Detwiler (Association Press).
I Like To Be Me (P, I), Barbara Bel Geddes (Viking).
I Like You (P), Sandel Warburg (Houghton Mifflin).
Jerry at School (P), Kathryn Jackson (Simon & Schuster).
Judy's Journey (I), Lois Lenski (Lippincott).
Just Me (P), Marie Hall ETS (Viking).
Learning to Say Goodbye (I), E. LeShan (Macmillan).
Let's Do Better (P, I), Munro Leaf (Lippincott).
Liam's Catch (P), D. D. Parker (Viking).
Love Is a Special Way of Feeling (P), J. Walsh (Harcourt Brace Jovanovich).
Mine for Keeps (P), Jean Little (Little, Brown).
Mr. Death: Four Stories (P), A. Moody (Harper & Row).
My Brother Stevie (I), Eleanor Clymer (Holt).
My Friend Johnny (P), Vane Earle (Lothrop).
My Grandpa Died Today (P), J. Fassler (Behavioral Publications).
My Twin Sister, Eureka (I), Margaret Vogel (Harper).
Noise in the Night (I), A. Alexander (Rand).
Nonna (I), J. Bartoli (Harvey).
North Fork (I), Doris Gates (Viking).
Old Can and Patrick (I), Ruth Sawyer (Viking).
Out to Win (I-Boys), M. G. Bonner (Knopf).
Peter's Treasure (I), C. I. Judson (Houghton).
Petunia (P), Roger Duvoisin (Knopf).
Play Fair (P, I), Munro Leaf (Lippincott).
Sad Day—Glad Day (P), Vivian Thompson (Holiday House).
Scat (P), A. Dobrin (Scholastic).
Shaken Days (I), Doris Gates (Viking).
Shelter from the Wind (I), M. D. Bauer (Seabury).
Something to Live By (I), Dorothea Kipplin (Doubleday).
Stories from a Snowy Meadow (P, I), C. Stevens (Seabury).
Switch on the Night (P), R. Bradbury (Pantheon).
Tales of A Fourth Grade Nothing (I), Judy Blume (Dutton).
Tell Me about Death (I), E. A. Corley (Grammatical Sciences).
The Elephant Who Liked To Smash Small Cars (P), Jean Merrill (Pantheon).
The Lion Twins (P, I), Elizabeth Stewart (Atheneum).
The Night the Storm Came (P), G. Relyea (Aladdin).
The Secret Name (I), Barbara Williams (Harcourt).
The Smallest Boy in the Class (I), M. Wohlberg (Morrow).
The Ugly Duckling (I), Hans C. Anderson (Harcourt).
The Very Little Girl (P), P. Krasilovksy (Doubleday).
The Wonderful Year (I), Nancy Barnes (Messner).
The Year the Dreams Came Back (I), A. M. Feagler (Atheneum).
Timid Timothy (P), G. Williams (W. R. Scott).
Understood Betsy (I), C. L. Judson (Houghton).
What Do They Say? (P), Ellen McKean (Vanguard).
What Every Kid Should Know (I), Ralb and Wescott (Houghton Mifflin).
What Is She Like? (I), Mary Brockman (Scribner).
What Mary Jo Shared (P), Jamie May Udry (Albert Whitman).
What's That Noise? (I), L. Kauffman (Lothrop).
Who Are You? Joan Bradfield (Whitman).
Why Did He Die? (P), A. Harris (Lerner).

9. Sex and Family Living Education

a. Films

(P) Primary Level, (I) Intermediate Level

Animals Hatched From Eggs (P), Coronet Films.
A Happy Family (P), Classroom Film Distributors. Family relations between a seven
    year old girl, her younger brother, older sister, and their parents. Depicts how
    members of the family have learned to live together.
Baby Animals (P), McGraw-Hill Book Company. Elementary.
Birth of a Colt (I), Thorne Films.
Birth of Puppies (P), Coronet Films.
Brothers and Sisters (I), National Instructional Television Center.
Farmyard Babies (P), Coronet Films.
Families (P), E. C. Brown.

Farm Babies and Their Mothers (P), Film Associates.

Friendship Begins at Home (P), Coronet Instructional Films.

Growing Up (P), Coronet Instructional Films. Elementary material.

Growing Up Day by Day (P), Encyclopaedia Britannica. Explains the principles of physical, mental, social, and emotional growth to children by comparing members of a group of eight year olds at a birthday party. Explains that actions should vary at different ages and that, as children grow older, they should learn to do more for themselves and others.

Happy Little Hamsters (P), Perennial Education, Inc.

Human and Animal Beginnings (P), E. C. Brown Trust. 22 minutes in color. Young children express their beliefs about origin of human life in drawings. Starts with newborn baby and compares with animal babies. Reviews egg development (human and animal) at one month, four months, six months, and nine months.

Human Growth (I), E. C. Brown.

Kittens—Birth and Growth (P), Bailey Films. Robin and Billy are present when their cat "Millie" gives birth to four kittens. Shows the kittens nursing, crawling, playing, and being weaned. Emphasizes the care the children give to the kittens.

Mike Finds out about Growing (P), Society for Visual Education. Elementary.

Mother Hen's Family (The Wonders of Birth) (P), Coronet Instructional Films. 10 minutes. Depicts how eggs are hatched by hens. Shows a small boy, with the help of his father, following the process from the laying of the eggs to the hatching of the chicks. The boy charts on a calendar the time of setting to the day of the hatching.

Our Family Works Together (P), Coronet Instructional Materials.

Boy to Man (I), Churchill Films. 16 minutes in color. Depicts the physical changes of the adolescent as well as complete glandular development. For boys 11–14; may also be used with girls. (Excellent for sixth or seventh grade.)

Everyday Courtesy (I), Churchill Films. Pupils arrange and present an exhibit on courtesy. Invitations are written by children to their parents and guests. Regards courtesy in connection with invitations, telephone introductions, and entertaining guests.

Growing Girls (I), Encyclopaedia Britannica.

Growing Up (Preadolescence) (I), McGraw-Hill Book Company. 10 minutes in color. Silhouette and animal photography regarding the development of twins. Discuss irregular growth, glands involved in growth, sex differences in growth. Emphasizes diet, relaxation, recreation, and rest.

Human Growth (I), Wexler Film Productions. 20 minutes, 16 mm, color. Shows a seventh grade class viewing and discussing animated film that traces human growth from conception to adulthood. Differences in male and female structural development are emphasized. (Revised.)

Human Reproduction (I), McGraw-Hill Book Company, 22 minutes, 16 mm. Stresses the biological normalcy of human reproduction. Models and animated drawings depict the anatomy and physiology of the male and female reproductive organs.

It's Wonderful Being a Girl (I), Personal Products Corporation. 20 minutes in color. This is an excellent film on menstruation. It presents a fine philosophy of being a girl.

Molly Grows Up (I), Personal Products Corporation. Upper elementary–junior high.

Story of Menstruation (I), Kimberly-Clark Corporation. 10 minutes in color. Animated drawings and diagrams present, in a direct and scientific way, the story of this natural phenomenon.

Tabby's Kittens (P), Kindergarten.

The Day Life Begins (I), Carousel Films. 23 minutes.

The Endocrine System (I), Encyclopaedia Britannica.

The Fable of He and She (I), Learning Corporation of America. Deals with male and female sex roles on a mythical island.

VD—Name Your Contacts (I), Coronet Instructional Films.

The Menstrual Cycle (I), Eli Lilly and Company.

The Story of Menstruation (I), Walt Disney Educational Media Company.

Tomorrow's Children (I), E. C. Brown Foundation.

You and Your Five Senses (I), Walt Disney Educational Media Company. Jimmy Cricket develops theme "All your pets are smart, but the only thinking animal is you. You use thought and reason with your five senses. Animals use their senses entirely by instinct."

You and Your Parents (I), Coronet Instructional Films.

Your Body During Adolescence (I), McGraw-Hill Book Company. Shows the seven glands that regulate human life and growth with emphasis on the pituitary and sex glands. Outlines changes that take place in the bodies of boys and girls.

Your Family (P), Coronet Instructional Films.

b. Filmstrips

About Your Life, Denver Public Schools. Denver, Col. (Grade 5).
After School Hours, Popular Science.
Becoming A Woman/Becoming A Man (I), Guidance Associates.
Confidence Because . . . You Understand Menstruation, Personal Products Corporation.
Especially for Boys (I), Wexler Film Productions.
Especially for Girls (I), Wexler Film Productions.
Families Around the World, Encyclopaedia Britannica.
Family Fun, Encyclopaedia Britannica.
Finding Out How Animals Grow, Society for Visual Education.
Fun at the Beach, McGraw-Hill Book Company.
Fun on a Picnic, Curriculum Films.
Getting Ready for School, Popular Science.
Growing Into Womanhood/Growing Into Manhood (I), Guidance Associates.
Growing Up, Walt Disney Educational Media Company.
How Babies Are Made, Creative Scope Inc. (Grades K–3).
Janet Helps Mother, Curriculum Films.
Let's Visit Our Friends, Society for Visual Education.
Miss Brown's Class Goes to the Zoo, Eye Gate House (Grades 2–3).
Reproduction in Flowers, Eye Gate House (Grades 4–6).
The Me I Want To Be, Kimberly-Clark Corporation.
Understanding Changes in The Family, Guidance Associates.

c. Posters

What Happens During Menstruation? Personal Products Corporation.

d. Charts

Baby's Bath, Scott, Foresman and Company.
Beginning the Human Story: A New Baby in the Family, Scott, Foresman and Co.
Female Anatomical Charts, Tampax, Incorporated.
How Baby Grows, Johnson and Johnson.
Physiology Chart, Kimberly-Clark Corporation.
What Happens During Menstruation? Personal Products Corporation.

e. Records

Talks With Growing Boys, Stanley Bowmar Co.
Talks With Growing Girls, Stanley Bowmar Co.
The Story of Growing Up, Stanley Bowmar Co.

f. Slides

Happy Vacation (H56), New York State University College of Agriculture, Cornell University.
House of Darkness, National Safety Council.
How Babies Are Made, Creative Scope, Inc., 509 5th Avenue, New York, N.Y., 10017.
Human Reproduction, Guidance Asociates.
Practical Considerations of Menstruation, Spenco Medical Corporation.
Stop–Look–Listen (H70), New York State University College of Agriculture, Cornell University.
The Story of Growing Up (Girls), Stanley Bowmar Co.
What It Means to Grow Up (Boys), Stanley Bowmar Co.

g. Transparencies

Babies From Eggs, 3M Company.
Frog's Life Cycle, 3M Company.
Mammal Babies, 3M Company.
Moth's Life Cycle, 3M Company.

h. Selected Stories for Children

(P) Primary Level, (I) Intermediate Level

A Baby Is Born (P), M. I. Levine and J. H. Seligmann (Golden Press).
A Baby Starts to Grow (P), Paul Showers (Crowell).
A Chimp in the Family (P), Charlotte Beeker (Messner).
A Doctor Talks to 5 to 8 Year Olds (P), D. Meilach (Budlong Press).
A Doctor Talks to 9 to 12 Year Olds (I), M. U. Lerrigo and M. Cassidy (Budlong Press).
A Father Like That (P), C. Zolotow (Harper and Row).
A Foal Is Born (P,I), Hannes-Jorg Anders (Putnam).

A Story about You (I), M. O. Lerrigo and M. J. Senn (American National Association).
About Eggs and Creatures That Hatch from Them (I), M. Uhl (Melmont).
All About Eggs and How They Change into Animals (P), Millicent Selsam (W. R. Scott).
All Kinds of Babies and How They Grow (P), S. E. Millicent (W. R. Scott).
Animal Babies (P), Ylla (Harper).
Animal Daddies and My Daddy (P), Barbara Sheek Hazen (Golden Press).
Animals As Parents (P), M. Selsam (Morrow).
Are You There, God? It's Me, Margaret (I), Judy Blume (Bradbury).
Baby Sister for Francis (P), R. Hoban (Harper & Row).
Bees and Beehives (P), Judy Hawes (Crowell).
Birthday of Obash (P), A. Chalmers (Viking).
Boo, Who Used to Be Scared of the Dark (P), Munro Leaf (Random House).
Daddies (P), L. Carton (Random House).
Daddy and Me (P), Monte Stein Jonathan (Scribner).
Daddy Is Home (P), D. Blomquist (Holt, Rinehart & Winston).
Did the Sun Shine Before You Were Born? (P), Sol Gordon (Third Press).
Exploring Home and Family Life (I), H. Fleck (Prentice-Hall).
Facts about Sex for Today's Youth (6th grade) (I), Sol Gordon (John Day).
Facts of Life for Children (I), (Child Study Association).
Finding Yourself (I), M. O. Lerrigo (American Medical Association).
Fine Eggs and Fancy Chicks (P), M. Marks (Dial).
Forever (I), Judy Blume (Bradbury).
Freddy's Book (I), John Newfield (Random House).
Girls Are Girls and Boys Are Boys (I), S. Gordon (John Day).
Growing Up (I), K. DeSchweitz (Macmillan).
Happy Little Family (P), R. Candill (Winston).
Hello, Aurora (I), A. Vestly (Crowell).
Holiday on Wheels (I), C. Wooley (Morrow).
How a Seed Grows (I), Helen Jordon (Crowell).
How Animals Live Together (I), M. Selsam (Morrow).
How Babies Are Made (P), A. Andry (Time-Life).
How Was I Born? (P), Lennart Nilsson (Delacorte).
How We Are Born (I), Julian May (Follett).
Hush Jon! (P), Joan Gill (Doubleday).
I Like to Be Me (P), Barbara Bel Geddes (Viking).
Johnny Jack and His Beginnings (P), Pearl Buck (John Day).
Kid Brother (P), J. Beim (Morrow).
Laurie's New Brother (P), M. Schlein (Abelard-Schuman, Ltd.).
Living Things and Their Young (I), Julian May (Follett).
Man and Woman (I), Julian May (Follett).
Mommies (P), L. Carton (Random House).
Mommies Are for Loving (P), R. Penn (Putnam's Sons).
Mommies at Work (P), J. Marian (Alfred A. Knopf).
Naomi in the Middle (I), N. Klein (Pantheon).
New Life (I), J. Jordon (Crowell).
Peter and Caroline (P), S. Hegeler (Abelard-Schuman Ltd.).
Possum (P), R. McClung (Morrow).
Red Bantam (P), L. Fatio (McGraw-Hill Book Company).
Seeds Are Wonderful (I), W. Foster and P. Queree (Melmont).
She Came Bringing Me That Little Baby Girl (P), E. Greenfield (Lippincott).
Sigurd and His Brave Companions (I), S. Undset (Knopf).
Sky Bed, a Norwegian Christmas (I), T. T. Grundrun (Scribner).
Squirrels in the Garden (P), O. Earle (Morrow).
Stepsister Sally (P), H. F. Daringer (Harcourt).
Tales of a Fourth Grade Nothing (I), Judy Blume (Dutton).
The Beginning of Life (I), Eva Knox Evans (Collier-Macmillan).
The Best Birthday (P), Quail Hawkins (Doubleday).
The Chosen Baby (P), V. P. Wasson (Lippincott).
The Growing Story (I), Ruth Grauss (Harper).
The Human Story (I), S. Hoftein (Scott-Foresman).
The Little Girl and Her Mother (P), Beatrice DeRiginier (Vanguard).
Then Again, Maybe I Won't (I), Judy Blume (Bradley).
The New Pet (P), Marjorie Flack (Doubleday).
The People Upstairs (I), Phyllis Cote (Doubleday).
The Stork Didn't Bring You (I), Lloyd Pemberton (Thomas Nelson & Sons).
The Story of a Baby (P), Marie Ets (Viking).
The Story of Life (I), M. O. Lerrigo and M. J. Senn (American National Association).
The Wonder of Life (I), M. I. Levine and J. H. Seligmann (Simon & Schuster).

The Wonderful Story of How You Were Born (P), J. Gruenberg (Doubleday).
The Wonderful Year (I), Nancy Barnes (Messner).
True Book of Health (P), O. V. Haynes (Children's Press).
Two Little Birds and Three (P), J. Kepes (Houghton).
Wait and See (P), C. Georgion (Harvey House).
Watching the New Baby (P), J. Samson (Atheneum).
We Are Having a Baby (P), J. Samson (Atheneum).
What Makes Me Tick? (I), H. Ruchlis (Harvey House).
What's Inside of Animals? (P), H. S. Zim (Morrow).
When Animals Are Babies (P), Elizabeth and Charles Schwartz (Holiday House).
When An Animal Grows (I), Millicent Selsam (William Morrow).
Where Do Babies Come From? (P), M. Sheffield (Knopf).
Whitefoot—the Story of a Wood Mouse (I), R. McClung (Morrow).
Window into An Egg: Seeing Life Begin (P), G. Lux Flanagan (W. R. Scott).
You and the World Around You (P), M. Selsam (Doubleday).

10. Environmental Health

a. Films

Adventuring in Conservation, Indiana University Audio-visual Center.
Bulldozed America, Carousel Films.
Choosing a Doctor, McGraw-Hill Book Company.
Communities Keep Clean, Coronet Instructional Films.
Community Health Is Up to You, McGraw-Hill Book Company.
Conservation and the Balance of Nature, International Film Bureau.
Defending the City's Health, Encyclopaedia Britannica.
Farm Animals, National Dairy Council.
Forest of Trees and Logs, American Educational Films.
Fun on the Playground, Encyclopaedia Britannica.
Lakes, Aging and Pollution, Centron Films.
Little Man, Big City, Center for Mass Communications, Columbia University Press.
Man's Natural Environment, Guidance Associates.
Mosquito, Encyclopaedia Britannica.
Of Time and a River, U.S. Department of Interior.
One Spring Day, American Educational Films.
Policemen—Day and Night, Charles Cahill and Associates.
The Animal Ark, American Educational Films.
The Doctor, Encyclopaedia Britannica.
The Endless Chain, Tribune Films, Inc.
The Fireman, Encyclopaedia Britannica.
The Ravaged Land, John Wiley & Sons, Inc.
The Second Pollution, U.S. Environmental Protection Agency.
The Water We Drink, Coronet Instructional Films.
To Live and Breathe, Aetna Life and Casualty Company.
Uncle Jim's Dairy Farm, National Dairy Council.
Vegetables for All Seasons, Arthur Barr Productions, Inc.
Your Friend the Doctor, Coronet Instructional Films.
Your Health in the Community, Coronet Instructional Films.
What Ecologists Do, Centron Films.
Within Our Reach, U.S. Environmental Protection Agency.

b. Filmstrips

Community Sanitation, Young America Films.
Concepts in Ecology, Centron Films.
Environmental Crisis, American Alliance for Health, Physical Education and Recreation.
Food, Clothing and Shelter, Society for Visual Education.
Fun at the Beach, McGraw-Hill Book Company.
Health Heroes (with transcription), Metropolitan Life Insurance Company.
I'm No Fool with Safety, Walt Disney Educational Media.
Keeping a Healthy Community, Harcourt Brace Jovanovich.
Keeping Sickness Away, McGraw-Hill Book Company.
Maintaining Community Health, Young America Films.
Learning to Be a Wise Consumer, Guidance Associates.
Making a Healthy Environment, Harcourt Brace Jovanovich.
Making Water Safe to Drink, Popular Science.
On the Road to the Country, Curriculum Films.

Our Health Department, Encyclopaedia Britannica.
Our Wounded Land: Land and Trash, Social Studies School Services.
Safeguarding Our Food, Young America Films.
Safety in the Community, Young America Films.
Sewage Disposal, McGraw-Hill Book Company.
The Beer Can by the Highway, Social Studies School Service.
The School That Learned to Eat, General Mills, Inc.
The Water We Drink, Young America Films.
Tommy and His Health Department, Educational Activities, Inc.
Tree Man: A First Adventure in Ecology, Coronet Instructional Films.
Vacation in the City, Curriculum Films.
Walter Reed and the Conquest of Yellow Fever (with transcription), Metropolitan Life
    Insurance Company.
Waste Disposal for the Community, Encyclopaedia Britannica.
Water and How We Use It, Coronet Instructional Films.
Water for the Community, Encyclopaedia Britannica.

c. Comics

Alfie Looks for Fire Trouble, National Fire Protection Association.
Sparky, National Fire Protection Association.
Sparky's Coloring Book, National Fire Protection Association.

d. Records

Fire on Thunder Hill, American Forest Products Industries, Inc.
The Constant Invaders, Wisconsin Anti-Tuberculosis Association.
Tommy and His Health Department, Educational Activities, Inc.

e. Radio Scripts

Fly Control, Bureau of Research in Education by Radio, University of Texas.
Home Safety, National Safety Council.
Keep Your Cold at Home, Bureau of Research in Education by Radio, University of
    Texas.
Know Your Traffic Laws, National Safety Council.
Make Your City Safer, National Safety Council.
Safe Water Supply, Bureau of Research in Education by Radio, University of Texas.
Swimming and Water Safety, Bureau of Research in Education by Radio, University of
    Texas.
To Walk in the Night, National Safety Council.

f. Slides

Leading Killers of Today, Spenco Medical Corporation.
Urban Slum Problems, J. Weston Walch, Publisher, Portland, Maine.
Water Conservation, J. Weston Walch, Publisher.
Water Pollution, J. Weston Walch, Publisher.

g. Selected Stories for Children

(P) Primary Level, (I) Intermediate Level

A Child's Book of Flowers (P), Kathleen Daly (Doubleday).
A Chimp in the Family (P), Charlotte Beeker (Messner).
ABC's of Ecology (I), Isaac Asimov (Walker),
About the Nature of Air (I), Harry Sootin (W. W. Norton).
And It Rained (I), Ellen Raskin (Atheneum).
A Walk in the City (P), Rosemary Dawson (Viking).
Brave Gives Blood (I), Philip and Mirina Eisenburg (Messner).
Camp-in-the-Yard (P), V. Thompson (Holiday).
Catch the Wind: A Book of Windmills and Windpower (I), Landt Dennis (Four Winds).
Come to the City (P), Ruth Tensen (Pertly & Lee).
Dangerous Air (I), Lucy Kavaler (John Day).
Experiences With Living Things for Five to Eight Year Olds (P), Katherine Wensberg
    (Beacon).
Fireman for a Day (I), Z. K. MacDonald (Messner).
First Book of Nurses (I), M. Etting (Watts).
Frog and Toad All Year (P), A. Lobel (Harper & Row).
Johnny Goes to the Hospital (P), J. Sever (Houghton).
Johnny Wants to Be a Policeman (P, I), W. J. Granberg (Aladdin).
Let's Go Fishing (I), Lee Wulff (Lippincott).
Let's Go to Stop Air Pollution (I), Michael Chester (G. P. Putnam's Sons).
Little Town (P), Bertrand Elmer Hader (Macmillan).

Our Insect Friends, (I), W. A. DuPuy (Winston).
Our Polluted World (I), John Perry (Franklin Watts).
Pat and Her Policeman (I), F. Friedman (Morrow).
Poems and Verses about the City (I), Nancy Varrick (Garrard).
Rain, Rain, River (P), Uri Shulevitz (Farrar).
Smoke (P), Ab Spang Olsen (Coward).
Strange Companions in Nature (I), I. Smith (Morrow).
Stu-Mei's Golden Year (I), M. H. Bro (Doubleday).
The City Book (P), L. Corcos (Golden).
The Discontented Village (I), Rose Dobbs (Coward-McCann).
The Fight to Save America's Water (I), U.S. Public Health Service.
The Last Free Bird (P), A. Harris Stone (Prentice-Hall).
The Life in the Forest (I), Jack McCormick (McGraw-Hill).
The Spirit of the Wild (I), Tom McGowan (Little, Brown).
The Water That Jack Drank (P), William R. Scott (W. R. Scott).
The Wonderful Farm (P), M. Ayme (Harper).
There Is a Seal in My Sleeping Bag (I), Lyn Hancock (Alfred A. Knopf).
This Vital Air (I), Thomas Hylesworth (Rand McNally).
True Book of Policemen and Firemen (P), I. Miner (Children's Press).
Tugboat (I), David Plowden (Macmillan).
Water (I), Luna Leopold (Time-Life).
Water, the Vital Essence (I), Peter Briggs (Harper & Row).
Weather (I), P. Thompson (Time-Life).
Where the Lilies Bloom (I), Vera and Bill Cleaver (Lippincott).
While Susie Sleeps (P), N. Schneider (W. R. Scott).

11. Tobacco, Alcohol and Drugs

a. Films

Alcohol—a New Focus, American Educational Films.
Alcohol in the Human Body, Sid Davis Productions.
Alcoholism, Encyclopaedia Britannica.
Alcoholism, the Hidden Disease, National Council on Alcoholism.
Barney Butt, American Heart Association.
Breaking the Habit, American Cancer Society.
Curious Alice, General Services Administration.
Donald's Better Self, Walt Disney Educational Media Company.
Drug Abuse—Everybody's Hang-up, American Alliance for Health, Physical Education
    and Recreation.
Drug Addiction, Encyclopaedia Britannica.
Drugs: A Primary Film, Arthur Barr Productions.
Drugs and the Nervous System, Churchill Films.
Drugs, Drinking and Driving, Aims Instructional Media Services.
Drugs—Use or Abuse, Instructional Media Services.
Drunk Driving, Teaching Film Custodians.
Flagged for Actions, National Film Board of Canada.
Focus on Drugs, American Educational Films.
From One Cell, American Cancer Society.
Huffless, Puffless Dragon, American Cancer Society.
Is Smoking Worth It? American Cancer Society.
Narcotics—Why Not? Charles Cahill and Associates.
99 Bottles of Beer, Norm Southerly & Associates.
Octopuff in Kumquat, American Lung Association.
One Day's Poison, National Film Board of Canada.
Out of Orbit, National Council on Alcoholism.
Should You Drink? McGraw-Hill Book Company.
Smoker's Lungs, Centron Films.
Smoking: A New Focus, American Educational Films.
Smoking and You, American Heart Association.
Smoking and Your Oral Health, American Dental Association.
The Drug Dilemma: A New Day Dawning, Coronet Instructional Materials.
The Tobacco Problem: What Do You Think? Encyclopaedia Britannica.
Tobacco and the Human Body, Encyclopaedia Britannica.
To Smoke or Not to Smoke, American Cancer Society.
To Your Health, Ideal Pictures.
Traffic with the Devil, Teaching Film Custodians.

What about Drinking? McGraw-Hill Book Company.
What Should I Do? Walt Disney Educational Media.

b. Filmstrips

Alcohol and Children (Gr 4–8), Educational Activities, Inc.
Alcohol and You, McGraw-Hill Book Company.
Alcohol and You, Young America Films.
Alcohol and Your Health, Society for Visual Education.
Algernon, the Ambulance, International Educational and Training, Inc.
Danger of Narcotics, Popular Science.
Drugs and Children (Gr 4–8), Educational Activities, Inc.
Drugs Helpful and Harmful, Wexler Film Productions.
Drug Misuse and Your Health, Society for Visual Education.
Drugs, Poisons and Little Children, Stanley Bowmar Co.
I'll Choose the High Road, American Cancer Society.
Junkie, Educational Activities.
Me, Myself–And Drugs, Guidance Associates.
Narcotics and You, Young America Films.
Nature's Filter, National Tuberculosis Association.
Only Sick People Need Drugs (K–3), Educational Activities, Inc.
Smoking and Children (Gr 4–8), Educational Activities, Inc.
The Champion, Image Publishing Corporation.
Tobacco and Alcohol, Guidance Associates.
Tobacco and Your Health, Society for Visual Education.
To Smoke or Not to Smoke, American Cancer Society.
What Are You Going to Do about Alcohol? Guidance Associates.
What Are You Going to Do about Smoking? Guidance Associates.
What Is Drug Abuse? Society for Visual Education.

c. Posters

Best Time to Stop Smoking, American Medical Association.
Best Tip Yet–Don't Start, American Cancer Society.
Break the Habit, American Medical Association.
I Don't Smoke Cigarettes, American Cancer Society.
The Family That Smokes Together Chokes Together, Spenco Medical Corporation.
This Chimp is No Chump . . . Don't Smoke, American Heart Association.
Where Have All the Smokers Gone? Spenco Medical Corporation.

d. Records

The Drugs You Use, American Medical Association.
The Most Frequently Asked Questions about Drug Abuse (3), The White House, Washington, D.C. 20506.

e. Comics

Dennis the Menace Takes a Poke at Poisons, U.S. Government Printing Office.
It's Best to Know, Connecticut State Department of Mental Health.
Where There Is Smoke, American Cancer Society.

f. Charts

Dial a Drug, Spenco Medical Corporation.
Drug Abuse Reference Chart, Pharmaceutical Manufacturers Association.
Drug Chart, Social Studies School Service.
Facts about Drugs, David C. Cook Pub. Co., Elgin, Ill., 60120.
Hazards of Drug Abuse, Spenco Medical Corporation.

g. Slides

Physical Dangers of Drug Abuse, Spenco Medical Corporation.
Smoking and Health, Spenco Medical Corporation.
The Problem of Drug Abuse, Pharmaceutical Manufacturers Association.

h. Kits

Audio-cassettes–Alcohol Abuse, Spenco Medical Corporation.
Drug Abuse Information Kit, Pharmaceutical Manufacturers Association.
Drug Education Package, Spenco Medical Corporation.
Smoking Education Package, Spenco Medical Corporation.

i. Selected Stories for Children

(P) Primary Level, (I) Intermediate Level

About Drugs (I), H. L. Bowen and L. Landen (Fearon).
Alcohol Talks from the Laboratory (I), H. Hamlin (The author, Columbus, Ohio).
Facts about Alcohol (I), Raymond McCarthy (Yale Center of Alcohol Studies).
Facts about Narcotics (I), V. A. Vogel (Science Research Associates).
Modern Medical Discoveries (I), I. Eberle (Crowell).
What You Should Know about Drugs (I), S. Christian (Harcourt Brace Jovanovich).

12. Consumer Health

a. Films

An Ounce of Prevention, Pharmaceutical Manufacturers Association.
Choosing a Doctor, McGraw-Hill Book Company.
Dress for Health, Encyclopaedia Britannica.
Folks, Facts, and Pharmacy, Lederle Laboratory.
Horizons of Hope, American Cancer Society.
How to Select Florida Oranges, Florida Citrus Commission.
I Have a Secret Cure for Cancer, American Cancer Society.
Medicine Man, American Medical Association.
More Food for Your Money, National Dairy Council.
Over-the-Counter Pills and Promises, Alfred Higgins Productions.
Pressure Steam Sterilization, Ideal Pictures.
Quacks and Nostrums, McGraw-Hill Book Company.
Read the Label and Live, Hank Newenhouse Films.
The Best Way to Eat, Florida Citrus Commission.
The Meanest Crime, U.S. Food and Drug Administration.
To Your Health, National Council on Alcoholism.
When It Comes to RX Medicines, Pharmaceutical Manufacturers Association.
Your Friend the Doctor, Coronet Instructional Films.

b. Filmstrips

Be a Balanced Wheel, National Dairy Council.
Buyer Beware, Guidance Associates.
Consumer Education, Centron Films.
FDA: A Nation's Watchdog? Guidance Associates.
Health Helpers, Encyclopaedia Britannica.
Merchandising Beef, National Livestock and Meat Board.
Nutrition: Foods, Fads, Frauds, Facts, Guidance Associates.
Project A. M., Cereal Institute, Inc.
Spending Your Food Dollars, Money Management Institute.
Tale of a Toothache, Society for Visual Education.
The Little Pink Bottle, National Foundation.
Tommy and His Health Department, Educational Activities, Inc.
You, the Consumer, Society for Visual Education, Inc.
You the Shopper, Money Management Institute.

c. Kits

Audio-Cassettes—Consumer Health Care Awareness, Spenco Medical Corporation.

d. Posters

What You Eat Can Make a Difference, Florida Citrus Commission.

e. Selected Stories for Children

(P) Primary Level, (I) Intermediate Level

Doctor John (P), F. Thompson (Melmont).
Doctors and What They Do (I), H. Coy (Watts).
Habits, Healthful and Safe (I), W. Charters (Macmillan).
Health Can Be Fun (P), M. Leaf (Stokes).
How Hospitals Help Us (P), A. Meeker (Benefic Press).
Linda Goes to the Hospital (P), N. Dudley (Coward).
Magic Bullets (I), L. Sutherland (Little).
The Hospital (P), M. Pyne (Houghton Mifflin).
We Went to the Doctor (P), C. Memling (Abelard-Schuman Ltd.).

13. Addresses of Film Sources

Aims Instructional Media Services, P.O. Box 1010, Hollywood, Calif., 90028.
Alfred Higgins Productions, Inc., 9100 Sunset Boulevard, Los Angeles, Calif. 90069.
American Educational Films, 132 Lasky Drive, Beverly Hills, Calif. 90210.
Arthur Barr Productions, Inc., P.O. Box 7-C, Pasadena, Calif. 91104.
Association Films, Inc., 25358 Cypress Avenue, Hayward, Calif.
Avis Films, 2408 W. Olive Avenue, Burbank, Calif. 91506.
Bailey Films, Inc., 6509 De Longpre Avenue, Hollywood, Calif, 90028.
BFA Educational Media, 2211 Michigan Avenue, Santa Monica, Calif, 90404.
Canadian National Film Board, 680 5th Avenue, New York, N.Y., 10019.
Carousel Films, 1501 Broadway, New York, N.Y. 10036.
Centron Films, 1621 West 9th St., Lawrence, Kan. 66044.
Center for Mass Communication, Columbia University Press, 562 West 113th St., New York, N.Y. 10025.
Charles Cahill and Associates, P.O. Box 3220, Hollywood, Calif., 90028.
Churchill Films, 622 No. Robertson Blvd., Los Angeles, Calif., 90069.
Classroom Film Distributors Inc., 5620 Hollywood Boulevard, Los Angeles, Calif. 90038.
Coronet Instructional Materials, 65 E. South Water Street, Chicago, Ill. 60601.
E. C. Brown Foundation, 1825 Willow Rd., Northfield, Ill. 60093.
Encyclopaedia Britannica Educational Corporation, 425 North Michigan Ave., Chicago, Ill. 60611.
Eye Gate House Inc., 146 Archer Avenue, Jamaica, N.Y. 11435.
Films Incorporated, 1144 Wilmette Ave., Wilmette, Ill. 60091.
Guidance Associates, 757 3rd Avenue, New York, N.Y. 10017.
Hank Newenhouse Films, 1825 Willow Rd., Northfield, Ill. 60093.
Harcourt Brace Jovanovich, 757 3rd Ave., New York 10017.
Ideal Pictures Corporation, 321 W. 44th Street, New York, N.Y. 10036.
Image Publishing Corporation, P.O. Box 14 North Station, White Plains, N.Y. 10603.
International Film Bureau, Inc., 322 S. Michigan Avenue, Chicago, Ill. 60604.
Knowledge Builders, 625 Madison Avenue, New York, N.Y. 10022.
Learning Corporation of America, 1350 Avenue of the Americas, New York, N.Y. 10019.
McGraw-Hill Book Company, Inc., 330 West 42nd Street, New York, N.Y. 10036.
Media Visuals, Inc., 342 Madison Ave., New York, N.Y. 10017.
Modern Talking Picture Service, 45 Rockefeller Plaza, New York, N.Y.
Moody Institute of Science, 12000 E. Washington Boulevard, Whittier, Calif., 90606.
National Instructional Television Center, Box A, Bloomington, Ind. 47401.
Norm Southerley and Associates, Box 15403, Long Beach, Calif. 90815.
Perennial Education, Inc., 1825 Willow Road, Northfield, Ill. 60093.
Popular Science, 330 West 42nd Street, New York, N.Y. 10036.
Sid Davis Productions, 2429 Ocean Park Blvd., Santa Monica, Calif. 90405.
Society for Visual Education, Inc., 1345 Diversey Park, Chicago, Ill. 60614.
Sunburst Communications, 41 Washington Avenue, Pleasantville, N.Y. 10570.
Teaching Film Custodians, 25 West 43rd Street, New York, N.Y. 10036.
Thorne Films, 1229 University Ave., Boulder, Col. 80302.
Tribune Films, Inc., 38 West 32nd St., New York, N.Y. 10001.
United World Films, 221 Park Avenue, South, New York, N.Y. 10022.
Walt Disney Educational Media, 500 South Buena Vista Street, Burbank, Calif. 91521.
Wexler Film Productions, 801 N. Seward Street, Los Angeles, Calif. 90038.
Young America Films, 330 W. 24th Street, New York, N.Y. 10011.

Evaluation in Health Education

11 _____

> To profess to have an aim and then neglect the means of execution
> is self-delusion of the most dangerous sort. When we take ends
> without means, we degenerate into sentimentalism. In the ideal,
> we fall back upon merely luck and chance and magic or exhortation
> and preaching.
>
> —John Dewey

Uncertainty about whether or not a health program is successful actually frustrates the conscientious teacher. Only through a continuous appraisal of the results of teaching can information be obtained to relieve frustration and doubt.

A few years ago, Havinghurst made a strong point concerning teachers' accountability for their students' learning process. He stressed that "the concept of accountability as a personal responsibility of the teacher is oversimplified and dangerous;" it overlooks joint accountability with parents and others, simply because young people live outside the school environment with their families, peer group, and other community influences that both limit and extend their interests, ambitions, and concept of self.[1]

Although this is a valid point of view, it is the teacher who is expected by both parents and school board members to take the leadership in appraising student progress toward preconceived educational goals. Under the educator's direction, in which parents and other local community people may become involved, accountability for pupil progress can be carried out in realistic fashion. This means, however, that the teacher must search for evaluative information beyond the walls of the classroom and the pencil and paper tests.

Purposes of Evaluation in Health

To evaluate, says Webster, is "to appraise carefully," and to appraise is "to set a value on." Value is determined by relative "worth, excellence, or importance." The process of evaluating, therefore, should be considered along with measurement. Measurement answers the questions how much, how many, and how often; it is concerned with quantities and qualities. Evaluation goes beyond

_____

[1]Havinghurst, Robert. "Joint Accountability: A Constructive Response to Consumer Demands," *Nation's School, 89*:45–46, May 1972.

the mechanics of testing and measuring to judgment in the light of aims and objectives. It answers the question of whether or not a particular experience has value. It is a continuous process.

Evaluation does several things when properly implemented.

It determines the health status of pupils. Learning in any area is limited by the presence of organic strains and drains, defects, and poor mental health.

It may be used to classify pupils for school activities. Pupils with chronic fatigue, faulty posture, or malnutrition often need a modified program.

It measures the efficiency of the total health program. The effective health services department, the healthful school environment, and the health teaching program all share in influencing the health status as well as the health practices of each pupil.

It measures teacher efficiency. Even the most elaborate health curriculum depends for its success on techniques and aids employed by the individual teacher.

It provides a basis for grading pupils in the instructional program; it is a means of reporting individual pupil achievement.

It contributes useful information relative to student knowledge, attitudes, and practices which may be of value when the curriculum or course of study is being updated.

EVALUATING THE TOTAL SCHOOL HEALTH PROGRAM

It is a major undertaking to appraise the effect of the total elementary school health education effort. The combined activity of many people is involved. The contributions of the classroom teacher are supplemented by those of the guidance and physical education personnel. In larger schools it involves not only the physician and nurse but also the school dentist, school nutritionist, and psychiatrist actively engaged in promoting child health. They may also be an active health council. These persons work in the three areas of health education: health services, healthful school environment, and health instruction. Any measure of pupil improvement in health understanding, awareness, and behavior must, therefore, relate to the cooperative efforts of several forces within the school.

As previously indicated in Chapter 3, there are many ways a pupil's health status can be appraised. Much of this appraisal, when understood by the student, has a beneficial effect on health attitudes and practices. By the same token, the example of a healthful school environment does much in a quiet, even subtle, way to influence the formation of desirable health behavior (Chapter 4). Usually, any formal health effort beyond this becomes one of specific instruction in the classroom.

It is sound educational practice to periodically evaluate the total elementary school program in health education. This may be acomplished every two or three years by employing a specially prepared evaluation instrument. Several such instruments are available for the use of elementary school administrators. Several of the more complete ones are as follows.

Criteria for Evaluating the Elementary Health Program (California State Department of Education, Sacramento, Calif.). This form is used to evaluate administration, health instruction, health services, and healthful school environment. Each of the criteria are set forth as desirable practices. The quality of each practice is judged for a particular school on a four-point scale: excellent, good, fair, and poor.

The Oregon State University *School Health Program Evaluation Scale* consists of checklist items about how the elementary school teacher uses health services information, and the nature of the health curriculum.[2] The scale has practical value, especially if employed for self-appraisal.

In this respect, the *Self-Appraisal Checklist for School Health Programs* of the Ohio Department of Health has immediate use in almost any school, as it pertains to health services, healthful school living, and health education.[3] Moreover, it is particularly concerned with the results of the evaluation being used as a basis for curriculum revision and program improvement.

An especially thorough instrument is the *Evaluative Criteria, Health Education* (NSSSE) prepared by the American Council On Education, 1785 Massachusetts Avenue, N.W., Washington, D.C. 20036. Health education criteria are presented in checklist form so that they may easily be applied to local health education programs as a self-testing activity or by an evaluating agency. Searching questions are raised about the extent of the instructional program.

Today the total school health program is focused on *output*—on achievement—on demonstrated results. We have moved from input to output. Thus the health services, curriculum content, materials, and grade placement of learning activities are viewed in terms of student output.

PROBLEMS IN EVALUATING THE HEALTH INSTRUCTION PROGRAM

In searching for ways in which to upgrade evaluation practices, Bedworth and Bedworth concluded that one of the difficulties is "the complexity of controlling all the relevant variables. As a consequence, interpretation of evaluative data may be biased by the existence of these variables. . . ."[4] It is reasonable to expect, therefore, that the effect of good health teaching on human activity may be difficult to measure. This is true for several reasons.

---

[2]Anderson, C. L. and Creswell, William H., Jr., *School Health Practice*. 6th ed., St. Louis: C. V. Mosby Co., 1976, p. 440.

[3]*A Self-Appraisal Checklist for School Health Programs,* Ohio Department of Health, P.O. Box 118, Columbus, Ohio 43216.

[4]Bedworth, David A. and Bedworth, Albert E. *Health Education: A Process for Human Effectiveness.* New York: Harper & Row, Publishers, 1978, p. 324.

The power of the human organism to adapt to the physical and psychological stresses placed upon it is most remarkable. All too often the apparently healthy person is harboring one or more potential killers. Heart disease, cancer, respiratory congestion, and kidney malfunction are all about us. The diseases of stress and the shades of malnutrition do not always manifest themselves so that they are easily observed. The line between adjustment and maladjustment is not always defined. Even "normality" is relative.

There is a "sleeper effect" in health teaching. What is learned today in terms of factual knowledge may not be applied until months or years later. Improved attitudes and practices make themselves known at a time when they do not seem to be directly related to anything—least of all to a health course taken at an earlier time.

Even under the most favorable conditions it will be difficult to fully appraise the health instruction program. Not all of the ramifications of a health lesson are statistically measurable. Very often health instruction goes far beyond the pupil and affects the behavior of parents and other members of the community. Frequently the support which the public gives to a health project is at least partially the result of effective school health teaching. Even such community items as improved disease reporting, increased circulation of health literature in public libraries, more adults taking regular exercise and controlling weight, reduced water pollution, the installation of additional sanitary facilities, the increase in dental and physical examinations, and even the increase in newspaper editors who speak out on consumer health—all of these may be related to the efforts of the classroom teacher.

An accurate measurement of health attitudes and practices is difficult under the best of circumstances. It has always been rather simple to test for health facts and considerably more difficult to sample attitudes or beliefs, or ascertain whether a pupil has shown the ability to apply health information in an effective manner. Further complicating attitude-behavior measurement is the validity of observations made by the teacher. Although the value in the observation is a child-structured response, there remains the difficulty that Piaget mentions "of distinguishing a child's play from his beliefs. . . . Pure observation is inadequate for distinguishing belief from romancing."[5] Piaget would couple observation techniques with opportunities for reasoning; this he does in his clinical method.[6]

Too many teachers through the years have simply handed out facts to their pupils and have received the facts back at examination time. Thousands of schoolchildren can spell, write, and recite the names of the vitamins and minerals found in specific foods; they can name the types of teeth and diagram how the blood circulates in the body. Yet many of them do not choose foods wisely; they do not own a toothbrush or appreciate the relationship of adequate rest and sleep to personal well-being in work and play. In short, they are rated as

---

[5]Piaget, J. *The Child's Concept of the World.* Paterson, N.J.: Littlefield, Adams, 1963, p. 7.
[6]Wadsworth, Barry J. *Piaget for the Classroom Teacher.* New York: Longman, Inc., 1978, p. 223.

good students of health because they have given teachers what they wanted to hear—health facts and figures.

These statements are not meant to imply that facts are unimportant in health teaching. Quite the opposite is true, for facts are always of value when it comes to specific knowledge and intelligent behavior. The quarrel comes when mere facts by themselves are the meat of the teaching and testing program. Personal involvement must be added. Students who *act* on facts during the teaching program are more apt to *behave* differently when habits and attitudes are appraised at a later date. One of the specific findings in the Los Angeles study was that "how people *feel* toward health education" determines to a great extent what they do about their health behavior. It takes time and a concentration of effort in school to develop *feelings* toward health. Research supports this view by showing that direct teaching is superior to integrated and correlated instruction.

The classroom teacher will evaluate health practices by noting readily observable items such as the increase in children having dental work completed, the number of improved practices relative to milk drinking, cleanliness, posture, and appearance, the increase in the sale of nutritious foods at the cafeteria, the reports by parents on changed behaviors, the increase in the number of parents attending school health examinations of their children, the increase in the percentage of physical defects remedied, and many more such specific items.

There is a shortage of valid and useful elementary health education tests, scales, and other appraisal devices. While local knowledge tests are not difficult to construct, homemade tests of attitudes and practices are harder to come by. Even when there are fairly good tests, their usefulness is reduced by the fact that many teachers fail to determine what a pupil or class knows about a health topic at the beginning of the study. In other words, some *pretesting* or early appraisal is necessary before a particular unit of work is started. The teacher's objective is simply to find out what the class knows and how it feels about the topic *before* instruction begins. There is tremendous variation in initial health knowledge, not only between individuals but also between classes and between schools. Pretesting provides the teacher with information relative to pupil inadequacies and strengths, and thus makes possible the selection of the most appropriate subject matter and the placement of emphasis to meet individual pupil shortcomings. In this connection, the Board of Regents of the New York State Education Department advocates basic competency tests for pretest and post-test purposes in order to demonstrate student mastery of specific skills.

APPRAISAL METHODS IN THE CLASSROOM

Health appraisal is not something that is done after the instruction has been completed; it occurs simultaneously with teaching and learning.

Bloom, Hastings, and Madaus have done much to advance the concept of concurrent teaching and appraising by stressing the need to broaden cognitive evaluations and *measure progress by the degree to which individual behavior conforms to the prearranged behavioral objectives.*[7] In keeping with what Bloom had done earlier in his *Taxonomy of Educational Objectives,* a considerable amount of attention is directed toward the application of knowledge. The student who is able to apply his or her knowledge uses abstractions in various situations. These may be in the form of general ideas or rules of procedure, or they may involve technical principles and theories. Bloom feels that if the student learns well it is partly due to the fact that the item learned is so serviceable—somehow important to the individual.

In his original work, Bloom set up six educational objectives in the *cognitive domain* that bear examining from the point of view of health education.[8]

No. 1 Knowledge

This is the recall of specifics—methods, processes, theories, structures or settings. Here one would test for knowledge relative to health terminology, definitions, and trends.

> *Example:* Which of the following is employed to prevent night blindness?
> 1. Vitamin C
> 2. Vitamin B
> 3. Vitamin A
> 4. Iron compound

No. 2 Comprehension

The lowest level of understanding, where the individual can make use of something without necessarily relating it to other things.

Included in this category is the ability to *translate* or paraphrase a communication.

> *Example:* While listening to the teacher you have heard the following terms frequently used: "alcohol," "drug," "alcoholic," "proof," and "social drinking." In a short paragraph tell in your own words what these terms mean to you.

No. 3 Application

Using abstractions or technical principles, ideas, and theories in some way. There is sufficient student understanding here in order to select and apply the abstraction. Application questions call for a show of practical ability where the student is able to match some already acquired concept with the phenomenon being considered.

> *Example:* a. Will this lightweight coat keep me comfortably warm in Alaska in the winter?
> b. Choose two pictures of automobile accidents from the local newspaper and compare them in terms of their being representative of what is happening on the highways today.

No. 4 Analysis

The examining of an idea, concept, or structure by breaking it down into its elements or parts so that the *relationship* between elements is clear.

> *Example:* The husband of a woman who died of lung cancer claimed

---

[7]Bloom, Benjamin S., Hastings, J. Thomas and Madaus, George F., *Handbook on Formative and Summative Evaluation of Student Learning,* New York: McGraw-Hill Book Company, 1971.

[8]For a fine elaboration on this see Solleder, Marion K. "Evaluation in the Cognitive Domain," *Journal of School Health, 42*:16–20, January 1972.

that the physican did not provide proper medical care during the several months in which he had the woman as a patient. Why is this accusation unfair?

    1. The woman was told several times by the physician to stop smoking but she paid no attention.
    2. Lung cancer cannot be cured unless the lungs are removed.
    3. The woman went to the physician too late for the cancer to be brought under control.
    4. The cancer appeared suddenly in the woman the week before she died.

No. 5 Synthesis

The bringing together of all parts and elements to form a whole. The student is able to work with pieces and make arrangements in such a manner as to create a structure or pattern not there before. Theorizing or making a firm statement on the basis of data on hand demonstrates the ability to synthesize.

    Example: Prepare an essay in which you consider the relationship between a human being and the plant-animal world and how this has a bearing on general health and well-being. This is explained in the Guidance Associates filmstrip, *Man's Nature Environment.*

    The filmstrip will be shown to you once as you begin to think about the assignment and once again ten minutes later. It is suggested that after the first showing you spend about ten minutes planning your remarks.

No. 6 Evaluation

This involves the making of judgments relative to the worth of materials, methods, and ideas.

    Example: Which of the following frequently is responsible for skin disorders in young people?

        1. Eating too many acid-type foods.
        2. Washing the skin too often.
        3. Changes in the chemistry of the body.
        4. Overexercise and extreme body fatigue.

In constructing health education tests, the *affective domain* is also important. Bloom points out that each cognitive behavior has an affective behavior and vice versa. The five part progression is as follows:

1. *Receiving:* Here there is a willingness on the part of the pupil to "tune in" and receive—to become *aware.*
2. *Responding:* This is active attending—doing something with the phenomenon and not just being aware of it.
3. *Valuing:* The concept of worth becomes part of the individual—consistent enough to take on the characteristics of a belief or an attitude. There is a commitment.
4. *Organization:* The internalized values become organized into the individual's value system and are related to other values.
5. *Characterization:* The organization of values into a total philosophy or world view. The peak of the internalization process.

Example (Through questioning):

The *action domain* is the culminating part of the whole process
of looking at pupil learning and evaluation. It is because of the
significance of this domain that stress has been put on competencies
and behavioral objectives. It is true that when behaviors are objec-
tified in terms of the verb "to do," clearly defined actions are set forth
and can be readily observed throughout the formal and informal
activities of the school day. One can ask almost anytime whether or

Figure 11–1. How would you
evaluate this situation? (Courtesy Gerber
Baby Foods.)

not a particular student is indeed able to "describe," "analyze," "investigate," "portray," "develop," "demonstrate," "identify," "distinguish," "select," "employ," "choose," "discriminate," etc.

For the teacher who has behavioral objectives on hand during the teaching of a major health topic, there is a reminder to look for changes. Critical observation, therefore, can be a fruitful measurement technique, especially if the observer has had some experience in deciding what to look for.

Recently the Michigan Department of Education developed Minimal Performance Objectives (MPO) for health education pupils in grades one through nine that related to ten content areas for each grade. Objective Reference Tests (ORT) were also developed for each grade. In one school district involving the first five grades, ORT scores improved considerably when teachers presented strategies and utilized teaching aids.[9]

Children of all ages have much to communicate if the teacher will simply question and observe. Written tests alone will not provide the answers. Answers to simple behavioral questions may be more enlightening. How do children get along with each other? Is there evidence of happiness?

Observing how children go about a task, how they work together, how they discuss and share information and ideas, how they report, and how well they manage the transition from one health activity to another are examples of situations which may be created to appraise their behavior. Some of the individual pupil practices that shed a good deal of light on the aplication of health knowledge that may readily be observed by the teacher are as follows.

Evidence of a cleaner and more attractive school building.

Increased cooperation in helping to maintain a healthful classroom.

Improved personal cleanliness—related to the use of the handkerchief, handwashing and toilet practices, condition of clothing, and eating.

Improved general appearance and posture, mental alertness, enthusiasm.

Better practices of oral cleanliness, e.g., rinsing mouth after meals.

Improved eating practices as observed at lunchtime: Increased consumption of milk during snack and lunch periods. Better lunches brought from home. Less food thrown away at lunchtime.

Evidence of attitude changes with respect to appreciation of the human body and its functions.

Evidence of practices to limit the use of sweets and carbonated drinks for class trips and parties.

Improved practices with regard to working and playing in good light.

Evidence of greater awareness of others, of social adjustment,

---

[9]Wantz, Molly S. and DuShaw, Martha. "A Cooperative Project to Evaluate Health Education at the Elementary Level," *Journal of School Health*, 47:462–465, October 1977.

personal friendliness, more willingness to share materials, and willingness to help when help is asked for.

Always Usually Seldom Never

Are the hands, face, neck, and ears clean?
Are the fingernails clean?
Are the clothes neat and clean?
Is the hair combed?
Is a handkerchief or tissue carried?
Are the hands washed before eating?
Is the shower enjoyed following the physical
    education period?
Is the mouth covered during coughing and
    sneezing?
Is there good sitting and standing posture?

Improved attitudes toward safety patrols, traffic officers, the handling of pets and animals, the handling of scissors, leaving materials and equipment where they may cause falls, and so on.

Improved behavior during safety and fire drills.

Evidence of increasing responsibility for planning a balanced school day by participating in rest, play, lunch, and work periods with decreasing assistance from the teacher.

Health Records

In practically every elementary school, health records are available for teachers to look over. Very often the school nurse will be able to interpret the physical examination in such a way that a good deal of meaningful information may be obtained. A review of individual pupil health records will reveal improvement in attendance, the extent to which remediable physical defects have been corrected, and the degree of personal illness. It will also show improvements in growth factors such as height and weight and the results of special screening examinations for vision, hearing, and mental health. Very often there is evidence of improvement in dental health status. Moreover, properly kept health records tell how much "follow-up" has been accomplished as a result of the discovery of organic drains, defects, or poor health practices and attitudes.

The cumulative record or anecdotal record has considerable value when it comes to pupil health evaluation. By making notations from time to time on the progress of a particular pupil, a record of lasting value is accomplished for others to use at a later date. Excellent examples of cumulative health record cards are found in California and New York.

Some classroom teachers prefer to keep a class chart which they call a Pupil Observation Chart. This lists the names of all class members in alphabetical order with space to the right for notations.

Each day when the attendance is checked the teacher may make a comment if it appears necessary. Such a chart tends to keep evaluation current with everyday teaching.

Another useful health record is one that may be kept by the pupils themselves and appraised periodically by the teacher. This includes diaries and other autobiographical records of pupils.

Performance Tests

One of the increasingly rewarding ways of appraising health status and health improvement in the elementary grades is to formally measure the *physical peformance* of boys and girls. Those pupils who generally demonstrate a high degree of vigor, strength, muscular endurance, and enthusiasm usually possess a high degree of physical fitness. When they appear to "slow down" and become less vigorous and enthusiastic, it is time to check more closely for hidden organic strains, physical defects, poor sleep and food habits, maladjustment, or something else.

In a number of elementary schools, tests of physical fitness are given by physical education teachers in cooperation with school health services personnel. The findings of such tests almost always reveal information of value to the classroom teacher of health. The pupil whose physical performance is sub-strength and below par is in need of special help, part of which may involve the classroom teacher.

TABLE 11–1. A. A. U. JUNIOR PHYSICAL FITNESS TESTS STANDARDS—BY YEARS

Event	Boys			Girls		
	6–7	*8–9*	*10–11*	*6–7*	*8–9*	*10–11*
Required events:						
1. Sprints	40 yd. 9 sec.	40 yd. 8 sec.	50 yd. 8 sec.	40 yd. 9 sec.	40 yd. 8 sec.	50 yd. 9 sec.
2. Walk and Run	¼ mile 5 min.	½ mile 8 min.	¾ mile 10 min.	¼ mile 5 min.	½ mile 8 min.	¾ mile 11 min.
3. Sit-ups	8	12	16	8	12	14
4. Pull-ups	(modified) 3	(modified) 7	(regular) 3	(modified) 3	(modified) 7	(modified) 8
5. Standing Broad Jump	3'	4'	5'	3'	4'	4'6"
Choose any one of these events:						
6. Push-ups	(modified) 5	(modified) 8	(modified) 13	(modified) 4	(modified) 7	(modified) 9
7. Playground Ball Throw for Distance	35'	65'	85'	20'	30'	40'
8. Continuous Hike for Distance	1 mile	2 mile	3 mile	1 mile	2 mile	3 mile
9. Running High Jump	1'6"	2'3"	2'9"	1'6"	2'3"	2'6"

A relatively simple screening device for physical fitness should be employed in schools where there is no physical education department or where the appraisal of physical capacity is a responsibility of the classroom teacher. Such a test can be most revealing in pointing out those pupils who lack the "work capacity" to put in a full day of study and play. Such pupils are frequently underachievers who are existing at a point far below their potential level of intelligence and effort.[10] The classroom teacher should be able to check boys and girls against the standards of the A.A.U. Junior Physical Fitness Tests (Table 11–1). These are adaptable to any school situation and can be used with little motivation as self-testing activities.[11] Ideally, every elementary school pupil should have his or her level of physical fitness routinely appraised three times during the school year by a regular teacher of physical education who is able to employ more sophisticated measures and work with health service personnel to interpret the findings.

There is one other performance test that is being used more and more in elementary schools. This is a motor skill *test for bicycle safety*. The children bring their bicycles to school and demonstrate how to turn, using appropriate hand signals. In the primary grades they demonstrate the method of getting on a bicycle, the means of guiding it, applying the brake, and the methods of stopping and parking. The National Safety Council has simple test suggestions to teach and appraise bicycle skills. An excellent bicycle skill test which may be set up on any elementary school playground is distributed free, complete with diagrams, by Aetna Life Insurance Company of Hartford, Connecticut. A guide entitled *Bicycle Safety* is also distributed for use with this test. These particular tests offer quite a challenge to youth and are a first-rate appraisal device for the teacher. (See bicycle safety section of Chapter 8 for a diagram of one of these tests.)

Oral-Individual Responses

A prestructured interview with a student or several students can be informative. So can an entirely unstructured interview in which the students react freely to certain ideas related to their health studies. Lewy makes a case for "hearings" and the "hearing technique" in which students appear before experts to respond to a variety of questions.[12] The appraisal process is popular in Swedish schools. Coupled with systematic observations of student practices, this technique could be quite productive for the teacher.

---

[10]Among the better screening tests for elementary school-age physical fitness are the Kraus-Weber, Physical Fitness Index, AAHPER Youth Fitness Test, Indiana Motor Fitness Test, Oregon Motor Fitness Test, and the Washington Elementary School Physical Fitness Test.

[11]Free copies with full directions may be obtained from the Amateur Athletic Union, 233 Broadway, New York, N.Y. 10007.

[12]Lewy, Arieh. *Handbook of Curriculum Evaluation,* New York: Longman, Inc., 1977, p. 177.

Reports

The results of good health teaching may sometimes be demonstrated by the reports of local physicians, ophthalmologists, nurses, and dentists regarding the increase in medical and dental treatment of school-age groups. Through interviews with these professional people, it is possible to become aware of the physical defects and other adverse health conditions that have been corrected or improved. Each year in the city of Cincinnati, Ohio, the school health director compiles an extensive breakdown of facts and figures relative to the health of the school-age children. This is used in a number of ways to improve health teaching at several grade levels.

Surveys

The survey is a formal approach to the topic of health appraisal. It may be community-wide and involve information secured from parents and others in the community or it may be limited to the confines of the school. In either case, it is an attempt to discover certain useful health information which may be related to health teaching. There may be a survey of the school cafeteria to check on the sale of milk, salads, fruits, whole-grain cereals, and enriched bread, or of a local restaurant, dairy, meat market, or grocery store. There are surveys of the school environment to determine such things as the cleanliness of shower and toilet rooms and whether there are appropriate rest and relaxation periods for young children. But more important from a health instruction viewpoint is the survey that seeks to determine *pupil behavior.* Environmentally, there may be an opportunity to wash the hands before eating, but what does the survey show? How many children using a lavatory actually wash their hands before eating? The survey, therefore, may make known a real need which calls for a different health teaching emphasis.

There are so many excellent items that lend themselves to being surveyed that care should be taken to select the ones most representative of changes in health behavior in a major health area. In surveying the class as a whole, the teacher will ask questions such as the following:

Are the children eating or at least tasting foods they never ate before? Are they eating more leisurely? What are the most popular breakfast cereals purchased in families? How frequent are colds among class members and their families? What is the most common kind of family recreation in the summer? Winter? How many hours of sleep do children average per night? How aware is the class of health news items as evidenced from newsclippings and other information brought to class? How frequently are the teeth brushed?

Does pupil absenteeism due to illness relate in any way to a lack of sleep? Is there any improvement in achievement and adjustment of pupils when sleep habits improve?

Do children willingly wear glasses after the physician recommends them? Is there any indication that children take more precautions regarding the prevention of physical injury to the eyes and ears?

Do children want to stay home from school at early signs of head colds or other illness?

Are there evidences of good manners while playing and sharing with others? Has there been an improvement in the respect shown for the feelings and viewpoints of others?

Is there evidence that the pupils are learning to accept their own limitations?

Is there less daydreaming, crying, timidity, "tattling," and hostility?

Do the results of a bicycle inspection indicate that adequate equipment is being used and that there is proper maintenance such as good brakes, lubricated chains, and proper air pressure in the tires?

How many class members have seen the dentist during the last six months?

It is becoming more and more common to ask pupils what they think about a certain happening or item of learning. When such questions are organized, they frequently take the form of a *pupil opinion survey*. Fifth and sixth graders sometimes have a very definite opinion about the nature of specific health instruction—techniques, materials, content, and whether or not it is effective in changing their attitudes and habits.

Parental Opinions

Very often when boys and girls apply their health knowledge, the alert parents are the first to notice it. Attitudes and practices relative to visits to doctor and dentist, foods, personal cleanliness, appearance, oral hygiene, and rest are concrete items that frequently cause parents a fair amount of concern. When children show increased cooperation along these lines at home, most parents will be aware of it and are happy to pass the information along to the teacher. One teacher in a small upstate New York town made it a point to talk to all 28 mothers of her second grade class. Using a simple check list, she asked pertinent questions relative to home improvement in specific areas where health instruction had been given. After reviewing all the evaluation techniques that she had previously used, it was her judgment that the interview with the parents was by far the most fruitful and enlightening. As a specific example, it was found that following several lessons on activity, rest, and relaxation, a rather large number of children willingly gave up television and radio programs that might interfere with their sleep and went to bed.

In the elementary schools of Los Angeles, a plan has been in operation whereby parents are asked to cooperate with the schools by keeping a check on the health behavior of their children at a very early age (kindergarten). Attached to the cover letter is a form consisting of 40 clear and straightforward questions which may be answered with "Yes" or "No." Here are a few examples selected at random:

		Yes	No
1.	Does your child wash his hands before eating?	☐	☐
2.	Does your child wash his hands after toileting?	☐	☐
8.	Does your child use his own toothbrush?	☐	☐
14.	Does your child go to bed at 7 o'clock?	☐	☐
18.	Is your child happy at mealtimes?	☐	☐
39.	Does your child stay away from strange animals?	☐	☐

Case Studies

Although it takes time to put together several case studies involving individuals and groups of pupils, they are nevertheless very useful when appraising the effectiveness of the health teaching effort. Consider the implications of a report such as the following:

I am a teaching principal in a small school. As we do not have a school nurse to visit us every day, it is my responsibility to take the children home when they are ill or when they are injured.

My primary teacher sent a small child to my room with a note. She believed the child had head lice. She wished me to check. I examined Linda and found that she did have head lice.

After making the necessary arrangements to leave my room, I drove Linda to her home. There I found the mother sick and in bed. Venice, who was a student in my room, was at home this day. It had been reported that she was ill; however this was not the case. She had stayed at home to care for the mother.

The house contained one room for the four members of the family. The small amount of furniture was old, dusty, dirty, and broken. The beds were not made and the linen was soiled. The table in the center of the room was piled with dirty dishes and food. It seemed to me that the dishes must not have been washed for several days. The sink and cupboard tops were piled high with dirty dishes, garbage was in evidence on the counter top and was splashed on the cupboards and so on to the floor. The room had not been swept recently. The chairs were covered with clothes so that one had to be unloaded so that I might sit down. There were new curtains at the windows.

Venice (age 12) was playing a game on the floor, oblivious to the condition of the room. The mother did not apologize for the room. She complained to me that her husband was "mad" about her being home, sick. She worked in a laundry and he thought she ought to go to work. (However, she was at home according to the doctor's orders.)

I explained the reason for my bringing Linda home. I gave her instructions for eliminating the lice. After telling her that the nurse would check both girls before they could return to school, I went back to my classroom. Several questions came to me as I was driving back to school. How could people live in such filth? How could that family be healthy? What could I do? How could I help? I had read about deplorable homes, but they were far away. This home life would be duplicated by these two girls if something was not done about the situation. I decided that this would be a good time for a unit on cleanliness. I called the school nurse, giving her the information and she promised to check on the girls.

We studied cleanliness in our classroom, talked about sanitation, clean clothes, clean bodies, and clean homes. The students were given opportunities to sweep and dust the floors. They washed dishes, emptied garbage, put clean linen on the bed in our infirmary. They learned how to scrub the floor using disinfectant in the water.

The mother came to the next Parent Teachers Association meeting. She was fairly clean. She told me that the girls were helping her so much, now. They were washing the dishes and cleaning the house for her before she came home from the laundry.

I visited the home a few days later. The house did have a different look. There was still room for improvement but a wedge had been made. There were no dirty dishes, no garbage to be seen. The beds were made. The floor had been swept.

Later in the year the father came to Parent Teachers Association with the mother. Both were clean and their clothes were neat. The father took an active part in the discussion on school safety. The next afternoon as I entered the sheriff's office to request some signs, I found Mr. "D." there for the same purpose.

The children now come to school with clean clothes. Their hair, which is very long, has been braided and looks neat. The father bought a television set and is going to buy a new living room suite this summer.

I know these children have benefited from this lesson and I hope that they will continue to strive for better conditions.

FORMAL TESTING IN HEALTH EDUCATION

A satisfactory test requires the student to think about the facts and *apply* them in a specific way. In so doing, the level of comprehension is demonstrated; also identified is an awareness and feeling so fundamental to ultimate commitment. In short, unless formal written and oral testing in health education adheres to the Bloom *Taxonomy*, very little valid information relative to pupil progress and teaching effectiveness will be determined.

Teacher-Prepared Tests. In view of the above it is important at the local level to consider the formulation of questions which will measure some degree of knowledge, comprehension, application, analysis, synthesis, and evaluation in the cognitive domain. (See pages 471–472.) Also, these should be mixed in with questions in the affective domain where feelings, beliefs, and attitudes can be expressed. This means that health instruction has to be concerned with concepts and behaviors rather than facts. How do pupils *feel* about a topic? What does it mean to them? An appropriate examination would be one in which pupils are asked to support certain concepts with their background of factual information. In this respect, the well-worded essay exam has a new potential value in many classrooms. This free-response type of test can be quite objective— particularly if the instructor knows what specific information is wanted from the examination.

Most elementary schoolteachers prepare their own test questions and ask them in a manner which benefits the local classroom situation. This is justified on the basis of varied pupil needs and individual differences at the local elementary level. However, test validity, reliability, and objectivity are sometimes sacrificed when local tests are employed. Frequently test item analysis has not been completed, thus reducing the amount of confidence that can be placed on the test as a whole.[13]

Teacher-made paper and pencil tests fall into two categories: *free-response* and *choice*. The essay question, in which the pupil explains what he or she knows about something, has already been mentioned. Much can be learned from this type of question, especially if the teacher will encourage the student to elaborate on "understandings" and "appreciations." This is sometimes hard to do when questions come out of a textbook. The textbook, say Read and Greene, "offers little opportunity for any mental activity except remembering," and to encourage thinking the teacher must present questions beyond the conventional textbook which would include "different interpretations, additional evidence, different line of measuring . . . or more recent and accurate materials."[14]

Another example of the free-response question is the short-answer type:

Short-answer question: In a sentence or two, express your understanding of each of the following terms:

alcohol	dentine
wheat germ	bacteria
vitamin A	obesity
sodium fluoride	mental health
calcium	overweight

Choice or guided-response questions are valuable because they do not depend upon skill in expression and handwriting. They provide a relatively wide sampling of knowledge in a short time. Once a key has been prepared, they encourage highly objective scoring.

Multiple choice questions are extremely adaptable and lend themselves to an unusually wide range of use. They have been used in many health knowledge and attitude tests. A carefully formulated multiple-choice question with several alternatives can provide the teacher with a basis for appraising errors in thinking. The following points apply to the construction of multiple-choice test items:

1. Preface the question with a short, clear set of directions.
2. State a single, definite problem in the lead statement.
3. Include as much of the item as possible in the lead statement.
4. Make the alternatives consistent with the lead.
5. Make the alternatives reasonably similar. The choices open to the student must be very much alike in order for the

---

[13]Shaw, Donald. "Evaluation—The Classroom Dilemma," *Health Education,* 8:5–7, March/April 1977.

[14]Read, Donald A. and Greene, Walter H. *Creative Teaching in Health,* 2nd ed., New York: Macmillan Publishing Co., Inc., 1975, p. 393.

discriminatory power of the student to be measured. In a five-choice question, at least three choices should be close so that only the student with real knowledge can select the most appropriate or best answer.

Example
Section 1—Multiple Choice: Read each question carefully. Select the one item which *best* answers the question. Put the number of the item selected in the space in front of the question.

18. At what time of year does the weight of schoolchildren increase more rapidly?
    (1) summer
    (2) winter
    (3) spring and late summer
    (4) fall and early winter
    (5) no set period

True-False questions have their limitations. They have been "worked to death" as a means of measuring factual knowledge. A proper true-false question should be written in the language of the pupil. It should be as nearly true or false as it can be made. Sweeping generalizations should be avoided. Directions should be clear.

Example
Section 2—True and False: The letters T and F have been placed before each statement given. Draw a circle around the letter T if the statement is *True* and around the letter F if the statement is *False* or *Partially False.*

T F 12. Accidents in the community are still the greatest threat to schoolchildren.

Matching questions are another variety of guided-response tests which, if properly prepared, will save the teacher time. The "stimulus" column should appear to the left and the "response" column to the right. There should be some five to 15 items listed with more response items than stimulus items. Directions regarding matching should be clear, preferably preceded by an oral discussion before the examination sheets are distributed. A matching test works quite well with health information.

Example
Section 3—Matching: Match the food elements listed in the left-hand column with the foods listed in the right-hand column. Put the number of the food element in the parentheses after each item.

1. Vitamin B	a. Roast pork ( )
2. Iron	b. Calves' liver ( )
3. Calcium	c. Bread ( )
4. Carbohydrates	d. Milk products ( )
5. Fats	e. Ham gravy ( )
	f. Onions ( )
	g. Oysters ( )
	h. Cabbage ( )

Standardized Tests. For several decades, standardized testing has been a growth industry. In view of this, one must ask how effective it is. And are there effective alternatives to standardized tests that will help to identify the great diversity of abilities and talents in the student population? Some of these tests are so impersonal and automatic that there is little opportunity to appraise qualities of what Lewis Mumford calls sensitiveness, consciousness, responsiveness, expressive intelligence, and human heartedness.

A limited number of standardized health and safety tests are available for elementary school use. Most of these are several years old and need up-dating, in terms of both current health information and the kinds of questions asked. There are no health education measures that embrace all of the Bloom *Taxonomy* requirements. Some are concerned with knowledge only and there are others which attempt to tie knowledge and its application together. Recommended are the following.

Cooperative Health Education Test (AAHPER) 1972. Form 4. Educational Testing Service, Box 999, Princeton, New Jersey 08540 and American Association for Health, Physical Education, and Recreation, 1201 16th St., N.W., Washington, D.C. 20036. Designed for grades 5 and 6 by a committee of health education leaders and test construction specialists from Educational Testing Service. After thorough country-wide testing the 50-multiple-choice-item test was distributed. It is a 40-minute test in which knowledge questions make up only about 20 per cent of the total; the others are as follows: application, 50 per cent; analysis, 20 per cent; and evaluation, 10 per cent. Questions asked relate to consumer health, community health, international health, disease and disorders, personal health care, growth and development, nutrition, mental health, drug use and abuse, and safety and first aid.

Los Angeles Health Education Evaluation Instruments. Los Angeles City School District, Calif. Excellent instruments for kindergarten and grades two, four, and six are available for the measurement of knowledge and attitudes. Contact Division of Educational Services, Los Angeles City Schools, P.O. Box 3307, Terminal Annex, Los Angeles, Calif. 90051.

Yellen, Sylvia. *Health Behavior Inventory,* Monterey, California: California Test Bureau, 1963. A 40-item picture-question inventory for pupils in Grades 3, 4, 5, and 6 which relates to the major health areas of personal health, personal cleanliness, nutrition, safety, community health, infection and disease, mental health, and dental health.

There are also a few useful tests for seventh grade pupils which may be of interest to sixth grade teachers and others employed in the middle school or the eight-year elementary school:

Veenker, Harold C. "A Health Knowledge Test for the Seventh Grade." *Research Quarterly, 30*:338–348, Revised. The two test forms of multiple-choice items are available from the author at Purdue University, Lafayette, Ind. The recent edition has been put together with the principles of the Bloom *Taxonomy* in mind.

Colebank, Albert D. *Health Behavior Inventory,* Monterey, Calif.: California Test Bureau, 1963. A 100-item test for grades seven, eight, and nine covering all major health topics. There are 24 health attitude items, 25 health behavior items, and 50 health knowledge items. All are multiple-choice.

The most complete set of health and safety tests are those developed by the Los Angeles City Schools for their evaluative survey. These were constructed for kindergarten and grades two, four, and six. In grade two, for example, health appraisal is made by means of a picture test—27 multiple-choice picture items. The teacher reads the item and asks the pupil to put an x on the picture which is the best answer. (A copy of the test pictures may be found in the appendix of the Instructional Guide, *Health in the Elementary Schools,* Los Angeles City School Publication No. EC-201, Revised.) As a result of using this test, the schoolchildren were found to be in need of more health instruction relative to sleep and rest, grooming, growth, and disease control. Here is an example of what the teacher says and what the pupils see.

Teacher says:

    3. Now let's look at the pictures in row 3. On a hot day, we play quietly in the shade, run around in a sweater, or climb a mountain. Mark the best answer and put your pencils up.

    In the area of safety education, there are some excellent sources of test materials for elementary school use. One test which gets at both understandings and application at the 5th grade level is *How Much Do Your Pupils Know About Safety?* It is available from the National Safety Council. The 130 questions cover home, traffic, school, playground, sports, bicycle, and holiday safety and can be used with classes anywhere from grades four through eight.

    A bicycle safety test that students can take by themselves is shown below. Another test, the *Bicycle Safety Quiz,* is a 20-question true-false test to be used in the classroom. (See next page.)

Is your bicycle 100 per cent safe? Take this test and see how you stand:

If your bike has: *Give yourself:*
    1. Good brakes .... 20 points
    2. A horn or bell that works..................... 20 points
    3. A light that works .... 20 points
    4. A reflector 1-1½ inches in diameter .... 20 points
    5. Tight seat and handlebars .... 10 points
    6. Solid front and rear fenders .... 5 points
    7. No loose spokes on wheels .... 5 points
                       Total .... 100 points

Bonus Points for:
    8. Carrier on back or basket for heavy loads .... 10 points
    9. Reflector tape on sides for added protection ..... 10 points

---

1. It is safe to learn to ride a bicycle on a busy street. (   ) True (   ) False

2. Bicycles, like autos, should keep to the right side of the road. (   ) True (   ) False

3. Bicycle riders should know and obey all traffic signs and lights. (   ) True (   ) False

4. People who are walking do not have the right-of-way on sidewalks and cross-walks. (   ) True (   ) False.

5. Bicycles should be walked across heavily traveled streets. (   ) True (   ) False

6. A bicycle in poor condition is safe if the rider is careful. (   ) True (   ) False

7. It is safe and proper for a bicycle rider to carry a passenger on an ordinary bicycle. (   ) True (   ) False

8. Bicycle riders may hitch to a moving truck if it is traveling less than 20 miles per hour. (   ) True (   ) False

9. Riding in a single line is the sensible thing to do. (   ) True (   ) False

10. Night riding with dark clothing and without a front white light and a rear reflector is dangerous. (   ) True (   ) False

11. When tired, the rider should rest by taking his feet off the pedals. (   ) True (   ) False

12. Bicycle riders should be very careful and give the proper hand signals before making turns or stopping. (   ) True (   ) False

13. It is only necessary to look straight ahead when crossing streets. (   ) True (   ) False

14. The size of the bicycle makes no difference if the rider is skilled. (   ) True (   ) False

15. All bikes should have a horn or bell, rear reflector, and front light. (   ) True (   ) False

16. As soon as you can balance your bike you are ready to ride in heavy traffic. (   ) True (   ) False

17. When passing a parked car, you should ride three feet away from it and give a warning with your horn or bell. (   ) True (   ) False

18. When entering a street from a driveway or sidewalk the bicycle rider has the right-of-way. (   ) True (   ) False

19. Bicycle riders should carry books or bundles in one hand if they must be carried on a bicycle. (   ) True (   ) False

20. Bicycles should be kept in good condition at all times and repaired by a mechanic when necessary. (   ) True (   ) False

NOTE TO TEACHER:

Allow five points for each question. Have each pupil correct any wrong answers.

The test was originally developed for elementary-age children by Aetna Life and Casualty. The company now distributes (free) a 10-item test in the colorful booklet *Bicycle Safety*. Acknowledging research findings that two out of three bicycle accidents occur to riders who have failed to follow the rules of the road, the Bicycle Institute of America, Inc. makes available (free) a very thorough *Bike Quiz Guide* which contains 50 in-depth true-false questions, a words test, and a safety matching test. As a public service the National Fire

Protection Association distributes free to school personnel their 20-item test for boys and girls relative to home fire inspection appraisal. This is part of the SPARKY program; the questions may be answered "Yes" or "No" and are particularly well written. Here are two examples from the battery:

3. Frayed electric cords often start fires. Are you sure all of the electric cords in your home are in safe condition?

Yes___No___

20. If there is a gas stove or gas heater in your home, do you know that you should call the gas company right away if you smell gas?

Yes___No___

The same organization makes available the *Home Fire Safety Quiz,* and the *Be-Prepared-For-Fire Quiz,* each of which consists of ten excellent multiple-choice questions for teachers to use in connection with safety education.

Knowledge testing may be made more revealing when the results are combined with teacher observations. The kind of classwork that pupils do—their drawings, projects, photographs, oral reports, and personal questions—provides evidence which, combined with formal test results, frequently gives a good appraisal of the health instruction efforts.

MEASURING ATTITUDES AND BEHAVIORS

As previously indicated, it is both important and difficult to readily appraise student responses in the affective and action domains. Where there are large numbers of schoolchildren assigned to teachers, it will always be hard to find out how everyone feels about a health issue and what they may be doing about it in their own community. How often do students at every age tell teachers *not* what they really feel and do, but what they believe the teachers *want* them to feel and do? This is why Gordon Allport, after decades of wrestling with the subject of human attitudes, concluded that it is most difficult to measure accurately in this area simply because attitudes are so personal and deep-seated and represent a latent predisposition to act.

In their review of knowledge/attitude studies, Iverson and Portnoy showed a positive relationship that also existed between attitude and behavior; however, knowledge appeared to function as a direct change agent for attitudes far more often than for behaviors.[15]

Working with smaller groups of children, it is possible to explore the affective and action domains by becoming more personally involved. A close relationship is required. Needed is a summative evaluation which means looking for side effects, prejudices, alienations, and other learner changes.[16] Seeking expressions of feelings,

---

[15]Iverson, Donald C. and Portnoy, Barry. "Reassessment of the Knowledge/Attitude/Behavior Triad," *Health Education,* 8:31–33, November/December 1977.

[16]See McNeil, John D. *Designing Curriculum: Self-Instructional Modules.* Boston: Little Brown and Co., 1976, Module 4.

convictions, beliefs, values, and judgments is much better accomplished on a one-to-one basis than it is in a mob scene. Small groups of children, taking their turn throughout the school year, can provide much evaluative information for the teacher. For example, in working on tobacco smoking and health with fifth, sixth, or seventh grade pupils, it is possible to sit in a small comfortable circle and discuss personal feelings about smoking. Test No. 2 from the U.S. Public Health Service's *Smokers Self-Testing Kit* may be obtained in quantity from the U.S. Government Printing Office (see Figure 11–2).

Again, in the small group exchange it is possible to get solid expressions of behavior by presenting well-defined decision making questions. Three statements that were employed in the experimentations of Schley and Banister were:[17]

1. As a result of studying this unit, my attitude toward the improvement of health practices in this area of health is (_____better, _____worse, _____unchanged).
2. As a result of studying this topic, my personal actions and/or activities in the area of health with which this topic deals are (_____better, _____worse, _____unchanged).
3. As a result of studying this topic, I (have, have not) helped someone else improve a personal health practice.

Interestingly, when students are asked to look into their lives for feelings, practices, and improvements, they begin to illustrate in a number of ways what is actually taking place. Moreover, as the personal approach to evaluation increases confidence, the validity of the process improves.

Self-Appraisal Activities

When pupils attempt to evaluate their own health improvement and actually enjoy doing so, there is an opportunity for a more accurate kind of appraisal and a more effective kind of teaching.

Self-testing activities provide pupils with a chance to measure progress in terms of their own potential, as well as to compare themselves with classmates. The child as well as the adult wants a certain amount of recognition, status, even prestige—all of which are dependent upon the acquisition of social poise, proper health practices, and mental well-being.

Adjustment or self-realization cannot be taught, except by providing materials, opportunities, conditions, and experiences whereby, *through self-activity,* the individual reaches the desired goals of achievement. It is not uncommon, therefore, to find that personal health inventories and self-rating charts have been used for some time with varying degrees of success. If the chart is one developed by the students themselves to measure their own advancement toward an accepted goal, or if the chart represents group decisions concerning items to be evaluated, it is likely to be more

---

[17]Schley, Robert A., and Banister, Richard E. "Behavioral Change in an Academic Setting: How It Works." *School Health Review,* 1:13–19, November 1970.

TEST 2

WHAT DO YOU THINK THE EFFECTS OF SMOKING ARE?

For each statement, circle the number that shows how you feel about it. Do you strongly agree, mildly agree, mildly disagree, or strongly disagree?

Important: Answer every question.

	strongly agree	mildly agree	mildly disagree	strongly disagree
A. Cigarette smoking is not nearly as dangerous as many other health hazards.	1	2	3	4
B. I don't smoke enough to get any of the diseases that cigarette smoking is supposed to cause.	1	2	3	4
C. If a person has already smoked for many years, it probably won't do him much good to stop.	1	2	3	4
D. It would be hard for me to give up smoking cigarettes.	1	2	3	4
E. Cigarette smoking is enough of a health hazard for something to be done about it.	4	3	2	1
F. The kind of cigarette I smoke is much less likely than other kinds to give me any of the diseases that smoking is supposed to cause.	1	2	3	4
G. As soon as a person quits smoking cigarettes he begins to recover from much of the damage that smoking has caused.	4	3	2	1
H. It would be hard for me to cut down to half the number of cigarettes I now smoke.	1	2	3	4
I. The whole problem of cigarette smoking and health is a very minor one.	1	2	3	4
J. I haven't smoked long enough to worry about the diseases that cigarette smoking is supposed to cause.	1	2	3	4
K. Quitting smoking helps a person to live longer.	4	3	2	1
L. It would be difficult for me to make any substantial change in my smoking habits.	1	2	3	4

HOW TO SCORE:

1. Enter the numbers you have circled to the Test 2 questions in the spaces below, putting the number you have circled to Question A over line A, to Question B over line B, etc.
2. Total the 3 scores across on each line to get your totals. For example, the sum of your scores over lines A, E, and I gives you your score on *Importance*—lines B, F, and J gives the score on *Personal Relevance*, etc.

Figure 11–2. Scores can vary from 3 to 12. Any score 9 and above is *high;* any score 6 and below is *low*. Included with the test is a section that explains the meaning of the scoring.

meaningful to the students involved than a printed or standardized chart.

As younger children learn to read, they help the teacher plan simple rating scales for evaluating group or individual health behavior. Primary grade children evaluate in simple ways, as when they select a food to eat, choose a story to hear, an activity, or a color to use in painting. They make such judgments as "We cleaned the room very well today" or "We liked playing with the other children." From such beginnings come standards and expectancies.

Pupils may rate themselves on posture skills, food habits, attitude toward others, personal appearance, and several other such items. The accompanying check list, simple as it is, was worked out by second graders.

HOW DO I LOOK?

Do I stand tall?	Yes	No
Do I smile?	Yes	No
Are my hands and face clean?	Yes	No
Are my clothes clean?	Yes	No
Am I happy?	Yes	No
Is there dirt under my fingernails?	Yes	No
Is my hair combed?	Yes	No
Are my teeth clean?	Yes	No

EVALUATING A HEALTH LESSON

There is another kind of evaluation that one should not lose sight of. This applies more to the teacher than it does to the pupils as such. It is concerned with appraising the actual instruction at any one time. The teacher should ask himself or herself some rather definite questions as to whether the health lesson was properly conceived and carried out. Students can be very helpful. Sally Kaizer at the Masconomet Regional School in Massachusetts asks the following probing questions:

1. Do you find my classes
   Boring   Interesting   Exciting
2. Do you think I do too much talking in class?
   Yes   No
3. Has anything I've done this year made you eager to learn more about the subjects we're studying?
   Yes   No
If your answer was yes, please state that activity which aroused your interest.
4. Do you think I'm
   too strict   easy going   about right
5. Do you feel comfortable about speaking up in class?
   or are you afraid you'll be laughed at or criticized?

6. Do you think that the material we studied has any use in your life now, or will have any use in the future?

       Yes   No

7. Please check which of the following teaching techniques have been most interesting and helped you the most:

       Lectures or explanations by teacher
       Small group discussions
       Field trips
       Class projects in which the students were involved
       Demonstrations
       Other (Please fill in) _____

8. Would the use of more films, tapes, records, and overhead projectors help you to better understand the course material?

       Yes   No

9. Perhaps I could have helped you to learn more. Do you feel that I have failed you in any of the following ways:

       Didn't give me enough individual help
       Ignored me a lot of the time
       Were too interested in the bright kids in the class
       Other (Please fill in) _____

10. Do you think the textbooks and any other study materials we use are:

       Dull   Hard to read   Out of date

11. If you were teaching this class would you

       provide more work sheets and other learning aids
       expect students to use more out of class reference materials
       have more class discussion
       provide for more group work

THE ULTIMATE STATE OF WELLNESS

Evaluation is an ongoing process. So is education itself as it seeks ways to attain enlightenment and human fulfillment and thereby raise the spirit of the nation a few solid points.

Expressing this spirit may represent the ultimate state of wellness. Moreover, there is today an excellent chance of it happening, because comprehensive school health programs, community health education efforts, and federal health legislation are all showing signs of maturation. What Trow said about the strivings of human beings almost five decades ago is still appropriate.

If enough good food, rest, sunshine, and so forth, are obtainable, so that the physiological organism is strong and healthy; if there is sufficient opportunity for free activity, for strivings for ends which he considers desirable, and for the appreciation of things which are to him beautiful; and if in the eyes of his comrades, there is something of respect for him; and if there are those in whom he can confide and those whom he can in some way serve, man may experience that feeling of happiness which has been the goal of life for untold generations.[18]

QUESTIONS FOR DISCUSSION

1. A recent study indicated that 80 per cent of all families could not identify any source of free health care in their community. Do you think this is

---

[18]Trow, W. C. *Educational Psychology.* Boston: Houghton-Mifflin Co., 1931.

partially the fault of the schools? Should existing consumer health instruction be evaluated to ascertain its worth in the program? Are there other
variables that may be behind the findings of the study?

2. From your reading, do you see any compelling reason to keep behavioral
objectives near-at-hand when teaching in the classroom? What is the
relationship between behavioral objectives and instruction?

3. What seem to be the chief values obtained when grade school pupils
appraise their own health instruction program? How does this differ from
a typical self-testing activity?

4. What is the value of an individual pupil conference in appraising the
health instruction program? Would you say that it represents an economical use of time? Would a small group provide better information?

5. Why is learning in health education difficult to measure accurately?
Support your answer with specific illustrations.

SUGGESTED ACTIVITIES

1. With the enactment of Public Law 94–317 came the establishment of the
Office of Health Information and Health Promotion under the Assistant
Secretary of Health in HEW. Two years earlier the Bureau of Health
Education was set up as a part of the U.S. Public Health Service in Atlanta.
With such a public and professional commitment, there usually follow
new expectations for performance and accountability. Do you see any
evidence of a concern for appraising health education activities in the
school and community at large? Look over the Kreuter and Green article
(see *Selected References*).

2. Select a major health area in which to appraise pupil health practices.
Construct a check list of significant items which should help you identify
pupil strengths and weaknesses. The items included on the check list
should be "behavior items"—action evidences of health understandings.

3. In keeping with the Bloom *Taxonomy*, prepare a number of multiple-
choice questions on a health topic of your choice.

4. Meet with three or four of your classmates and discuss the difficulties
involved in appraising health practices in a given school-community
setting. Are the problems any different in an urban setting compared with
a rural or suburban location?

5. Program success is only partially measured when outcomes are related to
prescriptive behavioral objectives. Inquire of several elementary school
teachers as to how they measure success in the health curriculum area.
Are other teaching staff members involved in evaluation? Peer groups?
Parents? Schoolwide research? Community agencies?

SELECTED REFERENCES

Anderson, S. B., et al.: *Encyclopedia of Educational Evaluation,* San Francisco:
Jossey-Bass, 1973.
Bedworth, David A. and Bedworth, Albert E. *Health Education: A Process for Human
Effectiveness.* New York: Harper & Row, Publishers, 1978.
Bloom, B. S. *Taxonomy of Educational Objectives: The Classification of Educational
Goals. Handbook 1. Cognitive Domain.* New York: McKay, 1956.

Bruess, Clint and Gay, John E. *Implementing Comprehensive School Health Education.* New York: Macmillan Publishing Co., 1978, Chapter 16.

Dalis, Gus. "Effect of Precise Objectives Upon Student Achievement in Health Education," *Journal of Experimental Education, 39*:20–23, Winter 1970.

Greenberg, Jerrold S. *Student-Centered Health Instruction: A Humanistic Approach.* Addison-Wesley Publishing Co., 1978, Chapter 1.

Grosshans, Onie R. "Personal Behavior Change Projects," *Health Education, 8*:22–24, September/October 1977.

Gruijter, D. N. M. (ed.). *Advances in Educational and Psychological Measurement.* New York: John Wiley and Sons, 1977.

Hoover, Kenneth A. and Hollingsworth, Paul M. *A Handbook for Elementary School Teachers.* 2nd edition, Boston: Allyn and Bacon, Inc., 1978, Chapter 20.

Kime, Robert E., Schladt, Richard G., and Tritsch, Leonard E. *Health Instruction: An Action Approach.* Englewood Cliffs, N.J.: Prentice-Hall, Inc., 1977, Chapter 8.

Kirschenbaum, Howard, et al. *Wad-Ja-Get?* New York: Hart Publishing Co., Inc., 1971.

Kreuter, Marshall W. "School Health Evaluation," *Health Education, 8*:2–3, March/April 1977.

_____ and Green, Lawrence W. "Evaluation of School Health Education: Identifying Purposes, Keeping Perspective," *Journal of School Health, 48*:228–235, April 1978.

Lewy, Arieh. *Handbook of Curriculum Evaluation.* New York: Longman, Inc., 1977.

Mager, Robert F. *Preparing Instructional Objectives.* Belmont, California: Fearon Publishing, Inc., 1962, Chapter 7.

Olsen, Larry K. "A Suggested Model for Assessing Teaching Performance," *Journal of School Health, 42*:224–228, April 1973.

Read, Donald A. and Greene, Walter H. *Creative Teaching in Health.* 2nd ed., New York: Macmillan Publishing Co., 1975, Part 5.

Rich, John M. *Innovations in Education: Reformers and Their Critics,* 2nd ed., Boston: Allyn and Bacon, Inc., 1978, Chapter 10.

Solleder, Marion K. *Evaluation Instruments in Health Education.* Washington, D.C.: American Alliance for Health, Physical Education, and Recreation, 1969.

Sorochan, Walter D. and Bender, Stephen J. *Teaching Elementary Health Science,* Boston: Addison-Wesley Publishing Co., 1975.

Vannier, Maryhelen. *Teaching Health in Elementary Schools,* 2nd ed., Philadelphia: Lea & Febiger, 1974, Chapter 19.

Willgoose, Carl E. *Health Teaching in Secondary Schools,* 2nd ed., Philadelphia: W. B. Saunders Co., 1977, Chapter 12.

_____. "Providing for Change: New Directions," in Read, Donald A., ed. *New Directions In Health Education.* New York: Macmillan Publishing Co., 1971, Chapter 1.

Yarber, William L. "Accounting for Health Instruction," *Health Education, 8*:4–5, March/April 1977.

Graduated List of Behavioral Objectives for the Major Health Topics, Grades 1–6

PERSONAL CLEANLINESS AND APPEARANCE

Grade 1

Appears in school clean and well-groomed: hands, nails, face, hair and teeth.
Demonstrates ability to wash hands competently.
Hangs up clothing at school and at home.
Dresses appropriately for the climate and weather for school and play.

Grade 2

Exercises some concern and care for personal articles.
Carries a handkerchief and blows nose properly.
Demonstrates proper toilet practices.
Keeps reasonably clean and washes when dirty without being told.

Grade 3

Relates personal and community cleanliness to disease control.
Differentiates between being well and being sick.
Explains the necessity for regular bathing.
Evaulates the cleanliness of the skin and nails.

Grade 4

Chooses to keep the school environment clean and attractive.
Is aware of the variety of personal health practices having a bearing on personal appearance.
Practices standing, walking, and sitting and explains how feelings of the moment are reflected in posture.
Prevents skin and scalp infections.

Grade 5

Shampoos the hairs and takes frequent baths without being told.
Investigates hair styles for girls and boys.
Explains the relationship of appearance to success in everyday life.
Describes why the wearing of eyeglasses is sometimes necessary.
Takes part in the selection of clothes for durability and style.

Grade 6

Chooses to prevent illness by practicing individual and group cleanliness.
Exercises personal responsibility in maintaining proper health and is able to advise others.

495

Describes the process of eliminating body wastes and body odors.

Compares current practices of keeping clean to control disease with the practices in ancient civilizations

PHYSICAL ACTIVITY, SLEEP, REST, AND RELAXATION

Grade 1

Demonstrates how to play, rest, and sleep for proper growth.

Engages in enjoyable activities such as fundamental rhythms, movement exploration, singing games, dances, stunts, and games of low organization.

Grade 2

Sleeps an appropriate number of hours each night and acknowledges that parental guidance is frequently necessary to insure proper sleep and activity practices.

Investigates how sleep and rest as factors help one avoid disease and chronic fatigue.

Explains and practices appropriate evening recreation, especially before retiring.

Portrays how to exercise for fun and health; demonstrates several stunts, animal actions, and novelty relay races for fun.

Grade 3

Develops sound reasons for physical strength and endurance.

Demonstrates several different ways of building and maintaining physical fitness: rhythms, dances, games, rope climbing and jumping, swimming, hiking.

Illustrates through stories and situations the relationship between physical activity and well-being.

Grade 4

Measures own level of physical fitness in an elemental way.

Explains how vigorous physical exercise may be alternated with rest and relaxation.

Relates how it feels to be "physically fit."

Describes the place of physical fitness in total health and the interrelationship of variables such as exercise, diet, rest, and medical check-ups.

Grade 5

Demonstrates strengthening exercises to improve muscular efficiency for standing, walking, playing, and working.

Explains the several effects of exercise on sleep, rest, and the digestion of foods.

Plans recreation to relieve mental fatigue and promote sleep.

Selects activities to promote the wise use of leisure time.

Shows how to develop a wide variety of active and quiet recreational skills.

Employs a number of ways to illustrate the place of sports in the Western culture.

Enumerates the several reasons for participating in individual and team sports activities.

Investigates how to prevent injuries when engaged in vigorous physical activities.

Explains the fundamental physiology involved in attaining a high level of physical condition.

Selects and explains the several factors contributing to an adequate night's sleep.

NUTRITION AND GROWTH

Grade 1

Relates why people eat (energy, growth, pleasure).

Explains the importance of a good breakfast and lunch.

Drinks fruit juices and milk.

Describes a pleasant, happy mealtime.

Distinguishes clean foods and utensils.

Identifies a wide variety of foods common to the community.

Grade 2

Recognizes a number of foods for various occasions.

Identifies individual differences in the rate of growth.

Chooses foods that help you grow (build tissue).

Chooses foods that help you "go" (energy).

Appraises sweets in the diet.

Grade 3

Demonstrates proper practices of eating: chewing, tasting, eating leisurely.

Discusses clearly how appetite may be improved.

Explains the importance of well-balanced meals to mental and physical efficiency.

Illustrates the many ways in which foods may be used: milk, fruit, etc.

Describes regularity in eating and the eating patterns in various cultures.

Grade 4

Investigates the essential function of carbohydrates, proteins, and fats in the human system.

Analyzes foods for vitamin and mineral sources.

Relates food products and eating practices to proper body weight—presently and in the future.

Describes the effect of cultural differences, customs, and foods on eating practices.

Determines that physical growth and early mental capacity are influenced by a balanced diet.

Grade 5

Looks into the mechanics and elemental chemistry of digestion and elimination.

Acknowledges a variety of daily eating practices, most of which are within the acceptable range of eating behavior.

Illustrates how to promote good digestion by referring to before, during, and after mealtime activities.

Chooses foods of nutritional value because they contribute to physical fitness for games, sports, and work.

Relates food excesses and deprivation to animal and human growth, repair, energy, etc.

Grade 6

Analyzes animal and human nutrition requirements, noting differences and similarities.

Investigates the nature of malnutrition; its effect in dentition, bone growth, intellectual achievement, energy levels, etc.

Applies caloric measurements and food chart information to the building of selected menus.

Constructs menus for both young people (10–12 years of age) and old people that may be obtained in the home or in a restaurant.

Distinguishes fallacies, fads, and superstitions that distort the truth relative to foods and their use.

Cites elimination problems which relate to digestion and food choices.

DENTAL HEALTH

Grade 1

Brushes the teeth at the appropriate time and in the proper way.

Explains the loss of baby teeth and appearance of first 6-year molar.

Tells why people visit the dentist.

Grade 2

Demonstrates how to use powder or toothpaste.

Tells how the teeth contribute to appearance and help break foods down for swallowing.

Illustrates how raw foods help keep the teeth clean.

Shows what happens to the teeth when many sweets are a part of the diet.

Describes the need for regular dental inspections and care.

Grade 3

Shows how teeth may be cleaned without brushing.

Chooses foods that build strong teeth and bones.

Explains the value of clean, attractive teeth to relationships with others.

Describes the causes and prevention of toothache.

Grade 4

Draws the basic structure of the tooth and explains the parts.

Identifies the action of teeth in talking clearly and in the digestive process.

Describes the undesirable effects of tooth decay.

Portrays practices that may subject the teeth to injury.

Explains the functions of the school dental hygienist.

Grade 5

Describes the function and importance of orthodontics.
Explains the meaning and consequences of properly handled cases of malocclusion.
Illustrates modern dental practice and the need for regular dental visits.
Cites the benefits of the way fluoride is applied to the teeth to help prevent tooth decay.

Grade 6

Tells how progress is being made at the sixth grade level toward the development of a full set of teeth.
Develops a logical argument in favor of water fluoridation and the reduction of tooth decay.
Illustrates the relationship of nutrition, aging, and other variables to bone and tooth decay.
Evaluates dentifrice advertisements in several ways.

BODY STRUCTURE AND OPERATION

Grade 1

Depicts how children grow tall and strong.
Tells the reasons for health examinations and tests of seeing and hearing.
Names the primary body organs and systems and tells what they do.

Grade 2

Demonstrates how the body moves using bones and muscles stimulated by nerves.
Illustrates how the body maintains various postures and positions: sitting, standing, walking, running.
Demonstrates various stunts, exercises, and other movements to depict a wide range of human movements.

Grade 3

Explains how the eyes see and the ears hear using models, pictures, or diagrams.
Describes the cooperative action between the five senses.
Shows how eyeglasses help correct visual defects.
Shows how to protect the eyes and ears from injuries: in sports, while working, etc.
Demonstrates how the skeletal make-up functions to support the body and protect the organs.

Grade 4

Explains the body's need for fuel and how this works through the digestive system.
Cites the function of the skin, hair, and nails in terms of health and appearance.
Depicts the various structural elements of the respiratory system.

Relates the speech function to the condition of the nose, tonsils, adenoids, and teeth.
Illustrates how the larynx and epiglottis work.

Grade 5

Employs the means to cite the function of human cells, tissues, organs, and systems.
Shows the mechanics of growth through cell division.
Relates enzymes to digestion.
Analyzes the circulatory system and the composition of the blood.
Seeks interrelationships of circulation, respiration, digestion, and elimination.

Grade 6

Illustrates how the central nervous system, brain, and sense organs function and how this relates to feelings.
Tells how muscles, bones, nerves, and glands work together.
Explains elimination in relation to diet, constipation, and frequency of bowel movements.
Describes the reproductive structure and function of the body (referred to also under Sex and Family Living Education).

PREVENTION AND CONTROL OF DISEASE

Grade 1

Maintains clean hands and keeps them away from mouth.
Explains the need for regular health examinations.
Describes the importance of vaccinations and immunizations.
Refuses to share "bites," whistles, straws, glasses, etc.
Demonstrates how to drink from a water fountain.

Grade 2

Cites ways to protect self and others from colds, sneezes, and sore throats.
Illustrates how to stay healthy through adequate amounts of food, water, sleep, and exercise.
Tells what the hospital does for people who are ill.
Describes how disease organisms can travel from person to person.

Grade 3

Describes the germ theory and how people get sick.
Illustrates several ways in which various germs are spread.
Explains why some disease germs are contagious.
Avoids illness through practicing cleanliness, regular medical check-ups, and immunizations.
Tells how to prevent ear and eye infections.

Grade 4

Differentiates between harmful, harmless, and helpful germs.
Takes part in school activities designed to curtail disease.

Explains what can be done in the home to prevent the spread of disease.
Relates how several men and women of science have contributed to the
conquering of disease.

Grade 5

Analyzes the sources of infection: bacteria, viruses, fungi; people, animals,
climate, insects, water, food.
Describes how immunizations are kept up to date.
Investigates how the spread of infections can be controlled.
Develops suggestions for the prevention of illness owing to the faulty storage
of foods and medicines.

Grade 6

Describes the basic symptoms of common respiratory and childhood diseases. Explains controls.
Employs ways to care for sick in the home and to tell others what can be
done.
Cites ways in which the body builds its own immunity to disease.
Reorganizes several superstitions and evidences of quackery in relation to
the control and cure of disease.

SAFETY AND FIRST AID

Grade 1

Demonstrates how to proceed to and from school safely.
Shows a number of general safety practices in the classroom.
Explains how to prevent accidents during and after school hours.
Gives accurate statement of personal identity when lost.
Tells where to seek help for injuries or illness.

Grade 2

Tells how police and fire officers protect children.
Shows how to use playground equipment in a safe and fun fashion.
Treats strange animals and strange people in a proper way.
Demonstrates how to report accidents and illnesses.
Explains safety on the water, the school bus, and the family automobile.

Grade 3

Tells how to play safely in all seasons of the year.
Cites bicycle safety rules and how to maintain the bicycle in fine running
condition.
Rides the bicycle skillfully and can demonstrate this at the school for others to
see.
Describes eyes, ear, and face protection and shows personal responsibility
for his or her own safety.
Explains fire prevention and fire safety in the home and school.

Grade 4

Shows how questionable water can be purified for drinking purposes.

Demonstrates elementary first aid practices.
Practices safety out-of-doors (insect bites, sunburn, poison ivy, etc.)
Is aware of accidents in the community and can tell how they might have
    been prevented.
Assists younger children in accident prevention.

Grade 5

Practices fire prevention at home and about the community.
Performs artificial respiration properly and explains water safety practices.
Exercises leadership in safety patrols and school safety councils.
Shows how to prevent eye, ear, and other injuries from accidents stemming
    from sports participation.

Grade 6

Performs first aid for minor injuries (cuts, burns, etc.)
Discriminates accurately between safe and unsafe medicines.
Describes personal safety at home (medicines, automobiles, rugs, stairways,
    electrical outlets, etc.)
Practices safety in recreational pursuits and in the choice of food products.
Investigates the means of survival in a nuclear age.

MENTAL HEALTH

Grade 1

Knows a number of children and how to get along with them.
Develops new friends and new interests.
Shows feeling and consideration for others.
Enjoys caring for pets and discussing them.
Demonstrates ability to work by himself or herself.
Seeks help when needed and knows why.
Controls emotions of fear and anger.

Grade 2

Has a sense of humor.
Shares experiences with others and willingly tries new things.
Accepts new responsibilities.
Demonstrates how to win and lose fairly, while having fun with others in a
    variety of situations.
Expresses feelings in an acceptable manner.
Overcomes difficulties and adjusts reasonably to disappointments.

Grade 3

Gains pleasure and satisfaction in helping others.
Works and plays to build self-control and self-reliance.
Develops new interests in hobbies, books, skills, etc.
Accepts others and makes new friendships in a wholesome way.
Expresses personal feelings through speech, play, and dance.

Grade 4

Shows appropriate attitudes toward leadership and group participation.
Appraises personal capabilities and limitations.

Describes the variety of human emotions as they affect performance, personality, and health in general.

Solves personal problems and shows how to live with handicaps.

Receptive to the suggestions of others and open-minded when dealing with others.

Grade 5

Contributes to group activity in school by exercising appropriate leadership and fellowship.

Makes a number of plans and carries them out.

Registers pleasure in solving pertinent class and individual problems.

Describes both pleasant and unhappy attitudes and tells how to overcome worry.

Investigates the building of confidence and the reduction of tension through successful accomplishments.

Is concerned for the feelings of others.

Obtains satisfaction from acceptable social behavior.

Grade 6

Portrays examples of the relationship of physical health to mental health.

Explains the meaning of recreation and how it along with rest contributes to mental health.

Shares ideas and experiences with others and understands their inherent values.

Describes the nature of mental illness.

Exercises emotional control and self-confidence in difficult school and home situations.

Identifies the relationship between the setting of personal goals and the attainment of good mental health.

SEX AND FAMILY LIVING EDUCATION

Grade 1

Describes how a happy home life depends upon the contributions of each member of the family.

Cooperates in the home, sharing work as well as fun.

Cares for the pets in the family or at school.

Accepts animals as part of family life.

Grade 2

Shows how several animals protect and feed their babies.

Recognizes that animals have babies like themselves.

Describes the many ways that happy families work and play together.

Names a variety of occasions when there are good times in a home and family.

Appreciates that boys and girls can play together, but that boys also play with boys, and girls with girls.

Explains how the family prepares for, cares for, and loves the new baby.

Grade 3

Observes how parents make a home a pleasant place.

Describes elementary reproduction: all living things come from other living things—illustrated by baby animals, plant life, and mothers and babies.
Shows how animals protect and feed babies in different ways.
Helps with family chores and the caring of younger family members.

Grade 4

Describes the unique contributions of men and women to society.
Explains how children inherit the way they look from mother and father.
Describes the growth of the human being in the body of the mother—where life starts and develops.
Investigates the meaning of families as good neighbors.
Differentiates between the ovaries, testes, ovum, sperm, glands, hormones, etc.
Distinguishes inherited characteristics from characteristics not inherited.

Grade 5

Details the start of life and how body cells begin from a single cell, which divides into two cells; terminology and structure.
Explains reproductive and growth process: egg cells, sperm cells, from egg to baby.
Describes elemental function of menstruation.
Investigates growth differences from 10 to 14 years of age: boy and girl differences; more rapid maturation of girls.
Recognizes the contributions of both sexes to family life and society in general.

Grade 6

Describes the continuing process of physical growth and maturation toward manhood and womanhood.
Explains how social, intellectual, and emotional growth are essential parts of the maturation process.
Tells the several meanings of adolescence.
Describes puberty and is aware of the physical and mental occurrences which have a bearing on peer group relationships.

ENVIRONMENTAL HEALTH

Grade 1

Contributes toward keeping the school, home, and neighborhood clean.
Explains the services performed by physicians, dentists, nurses and other selected health personnel.
Describes how people are a part of the animal-plant world.

Grade 2

Relates how everyone is a member of the community.
Explains how items such as milk and water are kept clean, fresh, and safe to drink.
Investigates how the community water supply is protected.
Tells how pets should be cared for to protect their health and the health of others.

Grade 3

Examines the problems of controlling insect pests and by what non-polluting means.

Shows how meat and other foods are handled in order to protect the purchaser.

Names public health functions and describes how many people help protect the health of citizens: physician, dentist, hospital worker, automobile inspector, barber, etc.

Grade 4

Indicates how health personnel work together to control the pollutants in the environment and the spread of disease: local government, professional personnel, and voluntary health workers.

Describes how water is made safe for swimming and for ice skating, and how it is purified for drinking.

Illustrates the duties of food inspectors.

Explains how playgrounds, parks, and other recreational services help build health and maintain a healthful environment.

Grade 5

Explains the several roles of the voluntary health agency.

Describes how public health officials work with private citizens (even pupils) to control air, land, and water pollution.

Demonstrates how to purify water on a camping trip.

Cites the several important points associated with water fluoridation.

Investigates the problems associated with advancing technology while controlling thermal and nuclear pollution.

Grade 6

Relates school health service findings to the work of health care centers and other community agencies.

Interprets the hospital function as an essential service which is expensive but worth the cost.

Explains rescue and ambulance services—a cooperative activity involving police, firemen, and hospitals.

Identifies local health leaders in the professions, business, public health, public works, planning, etc.

Evaluates land and water conservation practices in a community by relating this to environmental well-being.

Describes the functions of the U.S. Environmental Protection Agency.

ALCOHOL, TOBACCO, AND DRUGS

Grade 4

Describes beverages which contribute to growth.

Avoids coffee, tea, and cola drinks and is aware of the reasons for this action.

Explains why smoking if started becomes habit-forming and is difficult to give up.

Describes inhalants and their effect on the body (glue sniffing, etc.)

Exercises precaution in taking any medicine without parental control and for prescription by a physician.

Investigates the life saving and beneficial uses of a number of drugs (aspirin, antibiotics, pain killers, etc.)

Grade 5

Describes in detail the effects of tobacco smoking: minor effects: throat, appetite, tooth stain, bad breath, taste, smell, skin, etc.; major effects: heart, lungs, endurance, blood pressure, longevity, bronchitis, cancer, new births, etc.
Explains the relationship between smoking and athletic performance.
Investigates the wisdom of not starting to smoke and how one lives with family peers who smoke and yet remains a non-smoker.
Describes the negative effects of using barbiturates, amphetamines, hallucinogens, and other mood-modifying drugs.
Relates the effects of alcoholic beverages to human problems: alcoholism, intoxication, etc.

Grade 6

Tells about the harmful effects of drinking alcohol—effects on digestion, circulation, nerves (thinking, acting, controlling), longevity, athletic performance, occupational performance.
Investigates alcoholism as a disease of the society and its culture.
Relates the use of alcohol in industry and medicine.
Investigates the difficulty of breaking the smoking habit.
Discusses the laws governing the sale of drugs.
Appreciates the need for discovering new drugs for the treatment of disease.

CONSUMER HEALTH

Grade 4

Relates how foods are purchased to provide well-balanced meals.
Describes the plight of the consumer and the need to understand the many health related products being sold.
Recognizes that everyone is a consumer of health products.
Reads newspaper and magazine articles relative to pure foods, proper labeling, food handling, and "truth in advertising."
Acknowledges that self-diagnosis and self-medication are poor practices and that there is sometimes danger in using items such as dietary supplements, cosmetics, and pep pills.

Grade 5

Cites scientific ways in which to purchase health items: consumer guides, medical-dental opinions, support from investigating agencies.
Relates the watchdog functions of agencies such as Food and Drug Administration, Federal Trade Commission, and the Post Office Department to fraudulent products.
Investigates how a careful consumer eventually helps to make a careful producer or manufacturer.
Discusses the special work of different kinds of doctors.
Relates misinformation and superstition to quackery and the resultant billion dollars a year loss to unwise consumers.

Develops ways to evaluate advertised health products: sports equipment, pain-killers, dentifrices, cold tablets, "health" foods, vitamin pills, dietary substances.

Realizes that personal decision-making comes from adequate information and feelings.

Cites laws that exist to protect the consumer.

Examines media advertising, investigates FDA findings, and exercises caution in using new non-prescription items.

Index

Billings, Josh, 29
Births, illegitimate, 27
Blood pressure, 12–13, 25, 66–67, 236
Bloom, B. S., 185, 186, 355, 471, 492
Blue Cross Association, 437
Body structure, 171, 229–240, 448, 499
Bogle, Marion W., 123
Borden Company, 438
Boredom, and mental health, 14
  occupation and, 25
Boyd, Velena, 35
Bragg, Mabel, 87, 144
Braun, Samuel J., 88
Breakfast studies, 206–208, 214
Brown, E. C. Trust Foundation, 465
Brown, George, 431
Brown, James D., 105, 432
Bruess, Clint E., 431, 492
Bruner, Jerome, 147, 154, 186, 277
Bucher, Charles A., 35
Buhl, Jeanne, 349
Building, school, 91–92, 101
Bulletin boards, 420–421
Buonomano, Louise, 35
Bureau of Health Education, 177, 333
Burnham, William H., 91
Burns, Robert, 249
Burt, John J., 4
Butler, Nicholas Murray, 32
Byler, Ruth, 139

Cahalan, Don, 328
Cahill, Charles, and Associates, 465
Calderwood, Deryek, 292
Callahan, Joseph F., 35
Cameron, Paul, 331
Canadian National Film Board, 465
Cancer, 16–18, 24, 122, 343
Cantril, Hadley, 365
Cardiopulmonary resuscitation, 257, 423
Cards, flash, 420
Carkhuff, R. R., 354
Carlton, William, 30
Carousel Films, 465
Carrell, Alexis, 35, 358
Carroll, Charles R., 350
Carson, Rachel, 312
Cartoons, 415–416
Case studies, in health education, 480–481
Cat-scratch fever, 120
Center for Mass Communication, 465
Centron Films, 465
Cereal Institute, 206–207, 208, 209, 219, 369, 412, 438
Characteristics, sex, 131, 133
Charts, 418
Cheffers, John T. F., 196, 358
Chickenpox, 118
Child Study Association of America, 280–281, 436
Childhood deaths, 11, 22
Churchill Films, 465
Cicero, 32

Civilization and health, 6–7, 195
Clarke, Vivian, P. J., 53
Classroom, safety in, 91, 92–93
Classroom Film Distributors, 465
Classroom teacher, 83–84. See also teacher.
Cleanliness, 171, 189–193
Cleveland Health Museum, 304–305, 426, 427, 429, 436
Colds, 113, 118
Colgate-Palmolive Company, 438
Collections, 423
Combs, Arthur W., 98, 187
Commercial organizations, and elementary education materials, 437–438
Commoner, Barry, 22, 35, 312
Communicable disease, 57, 118–120, 245–247
Community health, 90–105
Community safety, 20, 135–136
Community–school activities, 48, 79–80, 126, 252, 258, 262, 316, 395–396
Compensatory education, 182
Competency, in teaching, 142–144, 160
Competency-based programs, 160
Conant, James B., 142
Conceptual approach, in curriculum development, 153–156
Conley, John A., 152
Construction activity method, 388
Consumer health, 171, 343–348, 464, 506
Cook, David C., 337
Cook, Ron J., 177
Cooper, James A., 186
Cooper, James M., 145, 146
Cooperative Health Education Tests, 484
Coronet Films, 465
Correlation, 149, 215, 396–397
Cosper, Barbara A., 349
Counseling method, 394
Courses of study, 147
Cousins, Norman, 7, 124
Cox, Harvey G., 2
CPR, 257, 423
Crase, Darrell, 127
Cream of Wheat Corporation, 438
Creative activities, 364, 385–386
Creswell, William H., 88, 146, 168, 468
Crispin, David B., 358
Cubbage, Mary-Louise, 88
Curran, William J., 31, 35
Current events method, of health education, 394
Curriculum, activity, 141, 172. See also Health education curriculum.
  broad fields, 148–149
  defined, 147
  development, 147–184, 278
  elementary, 148–149
  health, 51, 153
    implementation of, 187–348
  humanistic, 149

INDEX

National Board of Fire Underwriters, 438
National Commission on Product Safety, 264
National Commission on Safety Education, 100
National Congress of Parents and Teachers, 104, 126, 436
National Council on Alcoholism, 330, 436
National Dairy Council, 209, 210, 218, 412, 414
National Education Association, 37, 41, 60, 367, 412, 436, 438
National Film Board of Canada, 465
National Fire Protection Association, 258, 262, 438
National Foundation, 425, 436
National Health Survey, 19
National Institute of Mental Health, 16, 330
National Instructional Television Center, 465
National Livestock and Meat Board, 438
National Multiple Sclerosis Society, 436
National Nutrition Education Clearinghouse, 436
National Recreation Association, 436
National Safety Council, 100, 102, 103, 104, 252–253, 267, 406, 436, 485
National School Lunch Program, 183
National Society for Crippled Children and Adults, 436
National Society for the Prevention of Blindness, 62, 231, 412, 436
Needs, individuals, 48, 129–133, 205, 277
Neighborhood Health Centers, 80–81
Nelson, Leslie W., 350, 380, 431
Nemir, Alma, 53, 89
Neurological examinations, 81
Neurotic behavior, 30
Nicotine content of cigarettes, 339
Noise pollution, 25
Nolte, Ann, 123
Nongraded classes, 181
Nonofficial health agencies, 434
Normal, concept of, 106–107
Normal health, 83, 107–108
North Dakota State Wheat Commission, 438
Nurse, 75–76, 180
Nurse practitioner, 76
Nutrition, 18, 47, 80, 114, 171, 184, 204–219, 443, 497

Oakley, Ray S., 336, 350
Oberteuffer, Delbert, 53, 186
Obesity, 18–19, 111
Objectives, educational, 31–32, 125, 355
Observation, 110–114, 134–135, 469
O'Casey, Sean, 279

Ocean Spray Cranberries, Inc., 385, 438
Odum, H., 214
Official health agencies, 434
Oglesby, Allan, 88
Oil pollution, 24–25
Olsen, Einar, 35
Opaque projector, 408
O'Reilly, Lawrence B., 105, 432
Organic fitness, 18–19, 203–204. See also *Physical fitness*.
Oschsner, Alton, 17
Overhead projector, 408
Overweight, 18, 78

Pads, writing, 418
Palmer, Beverley B., 141
Pamphlets, 411–412
Parcel, Guy A., 146, 350
Parents, 57, 60, 73, 85, 144, 194, 286, 292, 479
Patient education, 31
Pedestrian accidents, 252
Pediculi, 69, 113, 119
Peer group attitudes, 331
Perceptual problems, 82
Perennial Education, Inc., 465
Persky, Barry, 186
Personal appearance, 189–193. See also *Appearance, personal*.
Personal Products Corporation, 305, 308, 309, 438
Pet Milk Co., 438
Petchel, Karen A., 222
Pflaum/Standard, 280
Pharmaceutical Manufacturers Association, 341, 438
Phenix, Phillip H., 154, 186
Phonograph records, 409–410
Physical education, 39, 49–50, 78, 139, 166
Physical examination, 11, 51, 59–60, 137
Physical fitness, 12, 18–19, 39, 49, 193, 198, 203–204, 441, 476, 496
Physician, family, 82, 183
Piaget, J., 141, 277, 358, 469
Pictures, 412
Pigg, R. Morgan, 151, 186, 344
Pink, Dan, 126
Pinkeye, 119
Pinworms, 119
Planned Parenthood Federation of America, 437
Playground–gymnasium safety, 270–273
Playground, 270
Poisoning, 20–21, 253
Poliomyelitis, 119
Pollock, Marion, 155, 186
Pollution, 22–24, 315, 323, 381
Ponder, L. D., 105
Poolton, Martha A., 350
Popular Science, 465
Portnoy, Barry, 487
Posters, 413–414

Shart, Phillip A., 432
Shattuck, Lemuel, 1
Shaw, Donald B., 88, 96, 105, 127
Sheldon, William H., 107
Shepherd, Dell A., 123
Shepherd, Gene D., 129, 173
Shoobs, Dorothy, 75
Sickle cell anemia, 48, 79, 243, 250
Sid Davis Productions, 465
Silberman, Charles E., 90, 94, 105, 277, 353
Silver, Henry K., 89
Simon, Robert K., 334
Simon, Sidney B., 360, 363, 432
Simonds, Scott K., 35
Sinacore, John S., 350
Sketches, 417
Skin, 111–112, 231, 330
Sleep, 171, 193–197, 441, 496
Slides, 407–408
Sliepcevich, Elena M., 40, 152
Smoking, 325–342. See also *Tobacco smoking.*
    attitudes toward, 331
Smolensky, Jack, 314
Snellen Test, 62–63, 231
Snow, David L., 432
Society for Visual Education, 366, 465
Socioeconomic status, 47, 205, 351
Solleder, Marion K., 471, 493
Sorochan, Walter D., 350, 432, 493
Sources of aids, 439–464
South Carolina Health Education Study, 152
South Dakota Wheat Commission, 439, 465
Special examinations, 61–62
Specimens, 423
Spector, Manuel, 49
Speech defects, 113, 117
Spencer, Mary E., 165
Spenco Medical Corporation, 329, 340, 401, 439
Stanford, Leland, 32
Stanley Bowmar Co., 409
Starling, Kenneth A., 123
Stewart, Gary, 27
Stilkind, Jerry, 21
Stone, Donald B., 105, 186, 432
Stone, Stephen E., 35
Stories for children, 441–465
Storytelling method, 393
Strasser, Ben B., 431
Streptococcus infections, 119
Stress, psychological, 13–14, 99, 195, 276
Sugden, John H., 105
Suicide, 14–15, 127
Sunburst Communications, 465
Sunkist Growers Association, 209, 214, 439
Superstition, 5, 28, 343
Supervision, 101
Surveys, 478–479
Swabb, L., 181
Swift and Company, 439
Swisher, John D., 350
Sylvester, Robert, 280
Syphilis, 26

Taba, Hilda, 147
Tables, 418
Tampax, Inc., 306, 308, 439
Tape recordings, 410–411
Taub, Alyson, 53
Teacher, disease detection and, 83–84
    and health agencies, 180
    health instruction program and, 124
        in kindergarten, 163
    health of, 44–45, 98–99
    materials available to, 402
    personality of, 99, 142–144
    and physical education, 195
Teaching, competency in, 142–144, 160
    cycle plan of, 172, 173
    team, 180–181
Teaching aids, 190, 351–430, 433–464
    sources, 402–404
    units, 175–176
    variety in, 400–401
Teaching Film Custodians, 465
Team Teaching, 180–181
Teeth, 19–20, 112
Television, 409
Temperature, 94, 137
Tennyson, Alfred Lord, 106
Teper-Singer, Lynn, 383
Tests, attitude, 487–490
    bicycle safety, 267, 485
    free response, 483
    health knowledge, 471
    multiple choice, 482–483
    performance, 476
    self-appraisal, 488–489
    standardized, 484–486
    teacher-prepared, 481
Tetanus, 120
Textbook method, 370–371, 411
Thackeray, William Makepeace, 282
Thoreau, Henry D., 471
Thorndike, Edward Lee, 37
Thorne Films, Inc., 465
Tillich, Paul, 353
Time, allotment of, 162
Timmreck, Thomas C., 385
Tobacco smoking, attitude test about, 489
    behavioral objectives and, 325–342, 505–507
    cancer and, 15, 17–18
    children and, 17–18
    educational materials about, 462–464
    as health topic, 171
    illustration of effects, 382–383
    questionnaire about, 362
Toothbrushing, 221, 223–224
Torrance, E. Paul, 280, 432
Transparencies, 408
Travelers Insurance Company, 209, 233, 439
Trends in health, 50–52
Tribune Films, Inc., 465
Trifiletti, John D., 89
Tritsch, Leonard E., 431, 493
Trow, W., 491
True-false tests, 483

Tuberculosis, 9, 70, 120
Turner, Claire E., 39
Tussing, Lyle, 37–38
Tyler, Ralph, 195

Ulcers, 17
Understanding, 127–128, 355, 358
United Cerebral Palsy Association, 437
United Fresh Fruit and Vegetable
    Association, 213, 439
U.S. Beet Sugar Association, 439
U.S. Department of Health, Education
    and Welfare, 330
U.S. Environmental Protection Agency,
    314, 319, 320, 322, 324
U.S. Public Health Service, 242, 313,
    333, 406, 488
United World Films, 465
Units in health, 173–176
    resource, 174–175
    teaching, 175–176
Urban Problems, 47

Values, 8, 360
Value clarification, 360–364, 387
Value illness, 7–8
Van Andsdell, William, 55
Vannier, Maryhelen, 53, 493
Varicella, 118
Variety in teaching, 401–402
Veenker, Harold C., 484
Venereal disease, 25, 287
Ventilation, 90, 92, 94, 137
Vincent, Edith P., 255
Vincent, Ronald G., 35
Violence, 22
Vision, 62–64, 115
Voluntary health agencies, 51,
    436–437

Wadsworth, Barry J., 350, 358, 469
Walt Disney Educational Media, 465

Walton, Elizabeth G., 350
Wantz, Molly, 349
Washington Wheat Commission, 439
Water pollution, 24
Watts, Parren R., 151
Weighing and measuring, 110
Wellness, 1, 3, 170
Wells, H. G., 34
Werra, Elsie, 197
Wetzel Grid, 111
Wexler Film Productions, 465
Wheat Flour Institute, 439
White, Paul Dudley, 18
White, Phillip L., 350
White House Conference, 55, 206, 288
Whitehead, Alfred North, 52
Whooping cough, 119
Wiist, William A., 432
Willgoose, Carl E., 35, 53, 105, 123,
    146, 165, 186, 277, 312, 314, 350,
    432, 493
Williams, Roger J., 107
Wolfson, B. J., 186
Woodruff, Asahel D., 186
Woody, J. D., 292
Wordsworth, 1
Workbooks, 412
World Health Organization, 3, 335
Worldwide health conditions, 8
Writing pads, 418

Yarber, William L., 493
Yellen, Sylvia, 484
Young America Films, 465
Youth-to-youth method, 392–393

Zaichkowsky, Leonard D., 196, 350
Zaichkowsky, Linda B., 350
Zais, Robert S., 148, 186
Zinsser, Hans, 248